Clinical Cases in Cardiac Electrophysiology: Supraventricular Arrhythmias

Lucian Muresan

Editor

Clinical Cases in Cardiac Electrophysiology: Supraventricular Arrhythmias

Volume I

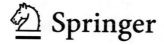 Springer

Editor
Lucian Muresan
Department of Cardiology
Centre Hospitalier de Mulhouse
Mulhouse, France

ISBN 978-3-031-07359-5   ISBN 978-3-031-07357-1   (eBook)
https://doi.org/10.1007/978-3-031-07357-1

This Springer imprint is published by the registered company Springer Nature Switzerland AG
The registered company address is: Gewerbestrasse 11, 6330 Cham, Switzerland

Preface

The field of interventional treatment of cardiac arrhythmias is continuously expanding. New diagnostic and therapeutic techniques are developed every year, improving our understanding and capabilities of offering better treatment options to our patients. In this regard, reading and learning remains a crucial step in keeping up with this rapidly evolving field.

This volume is a collection of 20 cases of supraventricular arrhythmias treated with catheter ablation, which we hope that our readers will find interesting. All these ablation procedures were guided by an electro-anatomical mapping system, some of them exclusively, some of them with the additional help of fluoroscopy. Our team strongly believes in the concept of "zero-fluoroscopy" procedures and, where this was possible to achieve, it was done so.

This book was created from the very beginning with a strong learning purpose. In this regard, each of the 20 cases contains a short presentation of the clinical context, relevant paraclinical examinations, and several multiple-choice questions related to the arrhythmia presented. The electrophysiological study and the catheter ablation procedure are then described, with additional questions addressed to the reader along the way. At the end, answers to the questions are provided, followed by a short commentary of the case, with comments and references to related articles from the literature. The most important aspects to be kept in mind are stressed out at the end of each presentation.

We hope that the readers will appreciate the format of the book and most importantly, that there will be something to learn for each of them, which will be able to improve their knowledge and most importantly, patients' care.

We would like to address our very warm and special thanks to our dear colleagues: Dr. Jorge Aventin, Dr. Gokhan Bodur, Dr. Narcisa Bors, Dr. Alexandrina Calatan, Dr. Jean-Pierre Chemouny, Dr. Claudine Cordier, Dr. Paul Klero de Rosbo, Dr. Daniel Franck, Dr. Stéphane Greciano, Dr. Francis Homatter, Dr. Jean-René Kieny, Dr. Patricia Magnus, Dr. Alvaro Pereira Zenklusen, Dr. John Philippe, Dr. Pedro Rodriguez, Dr. Olivier Roth, Dr. Elena Rugina, Dr. Antoine Wuillermin, Dr. Jean-Julien Stolz, Dr. Jean-Marie Reinbold, to our wonderful nurses: Catherine Paulus, Gaëlle Meyer, Jocelyne Scheibel, Sabine Bruckert, Elodie Gaullard, Natacha Meyer, Marie Ribstein, and to our hard-working radiology technicians: Anne Maresca, Michaël Wittiche, Anne Pelloux Gervais, Julie Welter, Marion Giannipatrani,

Françoise Furstenberger, and Valérie Luttenauer, whose dedication and implication in the patients' care made a significant difference. Without their effort, this project would have never been possible. Thank you!

Mulhouse, France   Lucian Muresan
June 2022

Contents

About the Authors

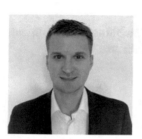

Romaric Bouillard   Biosense Webster France, Johnson & Johnson, Mulhouse, France

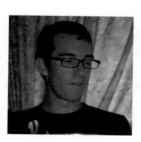

Nicolas Bourrelly   Cardiology Department, Emile Muller Hospital, Mulhouse, France

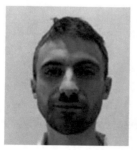

Didier Bresson   Cardiology Department, Emile Muller Hospital, Mulhouse, France

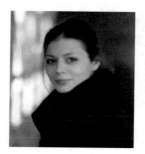

Mihaela Calcaianu   Cardiology Department, Emile Muller Hospital, Mulhouse, France

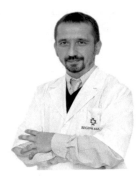

Gabriel Cismaru Cardiology Department, Rehabilitation Hospital, Cluj-Napoca, Romania

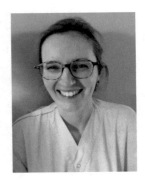

Robert Dallemand Cardiology Department, Emile Muller Hospital, Mulhouse, France

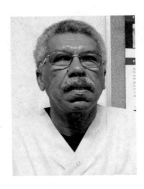

Charline Daval Cardiology Department, Emile Muller Hospital, Mulhouse, France

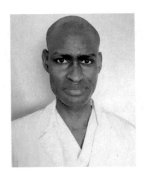

Lucien Leopold Diene Cardiology Department, Emile Muller Hospital, Mulhouse, France

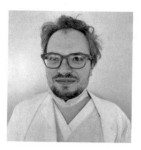

Laurent Dietrich Cardiology Department, Emile Muller Hospital, Mulhouse, France

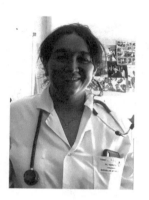

Yasmine Doghmi Cardiology Department, Emile Muller Hospital, Mulhouse, France

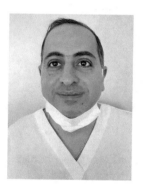

Tarek El Nazer Cardiology Department, Emile Muller Hospital, Mulhouse, France

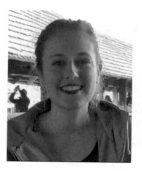

Emmanuelle Gain Biosense Webster France, Johnson & Johnson, Mulhouse, France

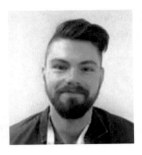

Matthieu George   Biosense Webster France, Johnson & Johnson, Mulhouse, France

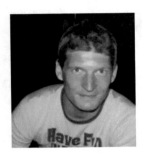

Frédéric   Halbwachs   Biosense   Webster France, Johnson & Johnson, Mulhouse, France

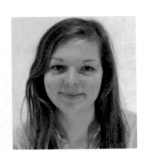

Justine Havard   Biosense Webster France, Johnson & Johnson, Mulhouse, France

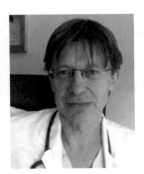

Laurent Jacquemin   Cardiology Department, Emile Muller Hospital, Mulhouse, France

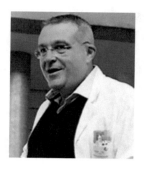
David Kenizou Cardiology Department, Emile Muller Hospital, Mulhouse, France

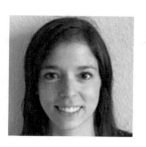
Marine Kinnel Cardiology Department, Emile Muller Hospital, Mulhouse, France

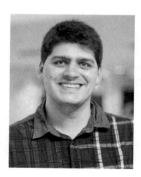
Arthur Kohler Biosense Webster France, Johnson & Johnson, Mulhouse, France

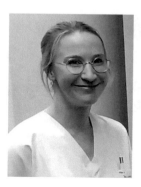
Aubrietia Lawson Cardiology Department, Emile Muller Hospital, Mulhouse, France

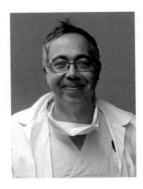
Ronan Le Bouar   Cardiology Department, Emile Muller Hospital, Mulhouse, France

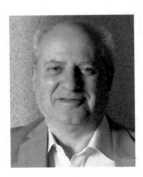
Jacques Levy   Cardiology Department, Emile Muller Hospital, Mulhouse, France

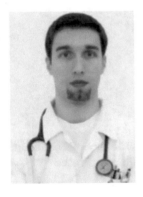
Lucian Muresan   Cardiology Department, Emile Muller Hospital, Mulhouse, France

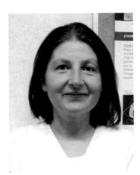
Crina Muresan   Cardiology Department, Emile Muller Hospital, Mulhouse, France

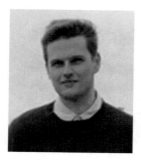

Thomas Robein   Biosense Webster France, Johnson & Johnson, Mulhouse, France

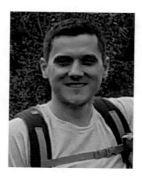

Serban Schiau   Cardiology Department, Emile Muller Hospital, Mulhouse, France

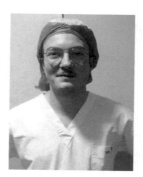

Maxime Tissier   Biosense Webster France, Johnson & Johnson, Mulhouse, France

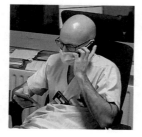

Jean-Yves Wiedemann   Cardiology Department, Emile Muller Hospital, Mulhouse, France

Abbreviations

AF	Atrial fibrillation
AP	Antero-posterior
ASD	Atrial septal defect
AT	Atrial tachycardia
AV	Atrio-ventricular
AVN	Atrio-ventricular node
AVNRT	Atrio-ventricular node reentry tachycardia
AVRT	Atrio-ventricular reentry tachycardia
BMI	Body mass index
BP	Blood pressure
BUN	Blood urea nitrogen
CABG	Coronary artery by-pass graft
CFAE	Complex fractionated atrial electrograms
COPD	Chronic obstructive pulmonary disease
cTnI	Cardiac troponin I
CX	Circumflex (coronary artery)
EDD	End diastolic diameter
EF	Ejection fraction
EP	Electrophysiology
EPS	Electrophysiological study
ESD	End systolic diameter
Hb	Hemoglobin
Hct	Hematocrit
HFpEF	Heart failure with preserved ejection fraction
HFrEF	Heart failure with reduced ejection fraction
HR	Heart rate
ICD	Implantable cardioverter defibrillator
ISV	Internal saphenous vein
IVC	Inferior vena cava
IVS	Interventricular septum
LA	Left atrium
LAD	Left anterior descending (coronary artery)
LAO	Left anterior oblique
LBBB	Left bundle branch block
LIMA	Left internal mammary artery
LIPV	Left inferior pulmonary vein
LL	Left lateral

LPSV	Left superior pulmonary vein
LV	Left ventricle
MI	Myocardial infarction
NT-pro BNP	N-terminal pro-Brain Natriuretic Peptide
ORT	Orthodromic reciprocating tachycardia
PA	Postero-anterior
PAC	Premature atrial contraction
PAF	Paroxysmal atrial fibrillation
PFO	Patent foramen ovale
PV	Pulmonary vein
PVC	Premature ventricular contraction
RA	Right atrium
RAO	Right anterior oblique
RBBB	Right bundle branch block
RCA	Right coronary artery
RIMA	Right internal mammary artery
RIPV	Right inferior pulmonary vein
RL	Right lateral
RSPV	Right superior pulmonary vein
RV	Right ventricle
SCD	Sudden cardiac death
sPAP	Systolic pulmonary artery pressure
SVC	Superior vena cava
TAPSE	Tricuspid annulus plane systolic excursion
TSH	Thyroid-stimulating hormone
VT	Ventricular tachycardia
WPW	Wolf-Parkinson-White

Case 1

Frédéric Halbwachs, Serban Schiau, Aubrietia Lawson, Mihaela Calcaianu, and Didier Bresson

1.1 Case Presentation

An 80-year-old male patient with a past medical history of remote myocardial infarction (NSTEMI) at the age of 68 years treated with medical treatment, chronic obliterant arteriopathy of the lower limbs with moderate bilateral atherosclerotic plaques at the level of the common femoral arteries, chronic venous insufficiency, was addressed to the Cardiology Department for an episode of chest pain accompanied by dyspnea at rest of sudden onset, 2 h prior to his presentation at the hospital. He recalled having presented intermittent pain in his left calf 2 days prior to his arrival at the hospital. His cardiovascular risk factors were represented by grade 1 obesity, dyslipidemia, and age >55 years. His medication at home consisted of atenolol 25 mg, clopidogrel 75 mg, pravastatin 20 mg, and omeprazole 20 mg.

At physical examination, his blood pressure was 132/71 mmHg, HR 142 bpm, SpO_2 89% breathing room air, $H = 180$ cm, $W = 104$ kg, $BMI = 32.09$ kg/m^2, heart sounds were rapid and regular, there was a mild systolic murmur in the mitral auscultation region, lung auscultation was clear, there were mild bilateral edema of the lower limbs. His CHA_2DS_2-VASc score was 3, his HAS-BLED score was 1.

Biological work-up revealed Hb 13.3 g/dL, leucocytes 12.3×10^9/L, platelets 247×10^9/L, CRP <3 mg/L, BUN 9.2 mmol/L, creatinine 107 µmol/L, glycemia 7.2 mmol/L, Na$^+$ 135 mmol/L, K$^+$ 4.3 mmol/L, TSH 0.97 UI/L, NT-proBNP 451 pg/mL, D-dimers 982 mcg/mL, and troponin I <0.015 ng/mL.

His ECG at presentation is showed in Fig. 1.1.

Transthoracic echocardiography showed a non-dilated left ventricle (ESD of 48 mm), with a preserved EF% of 58%, with a moderately dilated left atrium of 26 cm^2 (Fig. 1.2). It also showed LV filling pressure in the gray zone, E/e' of 9, mild septal LV hypertrophy, IVS of 12 mm, mild mitral regurgitation 1/4 of type 1 of the Carpentier classification, mild aortic stenosis with a mean transaortic gradient of 10 mmHg, mild aortic regurgitation, a non-dilated right ventricle, with 1–2/4 tricuspid regurgitation, mild pulmonary hypertension,

Supplementary Information The online version contains supplementary material available at [https://doi.org/10.1007/978-3-031-07357-1_1].

F. Halbwachs (✉)
Biosense Webster, Mulhouse, France

S. Schiau · A. Lawson · M. Calcaianu · D. Bresson
Cardiology Department, "Emile Muller" Hospital, Mulhouse, France

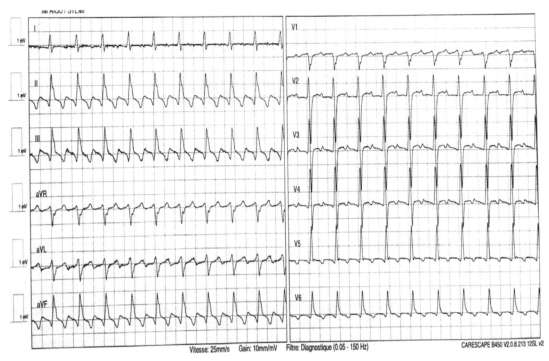

Fig. 1.1 Twelve lead ECG recording at admittance to the Cardiology Department showing atrial flutter with 2:1 AV conduction, with a heart rate of 140 bpm, QRS axis at +60°, absence of LV hypertrophy, negative T waves in V5, V6. The aspect of the flutter waves—negative in inferior leads, positive in V1, negative in V6—is in favor of a typical counterclockwise atrial flutter

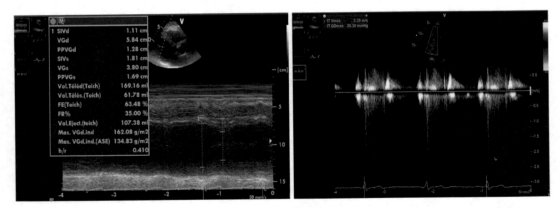

Fig. 1.2 *Left panel*: M-mode transthoracic echocardiography in parasternal long axis view, showing a non-dilated LV with an ESD of 58 mm and a LVEF of 63%, as well as absence of LV hypertrophy. *Right panel*: continuous Doppler at the level of the tricuspid valve in apical 4 chamber view showing mild tricuspid regurgitation with a RV—RA pressure gradient of 20 mmHg

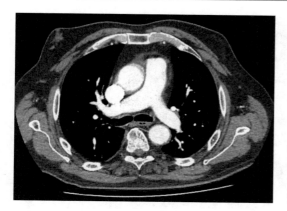

Fig. 1.3 CT angiography showing absence of pulmonary embolism at the level of the arterial pulmonary trunk and the main pulmonary arteries

sPAP of 45 mmHg, mild pericardial effusion, a mildly dilated ascending aorta (40 mm) with no visible sign of aortic dissection.

Given the patient's symptoms of pain in the lower left calf, dyspnea, chest pain, the mildly augmented D-dimers level, the presence of atrial flutter on the ECG, a CT angiography of the pulmonary arteries was performed (Fig. 1.3), which ruled out the presence of pulmonary embolism.

After acute treatment with oxygen, IV furosemide, beta blockers, and anticoagulation with IV heparin, the patient's symptoms improved. A catheter ablation of his atrial flutter was offered and, after informed consent was obtained, subsequently performed, after exclusion of a LAA thrombus by transesophageal echocardiography.

1.2 Electrophysiological Study and RF Catheter Ablation Procedure

The electrophysiological study was performed under local anesthesia and conscious sedation. Vascular access was obtained using the modified Seldinger technique, under Doppler ultrasound guidance. A 6F quadripolar steerable catheter (Dynamic Extrem, Microport®) was introduced in a 6F 20 cm vascular sheath and was subsequently advanced via the right common femoral vein up to the coronary sinus. A 5F steerable decapolar catheter (Livewire, Abbott©) was introduced in a 5F

20 cm vascular sheath and placed at the level of the lateral wall of the right atrium, with its distal poles at the level of the low lateral right atrium and the proximal poles at the level of the high lateral right atrium. A Biotronik® Alcath non-irrigated 8 mm tip catheter with black curve was introduced in a 7F 20 cm vascular sheath and was subsequently advanced via the right common femoral vein up to the CTI. Atrial pacing was carried out at twice the diastolic threshold using the EP-4™ Cardiac Stimulator (Abbott®) system. Surface ECG and intra-cavitary ECGs were recorded by the *WorkMate* Claris™ System (Abbott®).

The 12-lead ECG recorded at the beginning of the ablation procedure is presented in Fig. 1.4.

The atrial flutter cycle length was 260–270 ms. The depolarization sequence of the lateral wall of the right atrium was compatible with a typical counterclockwise atrial flutter (Fig. 1.5).

Entrainment maneuvers were performed at the level of the lateral wall of the right atrium, CTI, proximal and distal coronary sinus, confirming the presence of a counterclockwise macro-reentry around the tricuspid valve. RF ablation of the CTI was carried out with a target power of 60 Watts, applications of 60 seconds, with termination of atrial flutter (Figs. 1.6 and 1.7). Bidirectional conduction block at the level of the CTI was present at the end of the procedure (Figs. 1.8 and 1.9).

The 12-lead ECG recorded at the end of the ablation procedure is shown in Fig. 1.10.

Four days after the ablation procedure, the patient presented a new episode of dyspnea at rest, accompanied by chest pain, with a similar character to his symptoms present at admittance to the hospital. The ECG in Fig. 1.11 was recorded.

Question 1: What is the nature of the tachycardia from Fig. 1.11?
A. Recurrence of typical atrial flutter post RF ablation of the CTI
B. Atypical right atrial flutter
C. Atypical left atrial flutter
D. Focal atrial tachycardia originating in the right atrium
E. Focal atrial tachycardia originating in the left atrium

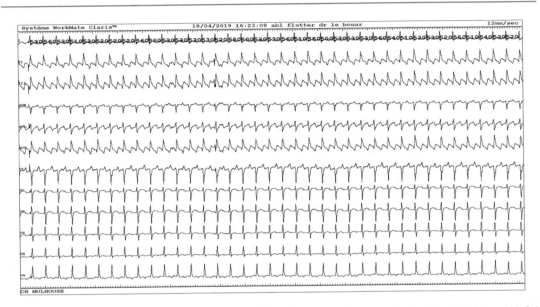

Fig. 1.4 Twelve lead ECG recorded at the beginning of the ablation procedure showing typical atrial flutter with 2:1 AV conduction, with a heart rate of 140 bpm

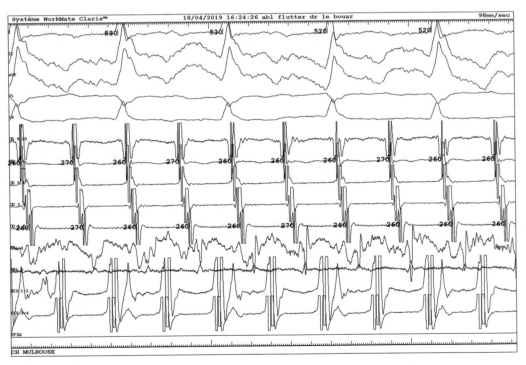

Fig. 1.5 Surface ECG leads I, II, aVF, V1, and V6 together with intracavitary leads recorded from the 10 poles of the Halo catheter (OD 1–2 to OD 9–10), from the distal and the proximal poles of the ablation catheter (ABL d and ABL p) and from the proximal and the distal bipolar electrodes of the coronary sinus catheter (named His 1–2, His 3–4) showing the atrial flutter cycle length of 260–270 ms and the depolarization sequence of the lateral wall of the right atrium, in a cranial to caudal direction (OD 9–10 to OD 1–2), sequence compatible with a typical counterclockwise peri-tricuspid macro-reentry circuit

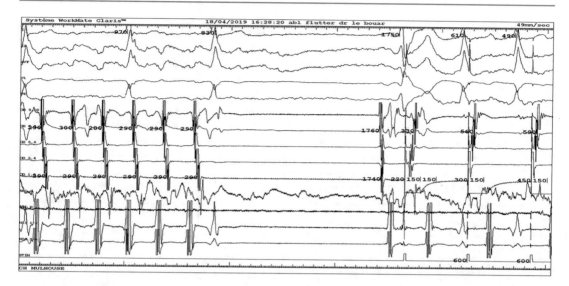

Fig. 1.6 Surface ECG leads I, II, aVF, V1, and V6 together with intracavitary leads recorded from the 10 poles of the Halo catheter (OD 1–2 to OD 9–10), from the distal and the proximal poles of the ablation catheter (ABL d and ABL p) and from the proximal and the distal bipolar electrodes of the coronary sinus catheter (named His 1–2, His 3–4) showing termination of atrial flutter during ablation of the CTI, with conversion to sinus rhythm

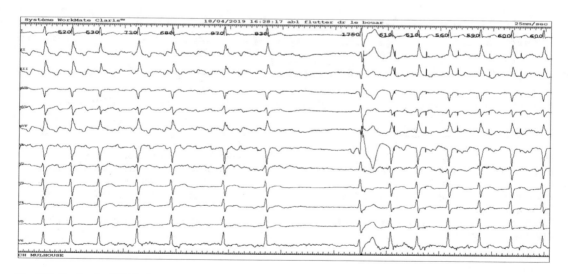

Fig. 1.7 Twelve lead ECG showing conversion of atrial flutter to sinus rhythm during RF ablation of the CTI

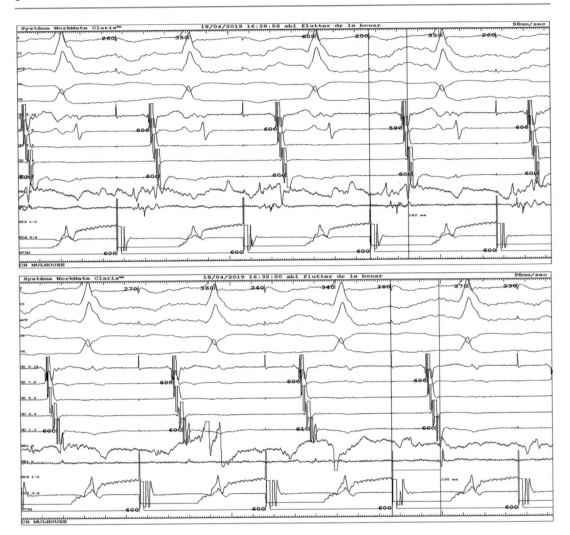

Fig. 1.8 Surface ECG leads I, II, aVF, V1, and V6 together with intracavitary leads recorded from the 10 poles of the Halo catheter (OD 1–2 to OD 9–10), from the distal and the proximal poles of the ablation catheter (ABL d and ABL p) and from the proximal and the distal bipolar electrodes of the coronary sinus catheter (named His 1–2, His 3–4) showing a counterclockwise conduc-tion delay of 182 ms at the level of the low lateral right atrium (upper figure) and a counterclockwise conduction delay of 230 ms just lateral to the RF line at the level of the CTI (lower figure), in favor of clockwise conduction block at this level. The delay of 230 ms is recorded by the roving/ablation catheter just lateral to the ablation line, during pacing from the proximal poles of the CS catheter

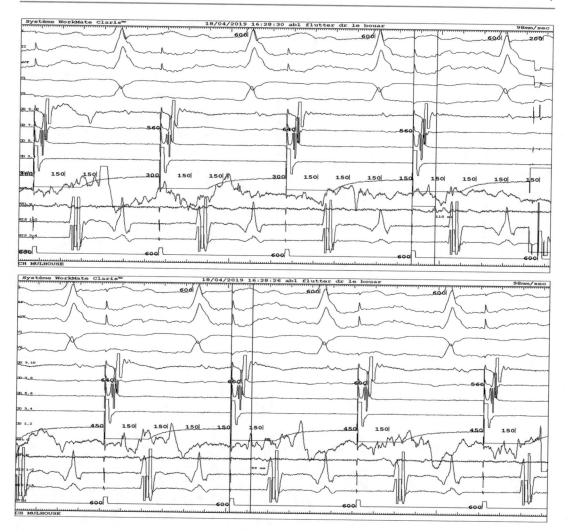

Fig. 1.9 Surface ECG leads I, II, aVF, V1, and V6 together with intra-cavitary leads recorded from the 10 poles of the Halo catheter (OD 1–2 to OD 9–10), from the distal and the proximal poles of the ablation catheter (ABL d and ABL p) and from the proximal and the distal bipolar electrodes of the coronary sinus catheter (named His 1–2, His 3–4) showing a clockwise conduction delay of 110 ms at the level of the low septal right atrium (upper figure) and a clockwise conduction delay of 150 ms just medial to the RF line at the level of the CTI (lower figure), in favor of counterclockwise conduction block at this level. The delay is recorded by the roving/ablation catheter just medial to the ablation line, during pacing from the distal poles of the decapolar catheter placed at the level of the lateral wall of the right atrium

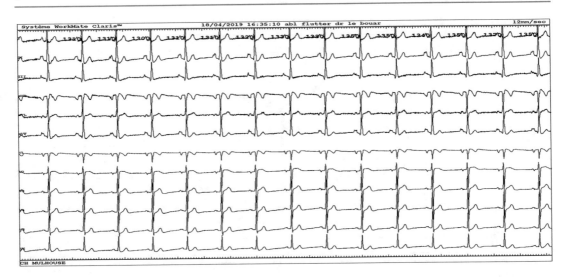

Fig. 1.10 A 12-lead ECG recorded at the end of the ablation procedure, showing sinus bradycardia with a heart rate of 44 bpm

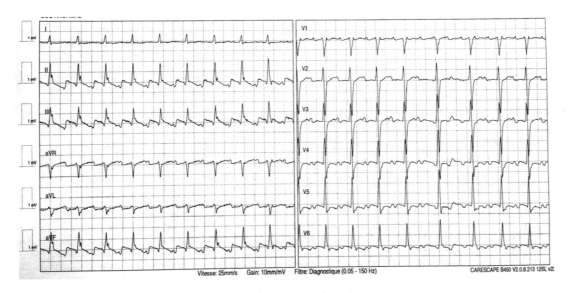

Fig. 1.11 A 12-lead ECG recorded 4 days after the ablation procedure

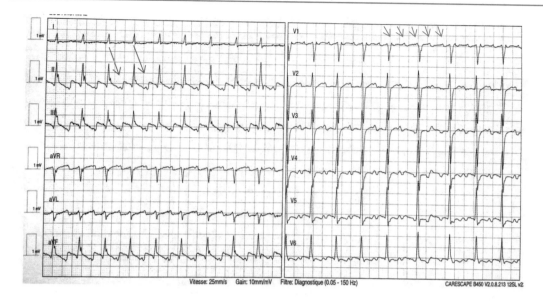

Figure 1.11 explained. A 12-lead ECG showing a narrow QRS complex tachycardia with 2:1 and 3:1 AV conduction (best seen in lead V1, indicated by the blue arrows), with a heart rate of 120 bpm, slightly lower than the ventricular rate during atrial flutter. At a first glance, the aspect in the inferior leads suggests a typical counterclockwise atrial flutter. However, a more careful analysis of the ECG allows observation of a reduced-amplitude P wave, indicated by the red arrows at the end of the negative slope of the "flutter wave," just before the upslope of the wave, suggesting a different mechanism than typical counterclockwise peri-tricuspid macro-reentry.

A second electrophysiological study in view of a catheter ablation procedure was scheduled and subsequently performed, this time with the help of the CARTO system.

1.3 Electrophysiological Study and RF Catheter Ablation Procedure 2

The electrophysiological study was performed under local anesthesia and conscious sedation. Vascular access was obtained using the modified Seldinger technique, under Doppler ultrasound guidance. A 6F quadripolar steerable catheter (Dynamic Extrem, Microport®) was introduced in a 6F 20 cm vascular sheath and was subsequently advanced via the right common femoral vein up to

the coronary sinus. A Biosense Webster® SmartTouch SF open-irrigated 3.5 mm tip with F curve was introduced in a 9F 20 cm vascular sheath and was subsequently advanced via the right common femoral vein up to the right atrium. Atrial pacing was carried out at twice the diastolic threshold using the EP-4™ Cardiac Stimulator (Abbott®) system. Surface ECG and intracavitary ECGs were recorded by the *WorkMate* Claris™ System (Abbott®).

The 12-lead ECG recorded at the beginning of the ablation procedure is shown in Fig. 1.12.

The tachycardia cycle length was 260 ms. The depolarization sequence of the CS catheter was proximal to distal (Fig. 1.13).

An anatomical map of the right atrium was initially created. The right atrium was mildly dilated, with a volume of 119 mL.

An activation map of the right atrium during tachycardia was subsequently created, which is shown in Figs. 1.14 and 1.15.

> **Question 2: What is the nature of the tachycardia from** Figs. 1.14 and 1.15**?**
> A. Recurrence of typical counterclockwise atrial flutter
> B. Typical clockwise atrial flutter
> C. Focal atrial tachycardia originating from the coronary sinus ostium
> D. Intra-CTI reentry
> E. Left atrial tachycardia

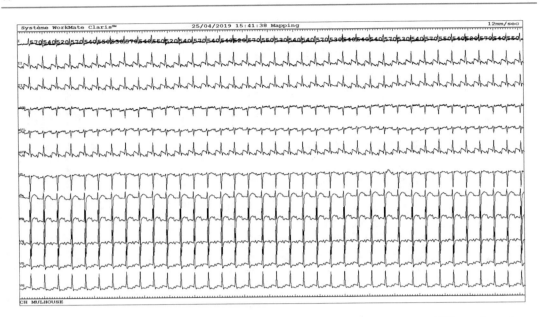

Fig. 1.12 A 12-lead ECG at the beginning of the second ablation procedure showing a narrow QRS complex tachycardia with a heart rate of 140 bpm

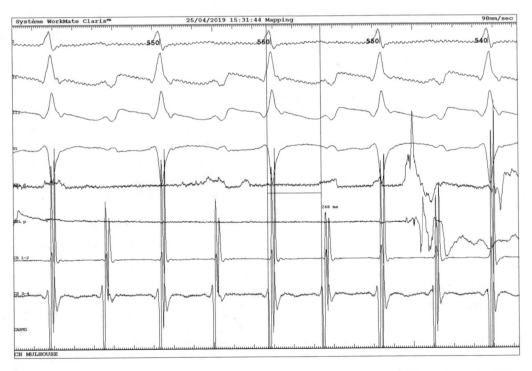

Fig. 1.13 Surface ECG leads I, II, III, and V1, together with intracavitary leads recorded from the distal and the proximal poles of the ablation catheter (ABL d and ABL p) and from the proximal and the distal bipolar electrodes of the coronary sinus catheter (named CS 1–2 and CS 3–4) showing a tachycardia with a cycle length of 260 ms, with 2:1 AV conduction, and with a depolarization sequence of proximal to distal at the level of the CS catheter

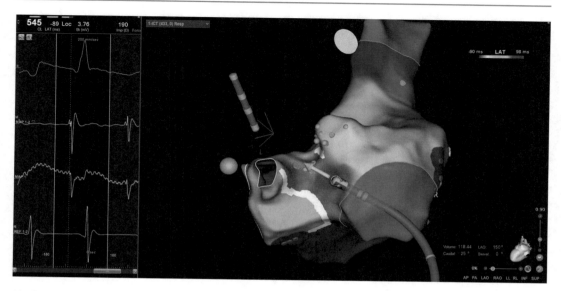

Fig. 1.14 CARTO image in postero-septal view showing the activation map of the right atrium during atrial tachycardia. The right atrium is mildly dilated, with a volume of 119 ml. The activation map is in favor of a focal atrial tachycardia with an origin posterior to the CS ostium. From this site, the depolarization of the right atrium takes place in a radial manner, compatible with a focal mecha-nism. Of note, only 70% of the tachycardia cycle length could be recorded in the right atrium, argument also in favor of a focal mechanism. The earliest local bipolar electrogram (blue dot) precedes the onset of the P wave on the surface ECG by 25 ms. The local unipolar electrogram has a "QS" aspect (MAP 1, left side of the image)

The activation map from Figs. 1.14 and 1.15 is compatible with a focal atrial tachycardia arising from the area just posterior to the coronary sinus ostium. From this area, the activation spreads in a radial manner, in several adjacent areas of the right atrium and towards the CTI. Of note, there was persistent conduction block at the level of the CTI as a result of the previous ablation procedure, best seen in Fig. 1.15.

Figure 1.16 shows the presence of double potentials along the previously ablated CTI-line, also in favor of conduction block at this level.

The ablation catheter recorded fragmented potentials at the level of the earliest atrial activation site, situated at the ostium of the coronary sinus, with duration of up to 187 ms, which represented 69% of the tachycardia cycle length (Fig. 1.17). Of note, only 69% of the tachycardia cycle length was recorded in the right atrium.

Question 3: Is this a good ablation site?
A. Yes. The earliest local bipolar electrogram precedes the onset of the P wave on the surface ECG by 25 ms
B. Yes. The local unipolar electrogram has a "QS" aspect
C. Yes. The activation map is in favor of a focal atrial tachycardia originating in this region
D. No. This is an atrial tachycardia probably originating in the left atrium

No. No atrial tachycardia can originate in this region.

Given the activation map of the right atrium during tachycardia, the "QS" aspect of the local unipolar electrogram, and the 25 ms difference between the local atrial electrogram and the P

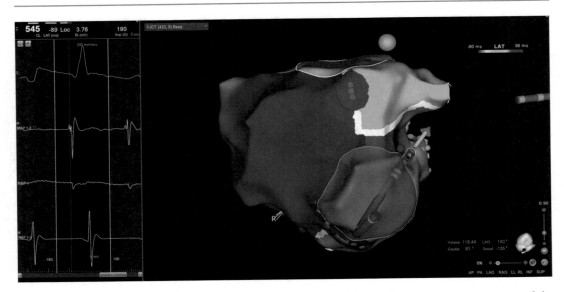

Fig. 1.15 CARTO image in inferior view showing the activation map of the right atrium during atrial tachycardia. The activation sequence of the CTI is compatible with conduction block at this level, as a consequence of the previous ablation procedure

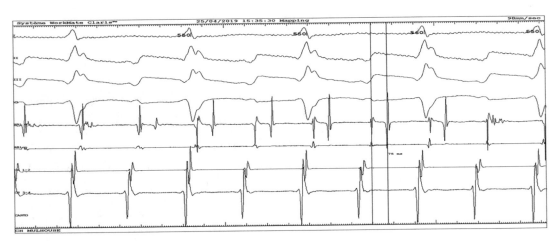

Fig. 1.16 Surface ECG leads I, II, III, and V1, together with intracavitary leads recorded from the distal and the proximal poles of the ablation catheter (ABL d and ABL p) and from the proximal and the distal bipolar electrodes of the coronary sinus catheter (named CS 1–2 and CS 3–4) showing the presence of wide double potentials (of 78 ms) along the previously created RF ablation line at the level of the CTI, in favor of conduction block at this level

wave onset on the surface ECG, a diagnosis of focal atrial tachycardia with origin just posterior to the coronary sinus ostium (Fig. 1.17) was established. The fact that 69% of the TCL was recorded in the right atrium in a very small area was an argument in favor of a micro-reentry focal atrial tachycardia with origin at this level.

RF ablation was carried out at this site, with a target power of 30 Watts, duration of application of 45 seconds, with prompt interruption of the tachycardia and restoration of sinus rhythm (Figs. 1.18, 1.19, and 1.20).

There were no complications related to the procedure.

The ECG recorded after the ablation procedure is shown in Fig. 1.21.

The patient was discharged home 48 h later on anticoagulant treatment.

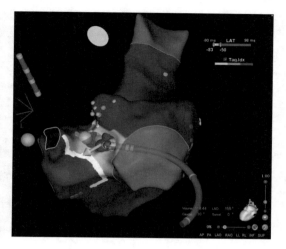

Fig. 1.18 CARTO image in postero-septal view (same as in Fig. 1.16), showing the position of the ablation catheter at the successful ablation site, with superposed RF ablation lesions (pink and red dots). The yellow dot represents the bundle of His

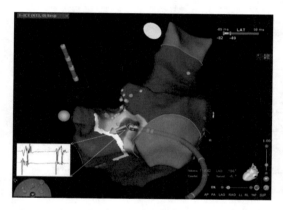

Fig. 1.17 CARTO image in postero-septal view, showing the position of the ablation catheter at the earliest atrial activation site during tachycardia, before RF delivery. The yellow dot represents the bundle of His

1.4   Commentary

The present case illustrates a catheter ablation procedure of a focal atrial tachycardia with origin in the low right atrium in an 80-year-old male patient with a previous catheter ablation procedure of the CTI for typical atrial flutter. Several observations can be made about the present case.

The tachycardia origin close to the CS ostium and the previously existing conduction block at the level of the CTI obtained during the previous RF procedure determined an ECG aspect mimicking the presence of typical counterclockwise atrial flutter. However, a close analysis of the ECG during typical atrial flutter and that of the ECG during atrial tachycardia raised suspicion of a different tachycardia mechanism and not typical atrial flutter recurrence. This underlines the importance of a careful and systematic ECG interpretation before a catheter ablation procedure. The tachycardia mechanism was elucidated with the help of the CARTO electroanatomical mapping system.

Focal atrial tachycardias can originate either in the left or in the right atrium, with right atrium origin being predominant (63% vs 37%), according to Kistler et al. [1]. The most common origins in the right atrium are the crista terminalis, the tricuspid annulus, the right atrial appendage, the coronary sinus ostium, and peri-nodal. The coronary sinus ostium is the origin of focal atrial tachycardias in 6.7% of patients [2, 3]. Based on the P wave morphology on the 12-lead ECG, several algorithm have been currently published, conceived to help the clinician identify the tachycardia origin before the catheter ablation procedure, in order to properly prepare for the ablation (such as the need to gain access to the left atrium by anticipating the need to perform transseptal puncture) [1, 2, 4, 5]. The ECG

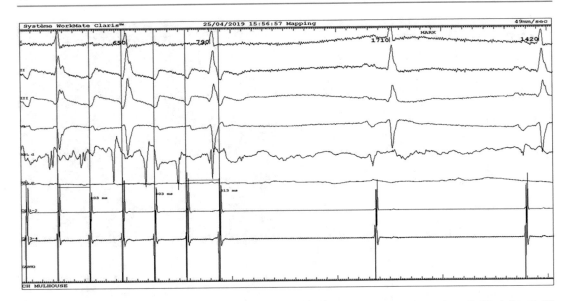

Fig. 1.19 Surface ECG leads I, II, III, and V1, together with intracavitary leads recorded from the distal and the proximal poles of the ablation catheter (ABL d and ABL p) and from the proximal and the distal bipolar electrodes of the coronary sinus catheter (named CS 1–2 and CS 3–4) showing the termination of the tachycardia with a slight prolongation of the cycle length just before restoration of the sinus rhythm

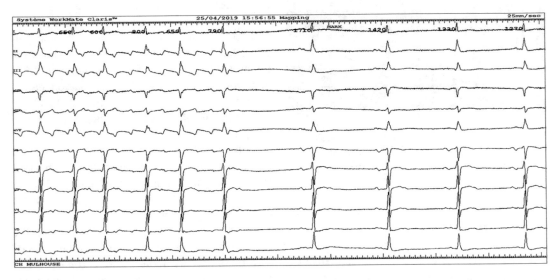

Fig. 1.20 A 12-lead ECG showing termination of the tachycardia during RF delivery at the earliest atrial activation site, just posterior to the coronary sinus ostium, and restoration of sinus rhythm

characteristics of focal atrial tachycardias originating from the CS ostium are negative P waves in leads II, III, aVF, isoelectric in lead I, positive in aVL and aVR, and usually negative in V6 [3]. RF ablation guided by an electroana- tomical mapping system is the most efficient way for the treatment of these patients [6].

Atrial tachycardias originating from the low interatrial septum masquerading as typical atrial flutter have been occasionally described

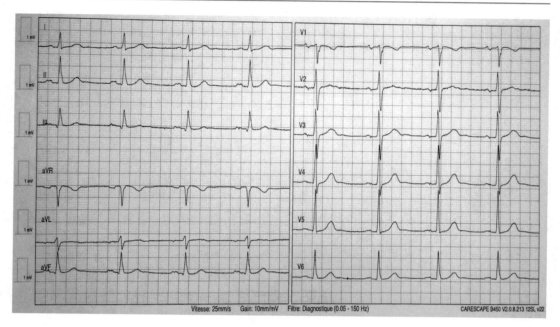

Fig. 1.21 A 12-lead ECG recorded after the ablation procedure, showing sinus bradycardia with a heart rate of 50 bpm, QRS axis at +60°, absence of LV hypertrophy, absence of ischemia

before [7]. RF ablation of the ectopic focus successfully eliminated the tachycardia in these cases.

The correct diagnosis in this specific patient was important, since this avoided unnecessary RF applications at the level of the CTI, for a possible misdiagnosis of typical counterclockwise atrial flutter recurrence.

Learning Point

- Atrial tachycardia originating in the right atrium occurring after ablation of the CTI may mimic typical atrial flutter on the 12-lead ECG.
- A careful analysis of the ECG is frequently able to suggest a different tachycardia mechanism.
- The correct diagnosis is established by the electrophysiological study.

References

1. Kistler PM, Roberts-Thomson KC, Haqqani HM, Fynn SP, Singarayar S, Vohra JK, et al. P-wave morphology in focal atrial tachycardia: development of an algorithm to predict the anatomic site of origin. J Am Coll Cardiol. 2006;48(5):1010–7.
2. Kistler PM, Kalman JM. Locating focal atrial tachycardias from P-wave morphology. Heart Rhythm. 2005;2(5):561–4.
3. Kistler PM, Fynn SP, Haqqani H, Stevenson IH, Vohra JK, Morton JB, et al. Focal atrial tachycardia from the ostium of the coronary sinus: electrocardiographic and electrophysiological characterization and radiofrequency ablation. J Am Coll Cardiol. 2005;45(9):1488–93.
4. Lee JM, Fynn SP. P wave morphology in guiding the ablation strategy of focal atrial tachycardias and atrial flutter. Curr Cardiol Rev. 2015;11(2):103–10.
5. Uhm JS, Shim J, Wi J, Mun HS, Pak HN, Lee MH, et al. An electrocardiography algorithm combined with clinical features could localize the origins of focal atrial tachycardias in adjacent structures. Europace. 2014;16(7):1061–8.

6. Higa S, Tai CT, Lin YJ, Liu TY, Lee PC, Huang JL, et al. Focal atrial tachycardia: new insight from non-contact mapping and catheter ablation. Circulation. 2004;109(1):84–91.

7. Ito S, Tada H, Nogami A, Naito S, Oshima S, Taniguchi K. Atrial tachycardia arising from the right atrial inferoseptum masquerading as common atrial flutter. Circ J. 2007;71(1):160–5.

Case 2

Ronan Le Bouar, Frédéric Halbwachs,
Charline Daval, and Gabriel Cismaru

2

2.1 Case Presentation

A 62-year-old male patient with a past medical history of atrial flutter, type 1 aortic dissection complicated with hemomediastinum and hemothorax at the age of 45 years treated with emergency surgery, chronic obliterative arteriopathy of the lower limbs treated with bilateral aorto-iliac bypass graft at the age of 57 years, COPD, and depression was addressed to the Cardiology Department for repeated episodes of intermittent palpitations accompanied by dyspnea and fatigue, that had progressively aggravated during the past 3 months. The palpitations had a sudden onset and termination, were rapid and regular, and had a variable duration up to several hours.

His cardiovascular risk factors were represented by arterial hypertension and dyslipidemia.

His medication at home consisted of rivaroxaban 20 mg, bisoprolol 7.5 mg, telmisartan + hydrochlorothiazide 40/12.5 mg, atorvastatin 20 mg, esomeprazole 40 mg, formoterol + beclometasone 2 inhalations/day, bilastine 20 mg, paroxetine 20 mg, and alimemazine 5 mg.

At physical examination, his blood pressure was 115/84 mmHg, HR 90 bpm, SpO_2 95% breathing room air, $H = 165$ cm, $W = 62$ kg, BMI $= 22.77$ kg/m^2, heart sounds were irregular, there was a mild systolic murmur in the mitral auscultation region, lung auscultation revealed bilateral sibilant rales, there were mild bilateral edema of the lower limbs.

His CHA_2DS_2-VASc score was 2, his HAS-BLED score was 0.

His ECG at presentation is showed in Fig. 2.1.

His biological workup showed a Hb level of 11.9 g/dl, leucocytes 9.29×10^9/L, platelets 224×10^9/L, CRP < 3 mg/L, BUN 9.5 mmol/L, creatinine 83 µmol/L, glycemia 4.5 mmol/L, HbA1c 6.0%, Na$^+$ 138 mmol/L, K$^+$ 3.8 mmol/L, total proteins 79 g/L, D-dimers 965 ng/ml, TSH 1.61 IU/L, total cholesterol 155 mg/dl, HDL 57 mg/dl, LDL 79 mg/dl, and triglycerides 166 mg/dl.

Supplementary Information The online version contains supplementary material available at [https://doi.org/10.1007/978-3-031-07357-1_2].

R. Le Bouar (✉) · C. Daval
Cardiology Department, "Emile Muller" Hospital, Mulhouse, France
e-mail: LEBOUARR@ghrmsa.fr

F. Halbwachs
Biosense Webster, Mulhouse, France

G. Cismaru
Cardiology Department, Rehabilitation Hospital, Cluj-Napoca, Romania

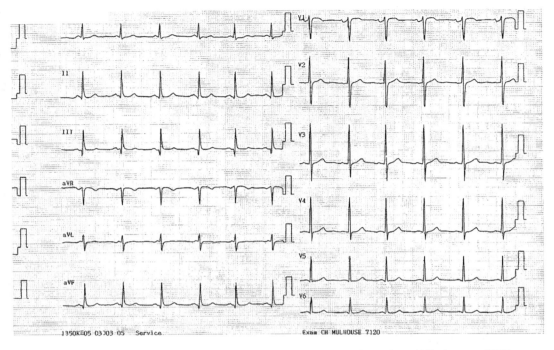

Fig. 2.1 A 12-lead ECG showing sinus rhythm with a heart rate of 75 bpm, QRS axis at +60°, absence of LV hypertrophy, absence of ischemia

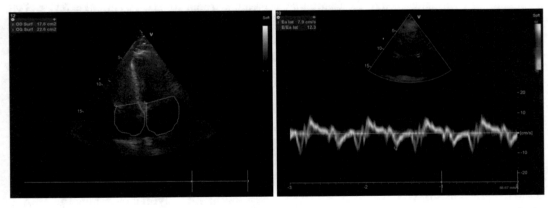

Fig. 2.2 *Left panel*: Echocardiography image in apical 4 chamber view showing a mildly dilated right and left atrium. *Right panel*: myocardial tissue Doppler image in apical 4 chamber view showing increased left ventricular filling pressure, with a ratio of *E/e'* >12

Transthoracic echocardiography revealed a non-dilated LV with a preserved LV EF%, mildly dilated left atrium with a surface of 22.6 cm^2, elevated LV filling pressure (*E/e'* of 12) (Fig. 2.2).

Given the history of intermittent palpitations, an electrophysiological study was offered and accepted by the patient.

2.2 Electrophysiological Study and RF Catheter Ablation Procedure

The electrophysiological study was performed under local anesthesia and conscious sedation. Vascular access was obtained using the modified

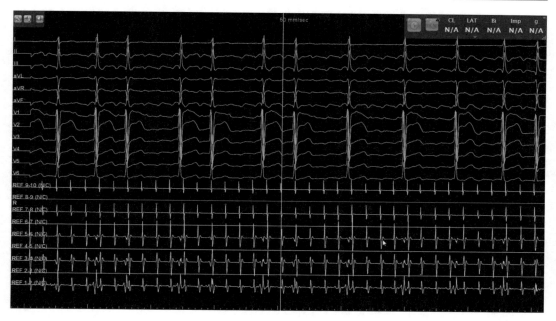

Fig. 2.3 A 12-lead ECG together with intracavitary electrograms recorded from the bipolar electrodes of the decapolar catheter placed inside the coronary sinus (REF 1, 2 to REF 9, 10) showing an irregular narrow QRS complex tachycardia, with an atrial cycle length of 240 ms and variable AV conduction. The F waves are negative in leads II, III, aVF, and V6, positive in lead V1, aVL. The depolarization sequence at the level of the coronary sinus catheter is proximal to distal. Paper speed at 50 mm/s

Seldinger technique, under Doppler ultrasound guidance. A 6F quadripolar steerable catheter (Dynamic Extrem, Microport®) was introduced in a 6F 20 cm vascular sheath and was subsequently advanced via the right common femoral vein up to the coronary sinus. A Biosense Webster® SmartTouch SF open-irrigated 3.5 mm tip with F curve was introduced in a 9F 20 cm vascular sheath and was subsequently advanced via the right common femoral vein up to the right atrium. Atrial and ventricular pacing were carried out at twice the diastolic threshold using the EP-4™ Cardiac Stimulator (Abbott®) system. Surface ECG and intracavitary ECGs were recorded by the *WorkMate* Claris™ System (Abbott®).

Baseline AH interval vas 97 ms, the HV interval was 36 ms.

Programmed atrial stimulation induced the tachycardia presented in Fig. 2.3.

> **Question 1: What is the tachycardia shown in Fig. 2.3?**
> A. Typical counterclockwise atrial flutter.
> B. Typical clockwise atrial flutter.
> C. Clockwise perimitral atrial flutter.
> D. Counterclockwise perimitral atrial flutter.
> E. Focal atrial tachycardia.

Figure 2.3 **explained:** this shows atrial flutter with negative F waves in leads II, III, aVF, V6 positive in aVL and V1, with variable AV conduction, QRS axis at +75°, absence of LV hypertrophy, absence of ischemia. This is compatible with typical counterclockwise atrial flutter.

An anatomical map of the right atrium was initially created. The right atrium was mildly dilated, with a volume of 110 ml. Next, an acti-

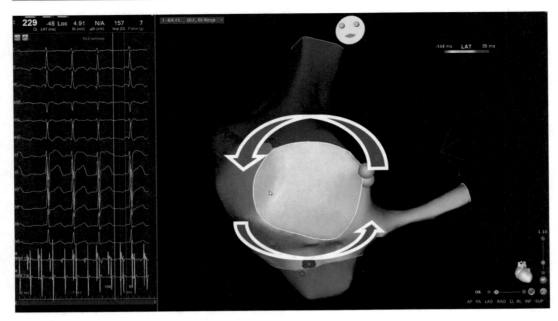

Fig. 2.4 CARTO image in LAO view showing the activation map of the right atrium during atrial flutter, showing a depolarization sequence in favor of typical counterclockwise atrial flutter. The activation wavefront proceeds from red to orange to yellow to green to blue to violet around the tricuspid valve, as shown in the upper right corner of the tracing. The left side of the tracing shows the 12-lead ECG together with the electrodes 7–8 from the coronary sinus catheter (REF 7, 8) ant the distal bipolar electrode from the roving/ablation catheter (MAP 1–2)

vation map of the right atrium was created during the arrhythmia, which demonstrated the presence of a macro-reentry circuit around the tricuspid valve, compatible with typical counterclockwise atrial flutter (Fig. 2.4).

RF ablation of the cavotricuspid isthmus was performed, and this terminated the atrial flutter with the patient converting to sinus rhythm. Bidirectional conduction block at the level of the CTI was confirmed. The confirmation of clockwise block is shown in Fig. 2.5.

After the RF ablation of the CTI and confirmation of conduction block at this level, during pacing from the coronary sinus catheter at a fixed coupling interval of 600 ms for verification of clockwise conduction block, a symptomatic narrow QRS tachycardia was initiated (Fig. 2.6).

> **Question 2: What is the tachycardia presented in Fig. 2.6?**
> A. Recurrence of typical counterclockwise atrial flutter
> B. Typical clockwise atrial flutter
> C. Atypical right atrial flutter
> D. Focal atrial tachycardia
> E. Atrial fibrillation

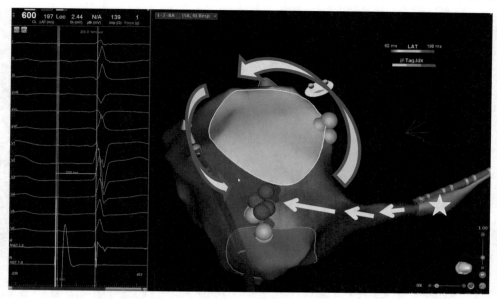

Fig. 2.5 CARTO image from a caudal view showing the activation map of the right atrium after RF ablation of the CTI (red and pink dots) during pacing form the proximal electrodes of the coronary sinus catheter (REF 7, 8), showing a depolarization sequence compatible with clockwise conduction block at the level of the CTI. During CS pacing at a fixed coupling interval of 600 ms, the roving/ablation catheter records a depolarization sequence around the tricuspid valve which travels from the CS ostium (red color) to the CTI (orange color), where conduction does not further propagate in a clockwise direc-tion but stops at the level of the ablation lesions (note the normal depolarization sequence presented in the upper right corner of the image); the depolarization wavefront travels in a counterclockwise direction from the CS ostium, around the tricuspid valve, activating the inter-atrial septum in a caudal-cranial fashion, the lateral wall of the right atrium in a cranial-caudal fashion (yellow curved lines), with the latest activation region being the area just lateral to the RF ablation line (purple). The delay from the pacing spike to the latest activation point just lateral to the ablation line is 200 ms

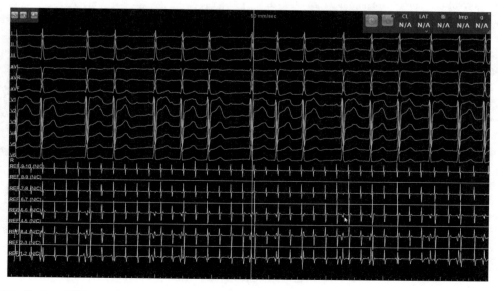

Fig. 2.6 Surface ECG leads together with intracavitary leads recorded from the 10 bipolar electrodes of the coronary sinus catheter (REF 9, 10) showing a narrow QRS complex tachycardia induced during programmed atrial stimulation after the RF ablation of the CTI for typical counterclockwise atrial flutter

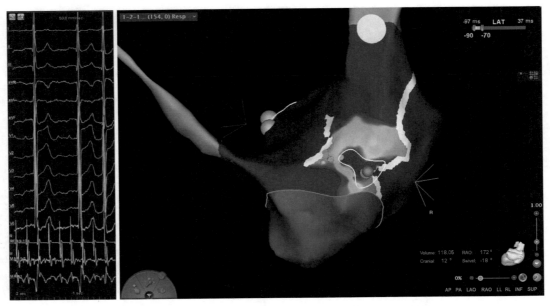

Fig. 2.7 CARTO image in postero-anterior view showing the activation map of the right atrium during the tachycardia, showing a depolarization sequence starting in the region of the lower part of the crista terminalis (red area), from where the depolarization wavefront travels in a centrifugal manner to the rest of the atrial tissue (red → orange → yellow → green → blue → violet). The described mechanism is compatible with a focal atrial tachycardia. The orange dot represents the site with the earliest activation during tachycardia. The left side of the image shows the 12-lead ECG during tachycardia together with intracavitary electrograms recorded by the proximal electrodes of the coronary sinus catheter (REF 9, 10), the distal electrodes of the roving/ablation catheter (MAP 1–2) and the unipolar recording from the distal electrode of the roving/ablation catheter (MAP 1). Note that the morphology of the P wave is negative in leads II, III, aVF, positive in aVL, flattened then positive in V1 and V2, suggesting an origin in the lower part of the right atrium, compatible with the activation map of the right atrium during tachycardia

An activation map of the right atrium was subsequently performed (Fig. 2.7). This was compatible with a focal atrial tachycardia originating in the lower part of the crista terminalis. The tachycardia cycle length was 200 ms.

Fig. 2.8 left panel shows the bipolar and the unipolar local signal recorded by the roving/ablation catheter at the earliest activation site in the right atrium. The local atrial activity preceded the onset of the P wave on surface ECG by 44 ms, and where the unipolar electrogram had a "QS" aspect

Question 3: Is this a good ablation site?

A. Yes. The earliest local bipolar electrogram precedes the onset of the P wave on the surface ECG by 44 ms.

B. Yes. The local unipolar electrogram has a "QS" aspect.

C. Yes. The activation map is in favor of a focal atrial tachycardia originating in this region.

D. No. This is an atrial tachycardia probably originating in the left atrium.

E. No. No atrial tachycardia can originate in this region.

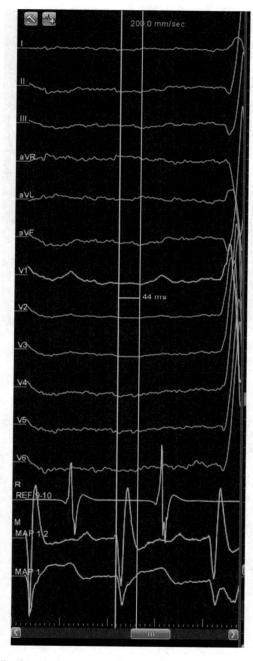

Fig. 2.8 A 12-lead ECG during tachycardia together with intracavitary electrograms recorded by the proximal electrodes of the coronary sinus catheter (REF 9, 10), the distal electrodes of the roving/ablation catheter (MAP 1–2), and the unipolar recording from the distal electrode of the roving/ablation catheter (MAP 1). The earliest local atrial activation precedes the beginning of the P wave on the surface ECG by 44 ms. The unipolar electrogram recorded by the distal pole of the roving/mapping catheter has a "QS" aspect, certifying the appropriate ablation site

The 44 ms difference between the local bipolar electrogram and the onset of the P wave, the "QS" aspect of the unipolar electrogram, and the activation map of the RA during tachycardia were all arguments in favor of a good ablation site. RF application with a power of 30 Watts terminated the tachycardia (Figs. 2.9 and 2.10).

There was no complication related to the procedure.

The patient was discharged from the hospital 24 h later. Given his CHA_2DS_2-VASc score of 1, anticoagulant treatment was continued.

> **ANSWERS TO:**
> **Question 1: A. Typical counterclockwise atrial flutter.**
> **Question 2: D. Focal Atrial Tachycardia.**
> **Question 3:**
> A. **Yes. The earliest local bipolar electrogram precedes the onset of the P wave on the surface ECG by 44 ms.**
> B. **Yes. The local unipolar electrogram has a "QS" aspect.**
> C. **Yes. The activation map is in favor of a focal atrial tachycardia originating in this region.**

2.3 Commentary

The present case presents an RF catheter ablation procedure of typical atrial flutter and of a focal atrial tachycardia in a 62-year-old male patient. Several comments can be made about the present case.

Typical atrial flutter is the most commonly encountered macro-reentry arrhythmia in clinical practice [1]. Atrial tachycardia, on the other hand, is a much rarer arrhythmia, with a prevalence of 10–15% of all SVTs [2]. Sometimes, such as in the present case, these 2 arrhythmias can coexist in the same patient.

Atrial tachycardia can have as underlying mechanism increased automaticity, triggered activity or reentry. It can be classified as focal or macro-reentry. From a clinical point of view,

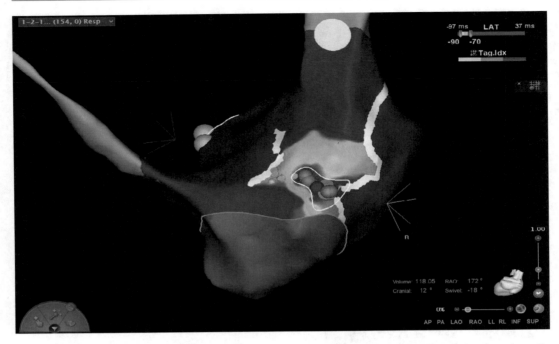

Fig. 2.9 CARTO image in postero-anterior view° showing the activation map of the right atrium during the tachycardia with superposed RF ablation lesions at the successful ablation site

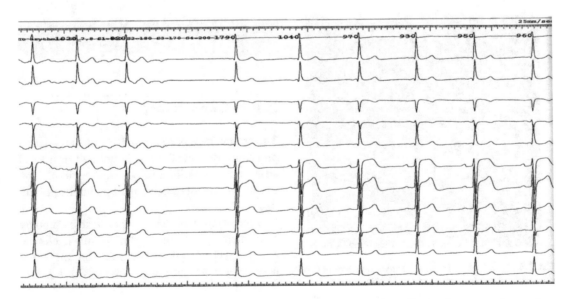

Fig. 2.10 A 12-lead ECG recorded during RF ablation of the focal atrial tachycardia showing conversion to sinus rhythm

it can be paroxysmal, persistent, or incessant. It can occur in patients with structural heart disease or in patients with structurally normal hearts. The most common origins of focal atrial tachycardia occurring from the left atrium include the pulmonary vein ostia, the left atrial appendage, and the mitral annulus. For focal atrial tachycardias occurring from the right atrium, the most common origins are the crista terminalis, the ostium of the coronary sinus, the right atrial appendage, and the tricuspid annulus [3, 4].

The diagnosis of atrial tachycardia is made from the 12-lead ECG, which shows the presence of P waves with a different morphology compared to the sinus P wave, separated by an isoelectric segment. In cases when the diagnosis is not straightforward, adenosine can be administered in order to produce transient AV block and unmask the P waves, for a more accurate analysis.

Focal atrial tachycardia is a rare atrial arrhythmia, with a prevalence of <1% [5]. It is equally found in men and women. The treatment of choice is catheter ablation, since it is superior to antiarrhythmic medication. It currently has a class I indication level of evidence B, according to the ESC Guidelines on the management of patients with supraventricular arrhythmias [6]. The reported success rate varies between 75% and 100% [7–9]. The recurrence rate varies between 2 and 20%, and the complication rate between 0.3% and 2% [6].

Catheter ablation of focal atrial tachycardias is usually performed using radiofrequency, but, in the case of ablating areas close to the normal conduction system, such as the case of peri-AV nodal atrial tachycardias, cryoablation can also be used, with good results [10]. An electroanatomical mapping system is very useful in reducing the fluoroscopy time and dose in the case of focal atrial tachycardia ablation. It also helps with accurate mapping and facilitates catheter placement in key positions inside the heart chambers, with reproducible results. In the case of contact force-equipped catheters, it also allows force application assessment before RF delivery. It also increases procedural success [11].

In the case of focal atrial tachycardias arising from the crista terminalis, it has been suggested that the patho-physiology of the arrhythmia is localized reentry caused by age-related local remodeling that determines conduction slowing [11]. Fluoroscopy-guided ablation can have an acute success rate as high as 92.2%, but this can increase to 98.5% if an electroanatomical mapping system is used [11]. Recurrences are rare, less than 10%. In the above presented-patient, the CARTO system identified the origin of the focal atrial tachycardia at the level of the low part of the crista terminalis. RF application at the earliest depolarization site during tachycardia terminated the arrhythmia. The patient remains arrhythmia-free more than 3 years after the procedure.

Learning Point

- Atrial flutter and focal atrial tachycardia can coexist.
- Performing programmed atrial stimulation after successful RF ablation of a supraventricular arrhythmia can sometimes induce a second arrhythmia, which can be treated during the same procedure.

References

1. Cosio FG. Atrial flutter, typical and atypical: a review. Arrhythmia Electrophysiol Rev. 2017;6(2):55–62.
2. Steinbeck G, Hoffmann E. 'True' atrial tachycardia. Eur Heart J. 1998;19 Suppl E:E10–2. E48–9
3. Balla C, Foresti S, Ali H, Sorgente A, Egidy Assenza G, De Ambroggi G, et al. Long-term follow-up after radiofrequency ablation of ectopic atrial tachycardia in young patients. J Arrhythm. 2019;35(2):290–5.
4. Huo Y, Braunschweig F, Gaspar T, Richter S, Schonbauer R, Sommer P, et al. Diagnosis of atrial tachycardias originating from the lower right atrium: importance of P-wave morphology in the precordial leads V3–V6. Europace. 2013;15(4):570–7.
5. Poutiainen AM, Koistinen MJ, Airaksinen KE, Hartikainen EK, Kettunen RV, Karjalainen JE, et al. Prevalence and natural course of ectopic atrial tachycardia. Eur Heart J. 1999;20(9):694–700.
6. Brugada J, Katritsis DG, Arbelo E, Arribas F, Bax JJ, Blomstrom-Lundqvist C, et al. 2019 ESC Guidelines for the management of patients with supraventricu-

lar tachycardia. The Task Force for the management of patients with supraventricular tachycardia of the European Society of Cardiology (ESC). Eur Heart J. 2020;41(5):655–720.

7. Kistler PM, Sanders P, Fynn SP, Stevenson IH, Hussin A, Vohra JK, et al. Electrophysiological and electro-cardiographic characteristics of focal atrial tachy-cardia originating from the pulmonary veins: acute and long-term outcomes of radiofrequency ablation. Circulation. 2003;108(16):1968–75.

8. Chen SA, Chiang CE, Yang CJ, Cheng CC, Wu TJ, Wang SP, et al. Sustained atrial tachycardia in adult patients. Electrophysiological characteristics, phar-macological response, possible mechanisms, and effects of radiofrequency ablation. Circulation. 1994;90(3):1262–78.

9. Spector P, Reynolds MR, Calkins H, Sondhi M, Xu Y, Martin A, et al. Meta-analysis of ablation of atrial flut-ter and supraventricular tachycardia. Am J Cardiol. 2009;104(5):671–7.

10. Chan NY. Catheter ablation of peri-nodal and pul-monary veno-atrial substrates: should it be cool? Europace. 2015;17(Suppl. 2):ii19–30.

11. Morris GM, Segan L, Wong G, Wynn G, Watts T, Heck P, et al. Atrial tachycardia arising from the crista terminalis, detailed electrophysiological fea-tures and long-term ablation outcomes. JACC Clin Electrophysiol. 2019;5(4):448–58.

Case 3

Frédéric Halbwachs, Ronan Le Bouar,
Jean-Yves Wiedemann, Jacques Levy,
and Laurent Jacquemin

3

3.1 Case Presentation

A 16-year-old male patient with no significant past medical history was addressed to the Cardiology Department for a first episode of malaise that occurred several days prior to his presentation to the hospital, after 2 h of cycling. He experienced an unusual state of fatigue and light-headedness that persisted for several minutes. He denied the presence of chest pain, dyspnea, or palpitations. He did not experience loss of consciousness. He had no family history of sudden cardiac death. He was on no chronic medication.

At physical examination, his blood pressure was 137/80 mmHg, HR 95 bpm, SpO$_2$ 99% breathing room air, $H = 165$ cm, $W = 85$ kg, BMI = 31.22 kg/m^2, heart sounds were irregular, there were no audible murmurs, lung auscultation was clear, there were no signs of right heart failure.

His CHA$_2$DS$_2$-VASc score was 0, his HAS-BLED score was 0. His ECG at presentation is showed in Fig. 3.1.

> **Question 1: What does the ECG show?**
> A. Sinus rhythm with grade 1 sino-atrial block.
> B. Sinus rhythm with grade 2 sino-atrial block.
> C. Sinus rhythm with runs of PAC.
> D. Atrial Fibrillation.
> E. Incessant atrial tachycardia.

His biological workup showed a Hb level of 15.7 g/dl, leucocytes 6.49 × 10^9/L, platelets 266 × 10^9/L, CRP <3 mg/l, BUN 3.9 mmol/l, creatinine76 µmol/l, glycemia 4.3 mmol/l, Na+ 141 mmol/l, K+ 4.7 mmol/l, cTnI <0.015 ng/ml, NT pro-BNP <30 pg/ml, TSH 1.97 IU/L, total cholesterol 160 mg/dl, HDL 52 mg/dl, LDL 92 mg/dl, and triglycerides 80 mg/dl.

Given the aspect of the 12-lead ECG at admittance, a 24-hour Holter ECG was performed. The result is presented in Figs. 3.2 and 3.3.

> **Question 2: What does the result of the Holter ECG from Fig. 3.3 show?**
> A. Sinus rhythm with grade 1 sino-atrial block.
> B. Sinus rhythm with grade 2 sino-atrial block.
> C. Sinus rhythm with runs of PAC.
> D. Atrial fibrillation.
> E. Incessant atrial tachycardia.

F. Halbwachs (✉)
Biosense Webster, Mulhouse, France

R. Le Bouar · J.-Y. Wiedemann · J. Levy
L. Jacquemin
Cardiology Department, "Emile Muller" Hospital, Mulhouse, France

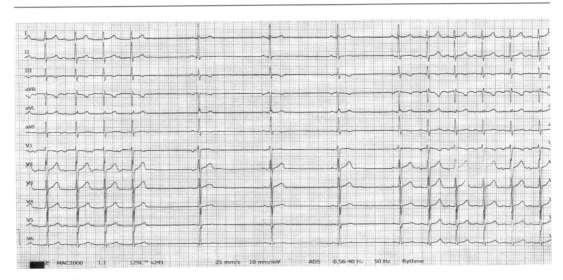

Fig. 3.1 A 12-lead ECG recorded at admittance to the Cardiology Department

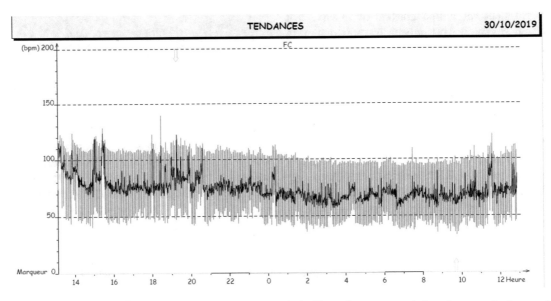

Fig. 3.2 A 24-hour Holter ECG showing the absence of significant heart rate variations between daytime and nighttime

Transthoracic echocardiography revealed a non-dilated LV with a normal systolic function, LV EF% of 77%, with non-dilated right and left atrium (Fig. 3.4). It also showed a normal diastolic function, absence of LV hypertrophy, trivial mitral regurgitation, a non-dilated right ventricle, absence of pulmonary hypertension, sPAP of 21 mmHg, absence of pericardial effusion, a non-dilated aorta.

An exercise stress test was performed, which was terminated for fatigue at 125 W, 9.5 METS, with a maximum heart rate of 200 bpm (98% of the maximum theoretical heart rate) which was negative for inducible myocardial ischemia and showed no significant ventricular arrhythmias, no conduction rhythm disorders (Fig. 3.5).

Figure 3.1 is explained below

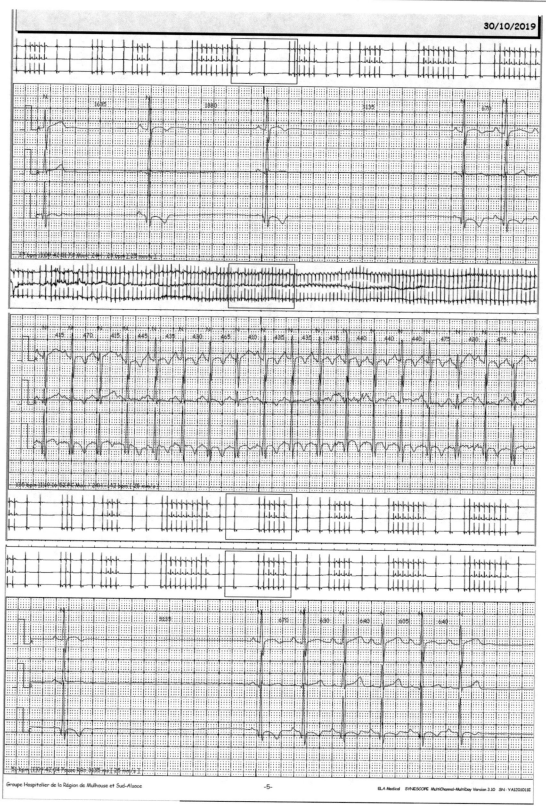

Fig. 3.3 Three excerpts from the 24-hour Holter ECG showing alternations between bradycardia and tachycardia

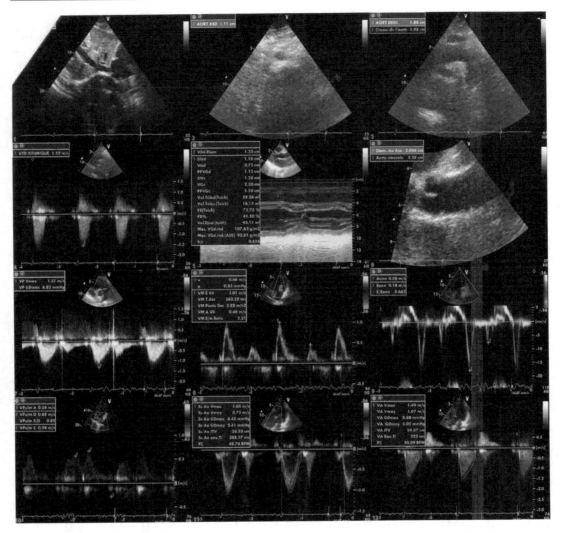

Fig. 3.4 Transthoracic echocardiography images showing a non-dilated LV with a preserved EF of 77%, normal diastolic function, no LV hypertrophy, absence of signifi-cant valve disease, non-dilated right heart chambers, a non-dilated aorta, absence of pericardial effusion

Question 3: What would be the appropriate management of this patient?

A. This is symptomatic sinus node disease. No other test is necessary. Pacemaker implantation should be performed.

B. This is symptomatic sinus node disease. Lyme disease should be suspected. If positive, antibiotic treatment should be started as soon as possible.

C. This is symptomatic sinus node disease. The likely cause is myocarditis. A cardiac MRI should be performed.

D. This is symptomatic sinus node disease. The most likely cause is cardiac sarcoidosis. A cardiac MRI should be performed to confirm the diagnosis.

E. This is incessant atrial tachycardia. Catheter ablation should be performed.

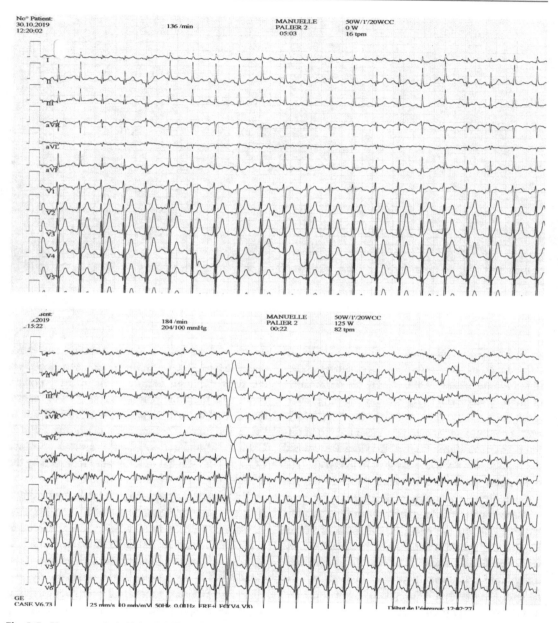

Fig. 3.5 *Upper panel:* A 12-lead ECG during exercise stress test at 50 W. *Lower panel*: 12-lead ECG during exercise stress test at 125 W, showing an isolated PVC

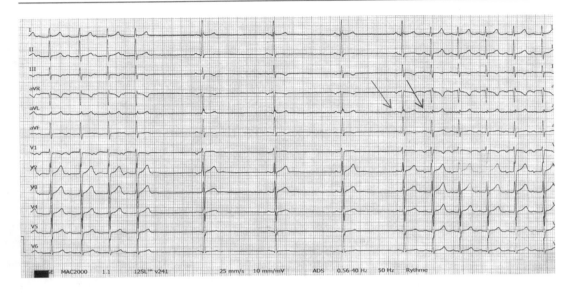

Figure 3.1 **explained.** A 12-lead ECG at Admittance to the Cardiology Department showing at the beginning of the tracing the termination of an incessant atrial tachycardia. Following this, 4 sinus beats can be seen, and then the atrial tachycardia resumes spontaneously. Note the slight differences in the morphology of the sinus P wave and the tachycardia P wave, best seen in lead aVL. The blue arrow indicates the sinus P wave, the red arrow indicates the tachycardia P wave.

Based on the ECG recorded at admittance to the hospital and on the result of the 24-hour Holter ECG, the diagnosis of incessant atrial tachycardia was established. Given the fact that long-term anti-arrhythmic treatment was not desired by the patient, a catheter ablation procedure was offered and subsequently performed.

3.2 Electrophysiological Study and RF Catheter Ablation Procedure

The electrophysiological study was performed under general anesthesia. Vascular access was obtained using the modified Seldinger technique, under Doppler ultrasound guidance. A 6F decapo-lar steerable catheter (Inquiry, Abbott®) was introduced in a 6F 20 cm vascular sheath and placed via the right common femoral vein in the coronary sinus, with the distal poles at the level of the lateral mitral annulus. Atrial pacing was carried out at twice the diastolic threshold using the EP-4™ Cardiac Stimulator (Abbott®) system. Surface ECG and intracavitary ECGs were recorded by the *WorkMate* Claris™ System (Abbott®).

Radiofrequency ablation was delivered using a Biosense Webster® SmartTouch SF open-irrigated 3.5 mm tip with D curve, which was introduced in a 9F 20 cm vascular sheath via the right common femoral vein at the level of the right atrium. The CARTO ® 3 electro-anatomic mapping System (Biosense Webster, Johnson & Johnson) was used to guide mapping and ablation of the accessory pathway.

Baseline ECG at the beginning of the procedure is shown in Fig. 3.6. The patient presented incessant runs of atrial tachycardia.

Baseline AH during sinus rhythm was 63 ms, the HV interval was 41 ms. Retrograde conduction was present, concentric, decremental. Parahisian pacing demonstrated an "AV nodal" response, showing no retrograde conduction over an accessory pathway.

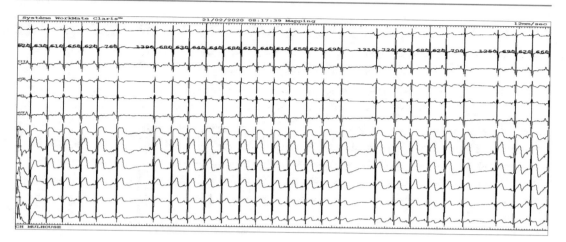

Fig. 3.6 A 12-lead ECG at the beginning of the electrophysiological study showing runs of incessant atrial tachycardia

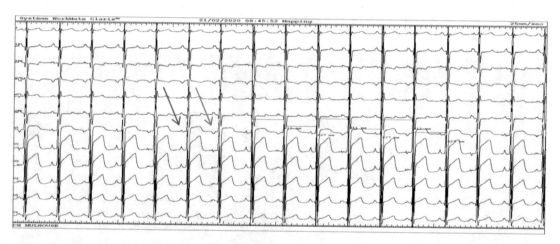

Fig. 3.7 A 12-lead ECG showing alternation between sinus P waves (red arrow) and ectopic atrial beats (red arrow) that have an identical morphology with that of the P wave during atrial tachycardia. Note the constant variation of the PP (and RR) intervals between 2 cycle lengths as a consequence of atrial bigeminy

The patient presented periods of alternating beats between sinus rhythm and those coming from an ectopic focus (Figs. 3.7 and 3.8).

An anatomical map of the left atrium was first created, showing a non-dilated right atrium, with a volume of 85 ml. Activation mapping of the right atrium was then performed during atrial tachycardia. The earliest local atrial activation was identified at the level of the superior part of the crista terminalis, where the local A preceded the surface P wave on the 12-lead ECG by 12 ms (Fig. 3.9). The unipolar atrial electrogram at this site had a "QS" aspect.

Before turning RF ablation on, the trajectory of the right phrenic nerve was identified, by pacing from the roving/ablation catheter in areas adjacent to the target ablation site, to assure lack of phrenic nerve capture. These sites were marked on the CARTO activation map (yellow and orange dots) (Fig. 3.9).

RF ablation was performed at this site with a target power of 25 W and an ablation index of 400. The tachycardia was terminated during the first RF application. The position of the ablation catheter at the successful ablation site is presented

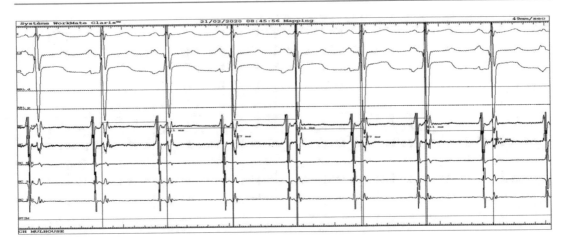

Fig. 3.8 Surface ECG leads I, II, V1, and V6 together with intracavitary leads recorded from the bipolar electrodes of the CS catheter (CS 1–2 to 9–10) showing the same depolarization sequence at the level of the coronary sinus electrodes during sinus beats and during ectopic beats, from proximal to distal, suggesting an origin of the ectopic beats in the right atrium

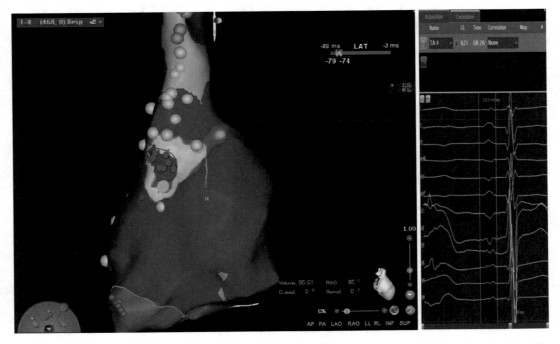

Fig. 3.9 *Left panel*: CARTO image in right lateral view showing the activation map of the right atrium during atrial tachycardia. The earliest endocardial atrial activation is recorded in an area measuring 28 mm², situated at the level of the superior part of the crista terminalis, on the high postero-lateral right atrium (red area). The orange and yellow dots represent the sites where local pacing from the roving/ablation catheter produces phrenic nerve capture, indicating its trajectory on the epicardial surface of the right atrium. *Right panel*: A 12-lead ECG showing the morphology of the P wave during atrial tachycardia

Fig. 3.10 CARTO image in right lateral view showing the activation map of the right atrium during atrial tachycardia with superposed RF ablation lesions at the successful ablation site (pink dots). The ablation catheter is positioned at the earliest endocardial atrial activation site during tachycardia

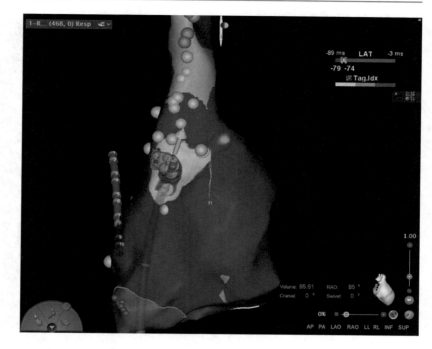

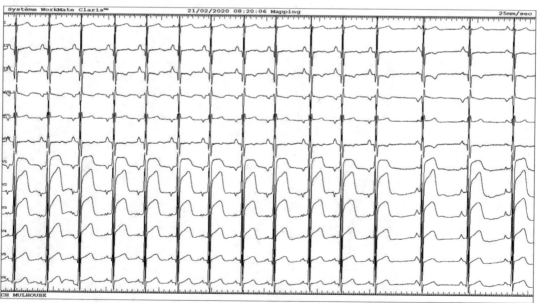

Fig. 3.11 A 12-lead ECG showing termination of the atrial tachycardia during RF ablation. The last 3 QRS complexes are preceded by sinus P waves

in Fig. 3.10 and the termination of the tachycardia in Fig. 3.11.

An activation map of the right and left atrium after the ablation of the tachycardia is presented in Figs. 3.12, 3.13, 3.14, and 3.15. As it can be observed, the sinus node area was situated just superior and slightly anterior to the successful ablation site of the tachycardia.

A comparison of the P wave morphology during atrial tachycardia and during sinus rhythm is presented in Fig. 3.16.

Fig. 3.12 CARTO image in RAO 45° showing the activation map of the right and left atrium recorded after the ablation of the atrial tachycardia. The earliest activation site is recorded at the antero-lateral and superior part of the right atrium, compatible with the sinus node region (red area, encircled by the yellow line). The yellow dot at the level of the tricuspid valve represents the bundle of His

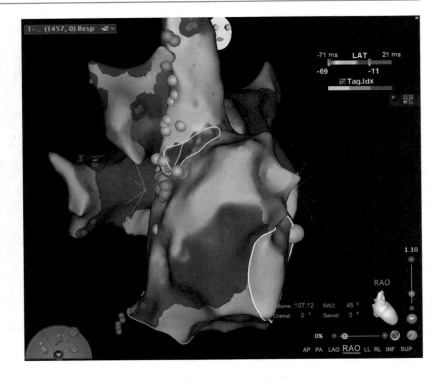

Fig. 3.13 CARTO image in LAO 5° showing the activation map of the right and left atrium recorded after the ablation of the atrial tachycardia. The earliest activation site is recorded at the antero-lateral and superior part of the right atrium, compatible with the sinus node region (red area, encircled by the yellow line). The yellow dot at the level of the tricuspid valve represents the bundle of His

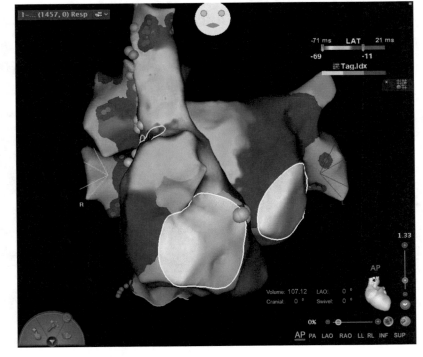

Fig. 3.14 CARTO image in RAO 1° cranial 42° showing the activation map of the right and left atrium recorded after the ablation of the atrial tachycardia. The earliest activation site is recorded at the antero-lateral and superior part of the right atrium, compatible with the sinus node region (red area, encircled by the yellow line). The yellow dot at the level of the tricuspid valve represents the bundle of His

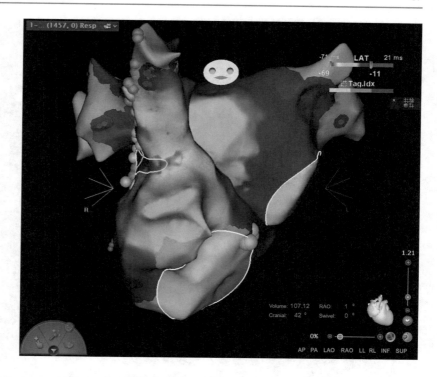

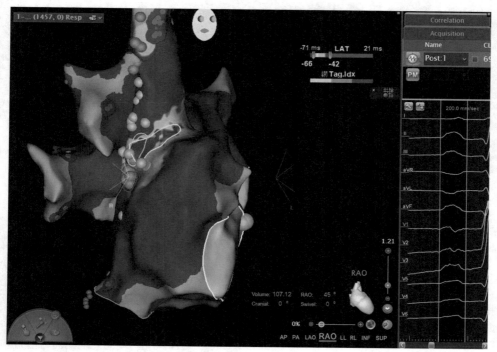

Fig. 3.15 CARTO image in RAO 45° cranial 0° showing the activation map of the right and left atrium recorded after the ablation of the atrial tachycardia. The earliest activation site is recorded at the antero-lateral and superior part of the right atrium, compatible with the sinus node region (red area, encircled by the yellow line). The yellow dot at the level of the tricuspid valve represents the bundle of His. The right side of the image shows the morphology of the sinus P wave on the 12-lead ECG

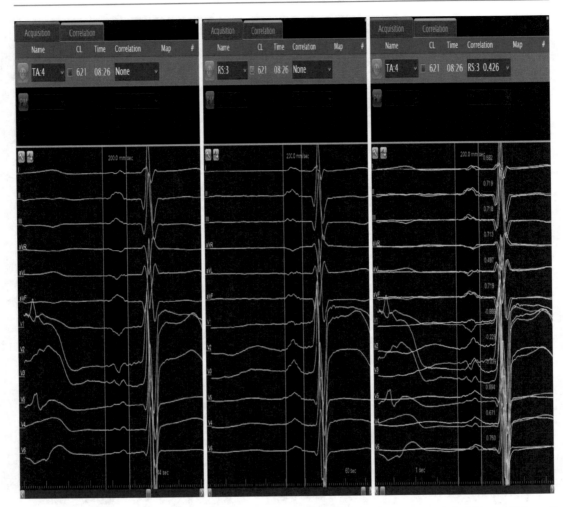

Fig. 3.16 CARTO image showing the comparison between the 12-lead ECG morphology of the P wave during atrial tachycardia (*left panel*) and sinus rhythm (*middle panel*). *Right panel*: the PASSO algorithm of the CARTO system showing a superposition coefficient of 71% between the sinus P wave and the P wave recorded during atrial tachycardia

The 12-lead ECG at the end of the ablation procedure is presented in Fig. 3.17.

There were no complications related to the procedure. The ECG recorded after the ablation procedure is presented in Fig. 3.18. The patient was discharged home 24 h later on no antiarrhythmic medication.

A 24-hour Holter ECG recorded 4 months after the ablation procedure showed no tachycardia recurrence (Fig. 3.19).

ANSWERS TO:
Question 1: E. Incessant atrial tachycardia.
Question 2: E. Incessant atrial tachycardia.
Question 3: E. This is incessant atrial tachycardia. Catheter ablation should be performed.

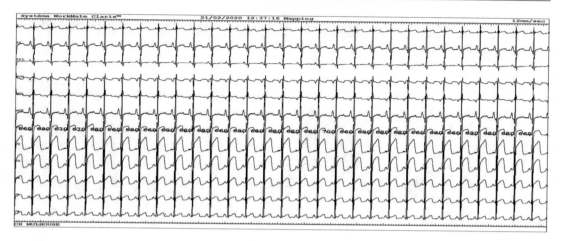

Fig. 3.17 A 12-lead ECG recorded at the end of the ablation procedure showing sinus rhythm with a heart rate of 88 bpm, QRS axis at +60°, no LV hypertrophy, absence of ischemia

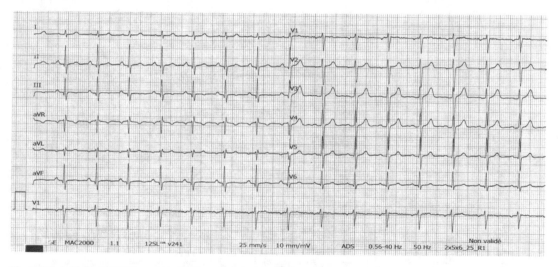

Fig. 3.18 A 12-lead ECG recorded after the ablation procedure showing sinus rhythm with a heart rate of 95 bpm, QRS axis at +60°, no LV hypertrophy, absence of ischemia

3.3 Commentary

The present case illustrates a catheter ablation procedure of a focal atrial tachycardia arising from the superior part of the crista terminalis in a young male patient without structural heart disease. Several observations can be made about the present case.

Atrial tachycardia represents less than 10% of SVTs, after AVNRT and AVRT [1]. Atrial tachycardias can be reentrant, caused by increased automaticity or due to triggered activity (such as in

digitalis intoxication). They can be macro-reentrant or focal. They can originate both from the right atrium and from the left atrium. For focal atrial tachycardias occurring from the right atrium, the most common origins are the crista terminalis, the ostium of the coronary sinus, the right atrial appendage, and the tricuspid annulus [2, 3].

The morphology of the P wave on the 12-lead ECG during focal atrial tachycardias arising from the right atrium is usually biphasic or positive in lead aVL. This marker has a sensitivity of 88% and a specificity of 79% [4]. If arising from the crista

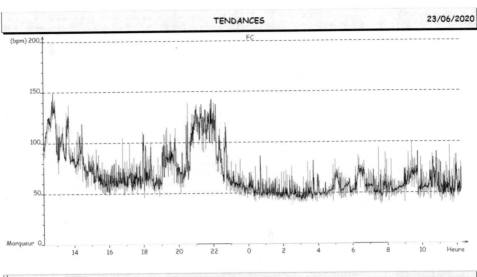

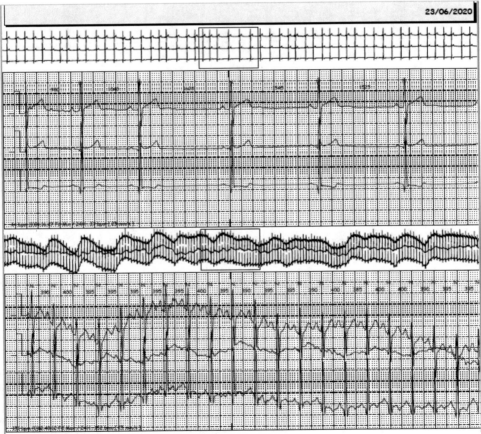

Fig. 3.19 Result of the 24-hour Holter ECG performed 4 months after the ablation procedure showing normal variations between daytime and nighttime heart rate (unlike the Holter ECG recorded before the ablation procedure presented in Fig. 3.2) and absence of atrial tachycardia

terminalis, the P wave is usually negative in aVR [4]. This is the case for the above-presented patient (see Fig. 3.19).

Like any SVT, focal atrial tachycardia can be asymptomatic, or can determine symptoms such as palpitations, dyspnea, chest pain, asthenia, fatigue, malaise, pre-syncope, or syncope. If present for more than 50% of the time, it is called incessant. Incessant atrial tachycardia merits special attention, since it can be complicated by tachycardia-induced cardiomyopathy, which is one of the causes of heart failure. The best treatment option is catheter ablation, since elimination of the tachycardia is accompanied by a significant reduction in heart rate and disappearance of congestive signs and symptoms. The alternative is antiarrhythmic medication, which is less effective and has the disadvantage of requiring long-term administration.

Catheter ablation has a high success rate for ablating focal atrial tachycardias with a relatively low recurrence rate [5]. Complications are rare, but 2 of these merit special attention.

First, when ablating focal atrial tachycardias arising from the crista terminalis, especially form its superior part, close to the junction of the superior vena cava—high right atrium, caution must be exercised not to injure the right phrenic nerve, which has a trajectory on the epicardial surface of the lateral right atrial wall and can be adjacent to the crista terminalis. When using an electroanatomical mapping system for catheter ablation guidance, the trajectory of the phrenic nerve should be identified and tagged before any RF application (such as presented in Figs. 3.9 and 3.10), in order to avoid its inadvertent lesion. For this, we recommend pacing from the distal electrode of the roving/ablation catheter at the tested site with at least 10 mA and a pulse duration of at least 2 ms and, if phrenic nerve capture is observed, the site should be marked and ablation should not be performed at this area. Sites where phrenic nerve capture is not observed should also be marked (with a different symbol) and ablation can usually be safely performed. However, even if phrenic nerve injury occurs, if RF delivery is immediately stopped, recovery is to be expected [6].

The second aspect that merits comment is ablating focal atrial tachycardias that originate in the right atrium, close to the sinus node, such in the above-presented case. Care should be taken not to damage the sinus node when ablating in the high lateral part of the right atrium. The sinus node is an epicardial structure situated at the junction of the superior vena cava with the lateral wall of the right atrium. In adults, it measures approximately 15 mm × 5 mm × 1.5 mm. Even though due to its subepicardial location and its relatively significant size, inadvertent irreversible damage to the sinus node is rare, we recommend caution, since sinus node dysfunction has been described as a complication of RF ablation, especially after ablation of inappropriate sinus tachycardia [7].

Right phrenic nerve injury is also a possible complication when ablating close to the sinus node area [8].

Learning Point

- Focal atrial tachycardia arising from the superior part of the crista terminalis may mimic inappropriate sinus tachycardia.
- Since the origin of these tachycardias is close to the sinus node region, the P wave morphology on the 12-lead ECG during tachycardia will resemble that of the sinus P wave.
- These tachycardias can be incessant and if left untreated, may induce tachycardia-mediated cardiomyopathy.
- Catheter ablation is the treatment of choice since response to antiarrhythmic drugs is sub-optimal.
- During catheter ablation, careful attention must be paid to the trajectory of the adjacent phrenic nerve, in order to avoid its inadvertent lesion.

References

1. Schmitt CPA, Schneider M. Catheter ablation of cardiac arrhythmias. 2006;Focal Atrial Tachycardia:165–81.
2. Balla C, Foresti S, Ali H, Sorgente A, Egidy Assenza G, De Ambroggi G, et al. Long-term follow-up after radiofrequency ablation of ectopic atrial tachycardia in young patients. J Arrhythm. 2019;35(2):290–5.
3. Huo Y, Braunschweig F, Gaspar T, Richter S, Schonbauer R, Sommer P, et al. Diagnosis of atrial tachycardias originating from the lower right atrium:

importance of P-wave morphology in the precordial leads V3-V6. Europace. 2013;15(4):570–7.

4. Kistler PM, Kalman JM. Locating focal atrial tachycardias from P-wave morphology. Heart Rhythm. 2005;2(5):561–4.

5. Morris GM, Segan L, Wong G, Wynn G, Watts T, Heck P, et al. Atrial tachycardia arising from the crista terminalis, detailed electrophysiological features and long-term ablation outcomes. JACC Clin Electrophysiol. 2019;5(4):448–58.

6. Bai R, Patel D, Di Biase L, Fahmy TS, Kozeluhova M, Prasad S, et al. Phrenic nerve injury after catheter ablation: should we worry about this complication? J Cardiovasc Electrophysiol. 2006;17(9):944–8.

7. Rodriguez-Manero M, Kreidieh B, Al Rifai M, Ibarra-Cortez S, Schurmann P, Alvarez PA, et al. Ablation of inappropriate sinus tachycardia: a systematic review of the literature. JACC Clin Electrophysiol. 2017;3(3):253–65.

8. Swallow EB, Dayer MJ, Oldfield WL, Moxham J, Polkey MI. Right hemi-diaphragm paralysis following cardiac radiofrequency ablation. Respir Med. 2006;100(9):1657–9.

Case 4

4

Frédéric Halbwachs, Serban Schiau, Crina Muresan, and Tarek El Nazer

4.1 Case Presentation

A 45-year-old female patient with a past medical history of rheumatoid arthritis, inappropriate sinus tachycardia diagnosed 1 year prior was addressed to the Cardiology Department for aggravating asthenia and fatigue. She had no cardiovascular risk factors. She was under treatment with methotrexate 15 mg/week, folic acid supplements 15 mg/week, prednisone 6 mg/day, potassium supplement 600 mg/day, calcium and vitamin D3 1000 mg/day, risedronate 35 mg/day, and bisoprolol 2.5 mg/day. She had observed a high resting heart rate for about 12 months prior, reason for which she consulted her family physician, who advised her to undergo a cardiology check-up. Her diagnosis was inappropriate sinus tachycardia, probably related to an autonomic nervous system dysfunction in the context of her rheumatoid arthritis. She was prescribed bisoprolol 2.5 mg/day, but her symptoms persisted. She was addressed to our cardiology department for a second opinion. At physical examination, her blood pressure was 117/77 mmHg, HR 86 bpm, SpO_2 96% breathing room air, $T = 36.1$ °C, H = 180 cm, $W = 62$ kg, BMI = 19.13 kg/m^2, heart sounds were irregular, there were no audible murmurs, lung auscultation was clear, there were no signs of left or right heart failure. Her CHA_2DS_2-VASc score was 1, her HAS-BLED score was 0. Her ECG at presentation is showed in Fig. 4.1.

A second ECG recorded a few moments later is presented in Fig. 4.2.

Her transthoracic echocardiography is presented in Fig. 4.3.

This showed a non-dilated LV with a normal systolic dysfunction, LV EF% of 62.7%, a non-hypertrophied LV with non-dilated left atrium. It also showed normal diastolic dysfunction, absence of mitral regurgitation, a non-dilated right atrium and ventricle, mild tricuspid regurgitation, absence of pulmonary hypertension, sPAP of 33 mmHg, absence of pericardial effusion, a non-dilated aorta.

Her biological workup showed a Hb level of 12.8 g/dl, leucocytes 8.46×10^9/L, platelets 235×10^9/L, CRP <3 mg/L, BUN 5.9 mmol/L, creatinine 62 µmol/L, glycemia 5.0 mmol/L, Na+ 144 mmol/L, K+ 3.5 mmol/L, cTnI <0.042 ng/ml, TSH 0.36 IU/L.

Given the aspect of the 12-lead ECG, a 24-hour Holter ECG was performed (Fig. 4.4).

Supplementary Information The online version contains supplementary material available at [https://doi.org/10.1007/978-3-031-07357-1_4].

F. Halbwachs (✉)
Biosense Webster, Mulhouse, France

S. Schiau · C. Muresan · T. El Nazer
Cardiology Department, "Emile Muller" Hospital, Mulhouse, France

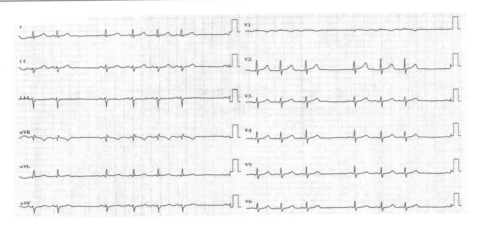

Fig. 4.1 A 12-lead ECG at the admittance to the Cardiology Department

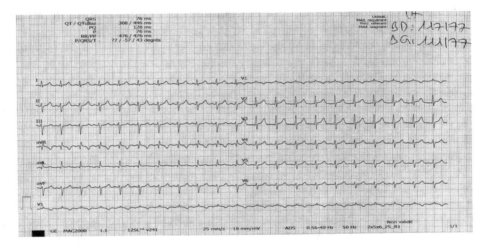

Fig. 4.2 A 12-lead ECG recorded 1 h after admittance to the Cardiology Department

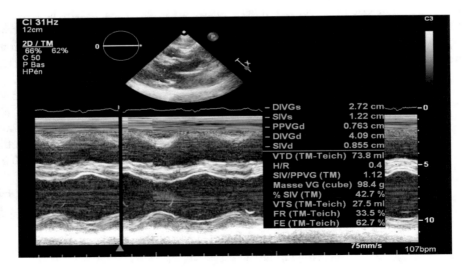

Fig. 4.3 M-mode transthoracic echocardiography image in parasternal long axis view showing a non-dilated LV with a preserved EF of 62.7%, absence of LV hypertrophy

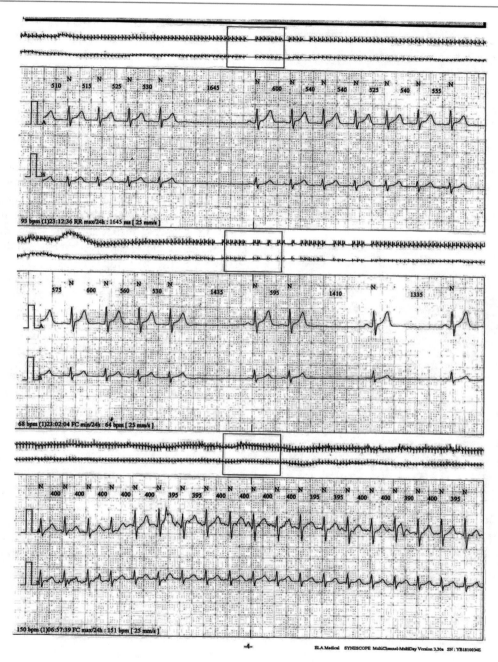

Fig. 4.4 Tracings obtained from a 24-hour Holter ECG

Question 1: What does the ECG in Fig. 4.1 show?

A. Atrial Fibrillation.

B. Atrial flutter.

C. Sinus rhythm with PAC of the same morphology.

D. "Tachycardia – Bradycardia" syndrome: sinus pauses alternating with runs of atrial fibrillation

E. Sinus rhythm with intermittent type 2 AV block.

Question 2: What does the ECG in Fig. 4.2 show?

A. Sinus tachycardia.

B. Atrial flutter.

C. Atrial tachycardia.

D. AVNRT.

E. AVRT.

Question 3: What does the 24-hour Holter ECG tracing show?

A. "Tachycardia – Bradycardia" syndrome: sinus pauses alternating with runs of atrial fibrillation

B. Sinus rhythm with intermittent type 2 AV block.

C. Sinus tachycardia with intermittent sinus pauses.

D. Sinus node dysfunction – sinus arrest.

E. Incessant atrial tachycardia.

Figure 4.1 **explained**: this shows sinus rhythm with a heart rate of 68 bpm, with a QRS axis at −60°, LAHB, absence of LV hypertrophy, absence of ischemia. The rhythm is irregular, due to the presence of runs of PAC, having the same morphology of the P wave, but slightly different from the morphology of the sinus P wave (best seen in lead aVL and V1). These P waves are positive in leads II, III, aVF, I, aVL, negative in lead V1, suggesting an origin in the superior part of the right atrium.

Figure 4.2 **explained**: this shows a regular narrow QRS complex tachycardia with a heart rate of 130 bpm, with a QRS axis at −60°. P waves are visible in all leads, preceding the QRS complex with a 1:1 AV relationship. The morphology of the P waves is positive in leads II, III, aVF, I, aVL, negative in lead V1, identical to the PAC present in Fig. 4.1, suggesting an origin in the superior part of the right atrium.

Figure 4.4 **explained**: the upper panel shows an incessant atrial tachycardia (which was present throughout all the recording). The atrial tachycardia stops abruptly, followed by a pause of 1.3–1.4 s, only to restart after one sinus beat. The mid-panel shows the spontaneous termination of the tachycardia, followed by a sinus beat and a PAC, then by 2 sinus beats. Of note, during sinus rhythm, the heart rate of the patient is around 45 bpm. The lower panel shows another episode of atrial tachycardia, with a heart rate of 150 bpm.

Given the patient's ECGs and the 24-hour Holter ECG, the diagnosis of incessant atrial tachycardia was established. An electrophysiological study in view of a catheter ablation procedure was offered and accepted by the patient.

4.2 Electrophysiological Study and RF Catheter Ablation Procedure

The electrophysiological study was performed under local anesthesia and conscious sedation. Vascular access was obtained using the modified Seldinger technique, under Doppler ultrasound guidance. A 6F decapolar steerable catheter (Inquiry, Abbott®) was introduced in a 6F 20 cm vascular sheath and was subsequently advanced via the right common femoral vein and placed in the coronary sinus, with the proximal poles at the level of the coronary sinus ostium and the distal poles at the level of the lateral part of the mitral annulus. Atrial pacing was carried out at twice the diastolic threshold using the EP-4™ Cardiac Stimulator (Abbott®) system. Surface ECG and intracavitary ECGs were recorded by the *WorkMate* Claris™ System (Abbott®).

Radiofrequency ablation was delivered using a Biosense Webster® SmartTouch SF open-irrigated 3.5 mm tip with D curve. The CARTO ® 3 electro-anatomic mapping System (Biosense Webster, Johnson & Johnson) was used to guide mapping and ablation.

Baseline ECG recorded at the beginning of the procedure is shown in Fig. 4.5.

The intracavitary ECG is presented in Fig. 4.6.

Baseline AH was 85 ms, and the HV interval was 50 ms.

The SmartTouch SF roving/ablation catheter was introduced in a 9F sheath and advanced at the level of the right atrium. An anatomical map of the left atrium was first created, showing a non-dilated right atrium, with a volume of 80 ml.

Activation mapping of the right atrium was then performed during the tachycardia. This showed an area of early activation at the level of the right atrial appendage, from where the depolarization spread in a radial manner, suggesting a focal mechanism (Fig. 4.7).

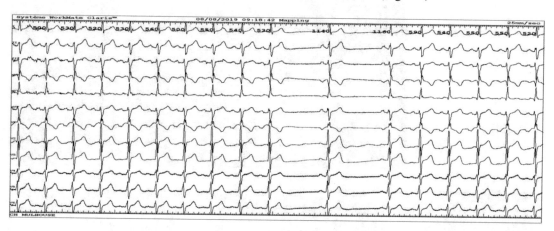

Fig. 4.5 A 12-lead ECG showing in the left part of the tracing a narrow QRS complex tachycardia with a heart rate of 115 bpm, with a 1:1 P to QRS relationship. The tachycardia stops spontaneously and, after 2 sinus beats, the tachycardia reinitiates. Of note, the morphology of the P wave is slightly different from the sinus P wave: it is positive in leads II, III, aVF, positive in I, aVL and negative in lead V1, suggesting an origin in the superior part of the right atrium. This is identical to the patient's clinical tachycardia

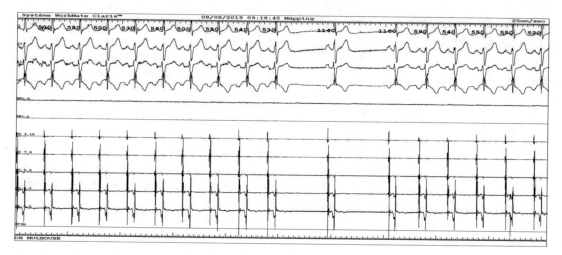

Fig. 4.6 Surface ECG leads I, II, III, V1, and V6 together with intracavitary leads recorded from the bipolar electrodes of the coronary sinus catheter (SC 1–2 to 9–10) showing the activation sequence of the coronary sinus during the narrow QRS complex tachycardia. The sequence is proximal to distal, suggesting an origin in the right atrium

Fig. 4.7 CARTO image in AP view showing the activation map of the right atrium during the tachycardia

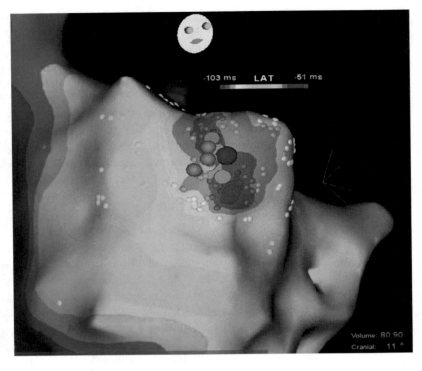

Question 4: What is the nature of the tachycardia shown in Fig. 4.7?

A. Sinus node reentry tachycardia.

B. Sinus tachycardia.

C. Focal atrial tachycardia originating in the right atrial appendage.

D. Atrial tachycardia originating in the crista terminalis region.

E. I don't know.

The earliest local atrial activation was identified at the level of the right atrial appendage, where the local A preceded the surface P wave on the 12 lead ECG by 19 ms (Fig. 4.8). The local unipolar electrogram recorded by the distal electrode of the roving/ablation catheter had a "QS" aspect at this site. These observations favored the diagnosis of incessant atrial tachycardia.

The local signal recorded by the roving/ablation catheter at the level of the earliest activation site is presented also in Fig. 4.9.

A decision to ablate the atrial tachycardia was taken.

RF energy was applied with a power of 25 W, which was subsequently augmented to 30 watts, with a target ablation index of 450.

RF application at this site immediately interrupted the tachycardia.

The interruption of the tachycardia is presented in Figs. 4.10 and 4.11.

An activation map of the right atrium was subsequently performed. This showed the earliest atrial activation at the junction of the superior vena cava with the antero-lateral superior part of the right atrium, compatible with the sinus node origin (Fig. 4.12). Of note, the distance between the successful ablation site and the region of the sinus node was 18 mm.

The ECG recorded at the end of the ablation procedure is shown in Fig. 4.13.

There were no complications related to the procedure. The ECG recorded the next day is shown in Fig. 4.14.

The patient was discharged the next day on no antiarrhythmic treatment.

She had no recurrence at her 1-year follow-up visit.

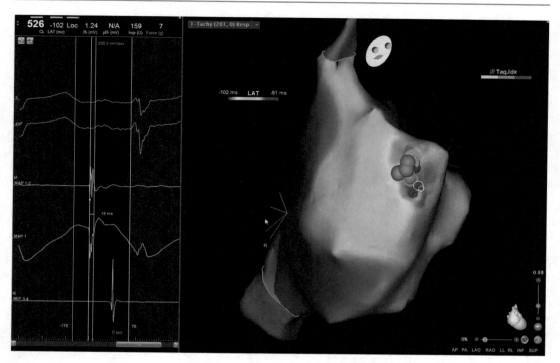

Fig. 4.8 Left part of the image: intracavitary lead recorded from the electrodes 3 and 4 of the decapolar coronary sinus catheter together with surface ECG leads II and aVF, and the intracavitary lead recorded from the distal electrode of the roving/ablation catheter, which is positioned at the level of the earliest activation site during the tachycardia, at the level of the right atrial appendage. Right part of the image: CARTO image in AP superior view showing the activation map of the right atrium during the tachycardia, with the earliest activation site (red zone, blue dot) at the level of the right atrial appendage

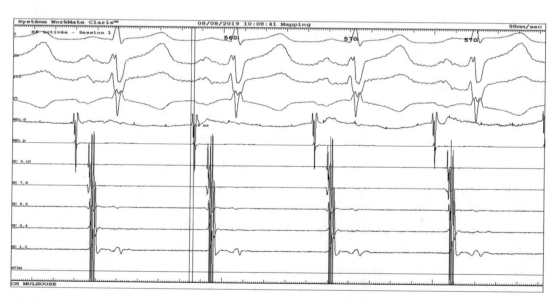

Fig. 4.9 Surface ECG leads I, II, III, V1, and V6 together with intracavitary leads recorded from the distal and from the proximal electrode of the roving/ablation catheter and the bipolar electrodes of the coronary sinus catheter (SC 1–2 to 9–10) showing the activation sequence of the coronary sinus during the narrow QRS complex tachycardia. The sequence is proximal to distal, suggesting an origin in the right atrium. The local signal recorded by the roving/ablation catheter (Abl d) at the level of the earliest activation site precedes the surface P wave on the 12 lead ECG by 19 ms

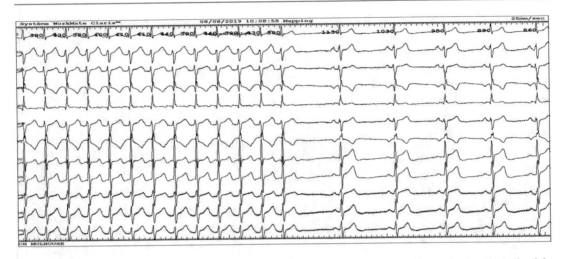

Fig. 4.10 A 12-lead ECG recorded during the first RF application at the level of the earliest activation site in the right atrial appendage during tachycardia showing its interruption and resumption of sinus rhythm

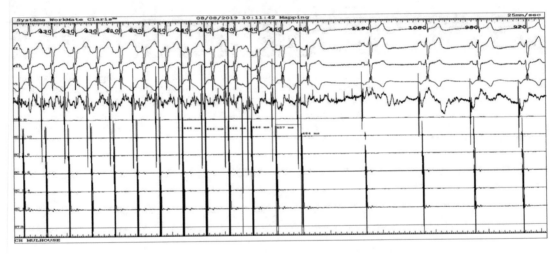

Fig. 4.11 Surface ECG leads I, II, III, V1, and V6 together with intracavitary leads recorded from the distal and from the proximal electrode of the roving/ablation catheter and the bipolar electrodes of the coronary sinus catheter (SC 1–2 to 9–10) showing the termination of the tachycardia during RF application

ANSWERS TO:

Question 1: C. Sinus rhythm with PAC of the same morphology
Question 2: C. Atrial Tachycardia
Question 3: E. Incessant atrial tachycardia
Question 4: C. Focal atrial tachycardia originating in the right atrial appendage

4.3 Commentary

The present case illustrates a catheter ablation procedure for a focal atrial tachycardia arising from the right atrial appendage in a 45-year-old female patient. Several observations can be made about the present case.

First, focal atrial tachycardias can be incessant in nature, determining dilated cardiomyopathy

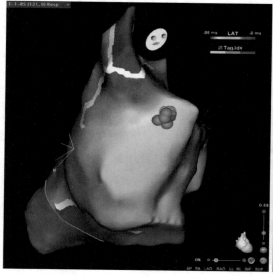
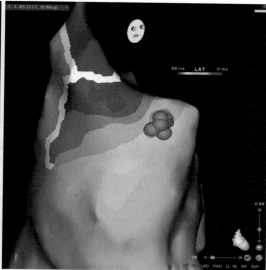

Fig. 4.12 *Left panel*: CARTO image in RAO view showing the activation map of the right atrium during sinus rhythm. The earliest atrial depolarization sequence is recorded in the region of the sinus node, in the superior anterior and lateral part of the RA. *Right panel*: same image, with zoom. The pink dots and the blue dot represent RF lesions at the successful ablation site of the atrial tachycardia

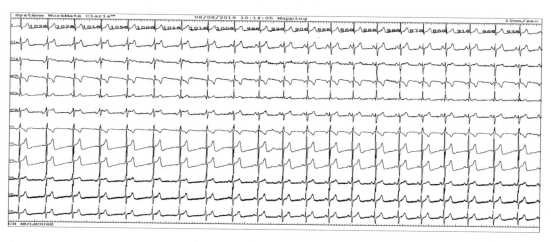

Fig. 4.13 A 12-lead ECG recorded at the end of the ablation procedure showing sinus rhythm with a heart rate of 98 bpm, QRS axis at −60°, LAHB, absence of LV hypertrophy, absence of ischemia

with severe alteration of the LV systolic function. Several case reports of atrial tachycardia-induced cardiomyopathy have been published [1–6], some presenting severe cases addressed for heart transplantation, when the LV systolic dysfunction was very severe and the diagnosis of tachycardia-induced cardiomyopathy was initially missed [7].

Second, the diagnosis of focal atrial tachycardia is sometimes challenging, since it can be wrongly interpreted as sinus tachycardia, such as in the present case, especially when the morphology of the P wave during atrial tachycardia is similar to that of the sinus P wave. This is especially true when the origin of the atrial tachycardia is close to the sinus node, as the case of

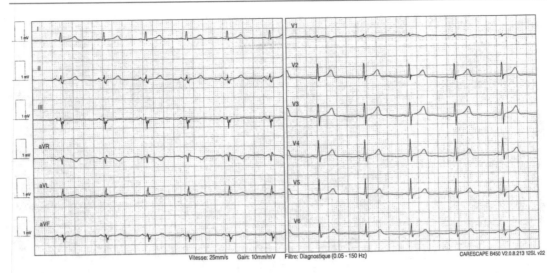

Fig. 4.14 A 12-lead ECG showing sinus rhythm with a heart rate of 66 bpm, QRS axis at +60°, absence of LV hypertrophy, absence of ischemia

tachycardias arising from the right atrial appendage.

Third, atrial tachycardia arising from the right atrial appendage is not that uncommon, with prevalence between 0.6% and 8% [8–10]. It is characterized by a higher prevalence in male patients compared to female patients (66% vs. 38%) and it have a higher likelihood of affecting younger individuals [8]. It can be incessant in nature and therefore it can induce tachycardia-related cardiomyopathy.

Forth, the ECG characteristics of focal atrial tachycardia arising from the right atrial appendage are a negative P wave morphology in leads V1, V2 with a mostly positive P wave in V3-V6. Such was the morphology of the P wave in the above-presented patient. This ECG pattern has been reported to have a very high sensitivity, specificity, PPV, and NPV, of 100%, 98%, 88%, and of 100%, respectively [8].

Treatment options include antiarrhythmic drugs [11], but these are mostly ineffective, and the treatment of choice remains catheter ablation. This is mostly done with radiofrequency [9, 10], but cryoablation for this type of tachycardia has been successfully reported [12]. The acute success rate is high, and recurrences are rare [8].

Learning Point
- Focal atrial tachycardia originating from the right atrial appendage can be misdiagnosed as sinus tachycardia.
- This type of tachycardia can be incessant in nature and, if left untreated, can determine tachycardia-induced cardiomyopathy.
- RF catheter ablation is the most efficient way of treatment.
- An electroanatomical mapping system is very useful in guiding the ablation procedure.

References

1. Chahadi FK, Singleton CB, McGavigan AD. Incessant atrial tachycardia: cause or consequence of heart failure, and the role of radiofrequency ablation. Int J Cardiol. 2013;166(3):e77–9.
2. Giorgi LV, Hartzler GO, Hamaker WR. Incessant focal atrial tachycardia: a surgically remediable cause of cardiomyopathy. J Thorac Cardiovasc Surg. 1984;87(3):466–9.
3. Bokhari F, Alqurashi M, Raslan O, Alama N. Right atrial appendage tachycardia: a rare cause of tachycardia induced cardiomyopathy with successful radiofrequency ablation using the 3D mapping system. J Saudi Heart Assoc. 2013;25(4):265–71.

4. Di Pino A, Caruso E, Gitto P. The limbus of the fossa ovalis: an unusual location for incessant focal atrial tachycardia in children. Europace. 2016;18(8):1251.

5. Femenia F, Arce M, Arrieta M, Baranchuk A. [Incessant focal atrial tachycardia arising from the right appendage: risk of tachycardia mediated cardiomyopathy. Role of the radiofrequency ablation]. Arch Argent Pediatr.2011;109(2):e33–e38.

6. Kiedrowicz RM, Podd S, O'Neill M. Focal automaticity manifesting as incessant right atrial tachycardia. Heart Rhythm. 2016;13(4):999–1000.

7. Driscoll D. Fundamentals of pediatric cardiology. Philadelphia, PA: Lippincott Williams & Wilkins; 2006.

8. Freixa X, Berruezo A, Mont L, Magnani S, Benito B, Tolosana JM, et al. Characterization of focal right atrial appendage tachycardia. Europace. 2008;10(1):105–9.

9. Guo XG, Zhang JL, Ma J, Jia YH, Zheng Z, Wang HY, et al. Management of focal atrial tachycardias originating from the atrial appendage with the combination of radiofrequency catheter ablation and minimally invasive atrial appendectomy. Heart Rhythm. 2014;11(1):17–25.

10. Walsh EP, Saul JP, Hulse JE, Rhodes LA, Hordof AJ, Mayer JE, et al. Transcatheter ablation of ectopic atrial tachycardia in young patients using radiofrequency current. Circulation. 1992;86(4):1138–46.

11. Page RL, Joglar JA, Caldwell MA, Calkins H, Conti JB, Deal BJ, et al. 2015 ACC/AHA/HRS guideline for the management of adult patients with supraventricular tachycardia: a report of the American College of Cardiology/American Heart Association Task Force on Clinical Practice Guidelines and the Heart Rhythm Society. J Am Coll Cardiol. 2016;67(13):e27–e115.

12. Amasyali B, Kilic A. Possible role for cryoballoon ablation of right atrial appendage tachycardia when conventional ablation fails. Tex Heart Inst J. 2015;42(3):289–92.

Case 5

Frédéric Halbwachs, Justine Havard, Tarek El Nazer, and Laurent Dietrich

5.1 Case Presentation

A 51-year-old male patient with a past medical history of coronary artery disease, acute myocardial infarction at the age of 49 years, treated with PTCA and stent implantation at the level of the proximal LAD (Fig. 5.1), obstructive sleep apnea treated with CPAP, was addressed to the Cardiology Department for repeated episodes of palpitations with sudden onset, at rest, with a rapid and regular rhythm, accompanied by dyspnea and anxiety.

His cardiovascular risk factors were represented by active smoking, grade 3 obesity, and dyslipidemia. His medication at home consisted of aspirin 75 mg, verapamil SR 240 mg, perindopril 2 mg, atorvastatin 40 mg, esomeprazole 40 mg, and sertraline 200 mg.

At physical examination, his blood pressure was 117/81 mmHg, HR 74 bpm, SpO_2 98% breathing room air, H = 173 cm, W = 125 kg, BMI = 41.76 kg/m^2, heart sounds were regular, there was a mild systolic murmur in the mitral auscultation region, lung auscultation was clear, there were mild bilateral edema of the lower limbs.

His CHA_2DS_2-VASc score was 1, his HAS-BLED score was 0.

His ECG at presentation is showed in Fig. 5.2.

Transthoracic echocardiography revealed a non-dilated LV with a mild systolic dysfunction, LV EF% of 48%, with non-dilated right and left atrium (Fig. 5.2). It also showed type 1 diastolic dysfunction, absence of LV hypertrophy, trivial mitral regurgitation, a non-dilated right ventricle, absence of pulmonary hypertension, sPAP of 32 mmHg, absence of pericardial effusion, a non-dilated aorta (Fig. 5.3).

A 1-lead ECG was recorded with the KardiaMobile (AliveCor©) device during an episode of paroxysmal palpitations (Fig. 5.4).

His biological workup showed a Hb level of 13.4 g/dl, leucocytes 7.12×10^9/L, platelets 243×10^9/L, CRP <3 mg/L, BUN 5.4 mmol/L, creatinine 78 μmol/L, glycemia 4.9 mmol/L, Na+ 138 mmol/L, K+ 4.1 mmol/L, cTnI <0.042 ng/ml, NT pro-BNP 298 pg/ml, TSH 2.34 IU/L, total cholesterol 158 mg/dl, HDL 40 mg/dl, LDL 67 mg/dl, triglycerides 155 mg/dl.

Given the patient's symptoms and the ECG recording from Fig. 5.4, an electrophysiological study was scheduled and subsequently performed.

Supplementary Information The online version contains supplementary material available at [https://doi.org/10.1007/978-3-031-07357-1_5].

F. Halbwachs (✉) · J. Havard
Biosense Webster, Mulhouse, France

T. El Nazer · L. Dietrich
Cardiology Department, "Emile Muller" Hospital, Mulhouse, France

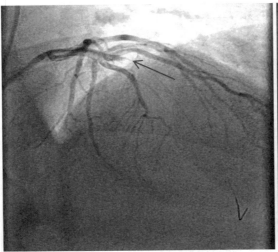
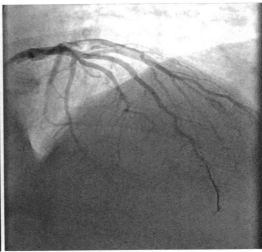

Fig. 5.1 *Left panel*: coronary angiography image showing acute occlusion of the proximal LAD artery (red arrow). *Right panel*: coronary angiography image show-ing the aspect of the LAD coronary artery after PTCA and stent implantation

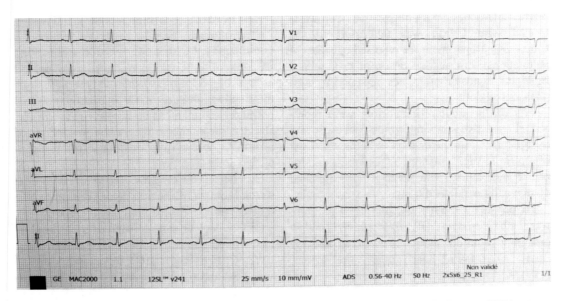

Fig. 5.2 A 12-lead ECG showing sinus rhythm with a heart rate of 74 bpm, QRS axis at +30°, absence of LV hypertrophy, absence of ischemia, no signs of ventricular pre-excitation

5.2 Electrophysiological Study and RF Catheter Ablation Procedure

The electrophysiological study was performed under local anesthesia and conscious sedation. Vascular access was obtained using the modified Seldinger technique, under Doppler ultrasound guidance. A 6F quadripolar steerable catheter (Dynamic Extrem, Microport®) was introduced in a 9F 20 cm vascular sheath and was subsequently advanced via the right common femoral vein up to the bundle of His. A 6F decapolar steerable catheter (Inquiry, Abbott®) was intro-

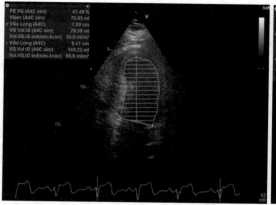
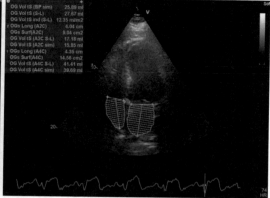

Fig. 5.3 *Left panel*: transthoracic echocardiography in apical 2 chamber view showing a non-dilated LV, with mild systolic dysfunction, EF% of 48% (Simpson biplane method). *Right panel*: apical 4 chamber view showing a non-dilated right and left atrium

duced in a 6F 20 cm vascular sheath and placed via the right common femoral vein in the coronary sinus, with the distal poles at the level of the lateral mitral annulus. A bipolar non-steerable catheter (Viking, Boston Scientific®) was introduced in a 6F 20 cm vascular sheath and was subsequently advanced via the right common femoral vein up to the right ventricular apex. Atrial and ventricular pacing were carried out at twice the diastolic threshold using the EP-4™ Cardiac Stimulator (Abbott®) system. Surface ECG and intracavitary ECGs were recorded by the *WorkMate* Claris™ System (Abbott®).

Radiofrequency ablation was delivered using a Biosense Webster® SmartTouch SF open-irrigated 3.5 mm tip with D curve. The CARTO® 3 electro-anatomic mapping System (Biosense Webster, Johnson & Johnson) was used to guide mapping and ablation of the accessory pathway.

Baseline ECG at the beginning of the procedure is shown in Fig. 5.4.

The AH interval was 83 ms, the HV interval was 43 ms. Anterior Wenckebach point was 320 ms. Retrograde conduction was present, concentric, decremental. Parahisian pacing demonstrated an "AV nodal" response, showing no retrograde conduction over an accessory pathway.

Programmed atrial stimulation (S1 = 600 ms, S2 = 360 ms) initiated of a narrow QRS complex tachycardia, with a cycle length of 500 ms, with the earliest atrial depolarization situated at the level of the His catheter, which reproduced the patient's symptoms. The AH interval during tachycardia was 105 ms, the HV interval was 41 ms, and the VA interval was 354 ms at the level of the His catheter.

The 12-lead ECG during tachycardia is shown in Fig. 5.5.

Question: What is the tachycardia shown in Fig. 5.6?
A. Sinus tachycardia.
B. AVNRT.
C. AVRT.
D. Atrial Tachycardia.
E. Fascicular ventricular tachycardia.

Patient :   (51 ans)   Balises :   À la maison   Kardia
Enregistré :   2020 à 9:20:57 PM   Notes :   such eighteen
Fréquence cardiaque :   135 bpm   Durée : 30s   Analyse instantanée   Tachycardie

Enhanced filter, Filtre secteur : 50 Hz   Échelle : 25mm/s, 10mm/mV

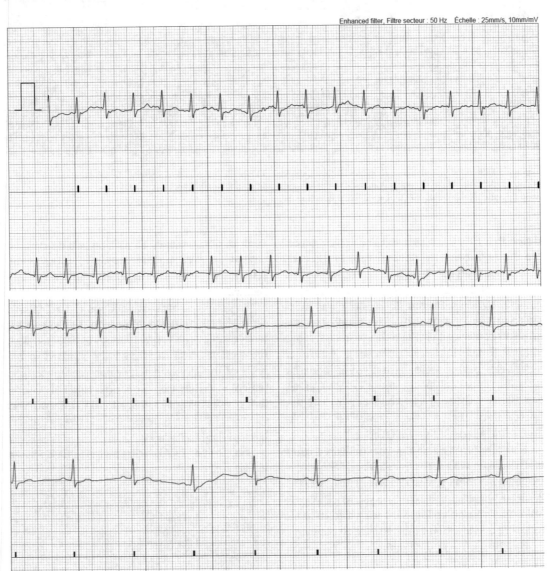

Fig. 5.4 A 1-lead ECG recorded with the KardiaMobile during an episode of palpitations showing a narrow QRS complex tachycardia with a heart rate of 135 bpm, with sudden offset, in favor of a paroxysmal SVT

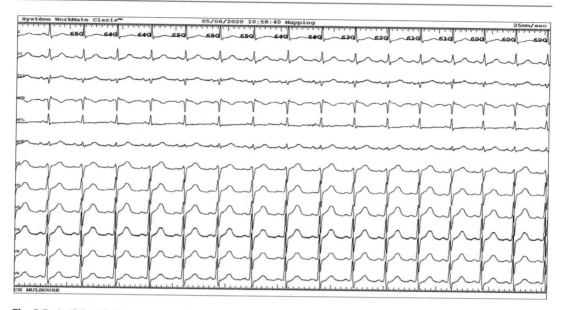

Fig. 5.5 A 12-lead ECG recorded at the beginning of the EP study showing sinus rhythm with a heart rate of 95 bpm, QRS axis at +30°, absence of LV hypertrophy, absence of ischemia, no signs of ventricular pre-excitation

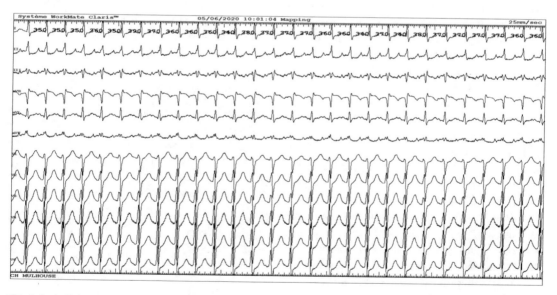

Fig. 5.6 A 12-lead ECG showing the tachycardia induced during programmed atrial stimulation, that reproduced the patient's symptoms

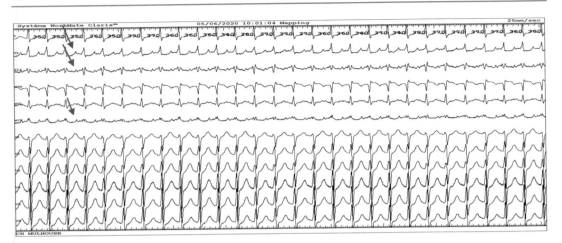

Fig. 5.6 explained. A 12-lead ECG showing a narrow and regular QRS tachycardia with a cycle length of 360–370 ms and a QRS morphology identical to that in sinus rhythm. Note the presence of positive P waves in leads II, III, and aVF (red arrows), that make the diagnosis of AVNRT and AVRT unlikely

A single ventricular extrastimulus during His refractoriness did not advance the tachycardia. At the end of burst ventricular pacing at a fixed cycle length of 470 ms, the return response was V-A-A-V. Short rapid burst ventricular pacing during tachycardia dissociated the A from the V with continuation of the tachycardia with an unchanged cycle length at the level of the atria.

All these observations favored the diagnosis of atrial tachycardia. A decision to ablate the atrial tachycardia was taken.

The SmartTouch SF roving/ablation catheter was introduced in the 9F sheath and advanced at the level of the right atrium. An anatomical map of the left atrium was first created, showing a non-dilated right atrium, with a volume of 70 ml. Activation mapping of the right atrium was then performed during tachycardia. The earliest local atrial activation was identified at the level of the tricuspid annulus at 8 o'clock position, where the local A preceded the surface P wave on the 12-lead ECG by 28 ms (Figs. 5.6 and 5.7).

The local unipolar electrogram recorded by the distal electrode of the roving/ablation catheter had a "QS" aspect at this site (Fig. 5.8). The activation map showed a depolarization sequence compatible with a focal mechanism.

Question 2: Is this a good ablation site?

A. Yes. The earliest local bipolar electrogram precedes the onset of the P wave on the surface ECG by 28 ms.

B. Yes. The local unipolar electrogram has a "QS" aspect.

C. Yes. The activation map is in favor of a focal atrial tachycardia originating in this region.

D. No. This is an atrial tachycardia probably originating in the left atrium.

E. No. No atrial tachycardia can originate in this region.

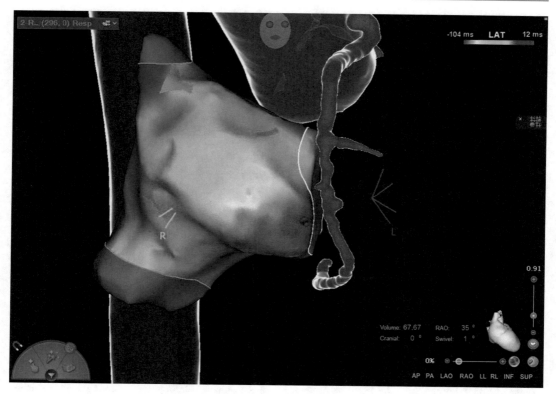

Fig. 5.7 CARTO image in RAO 35° CARTO showing the activation map of the right atrium during the tachycardia initiated by programmed atrial stimulation, showing a depolarization sequence starting in the region of lateral part of the tricuspid annulus (red area), from where the depolarization wavefront travels in a centrifugal manner to the rest of the atrial tissue (red → orange → yellow → green → blue → violet). The described mechanism is compatible with a focal atrial tachycardia. The red dot represents the site with the earliest activation during tachycardia. Note the proximity of the right coronary artery (superposed angiography CT image, in red), emerging from the right sinus of Valsalva and continuing around the tricuspid annulus

RF application at this site with a target power of 30 Watts immediately interrupted the tachycardia (Figs. 5.9 and 5.10). The ablation index target used was 450.

The relationship between the successful ablation site and the right coronary artery is shown in Fig. 5.11.

After a waiting period of 30 min, there was no arrhythmia recurrence. Programmed atrial stimulation performed after isoprenaline administration did not result in any arrhythmia induction.

There was no complication related to the procedure.

The 12-lead ECG recorded after catheter ablation is shown in Fig. 5.12.

The patient was discharged from the hospital 24 h later.

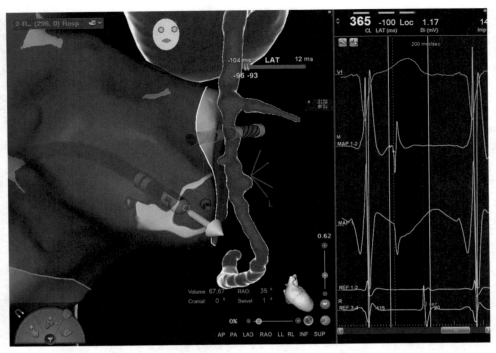

Fig. 5.8 The right side of the image shows the intracavitary electrograms recorded by the distal electrodes of the roving/ablation catheter (MAP 1–2) and the unipolar recording from the distal electrode of the roving/ablation catheter (MAP 1) and by the proximal electrodes of the coronary sinus catheter (REF 1–4). Note the "QS" aspect of the unipolar electrogram, indicating a good ablation target

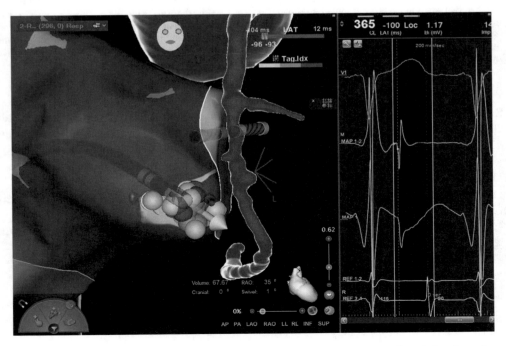

Fig. 5.9 CARTO image in RAO 35° CARTO showing the activation map of the right atrium during the tachycardia (same as in Fig. 5.6) with ablation lesions superposed at the site of the earliest endocardial activation (pink and red dots)

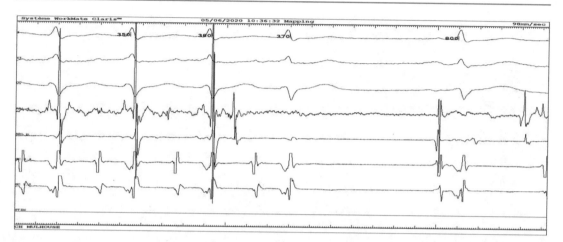

Fig. 5.10 Surface ECG leads I, II, V1 and intracavitary leads recorded by the distal and proximal electrodes of the ablation catheter positioned at the level of the earliest endocardial activation during tachycardia, corresponding to the lateral part of the mitral annulus (T8) showing the termination of the tachycardia during RF delivery and conversion to sinus rhythm

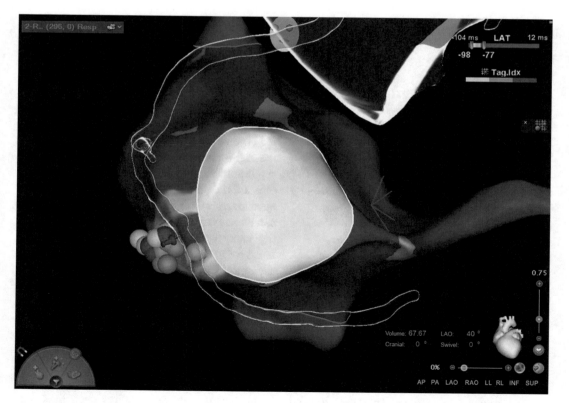

Fig. 5.11 CARTO image in LAO view 40° showing the earliest endocardial activation during tachycardia corresponding to the lateral part of the tricuspid annulus (T8), with superposed RF ablation lesions (pink and red dots). Note the proximity of the right coronary artery (superposed angiography CT image, in red), emerging from the right sinus of Valsalva and continuing around the tricuspid annulus

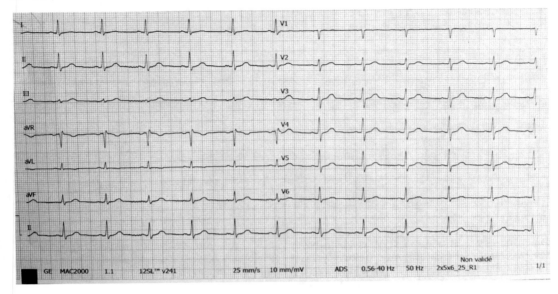

Fig. 5.12 A 12-lead ECG showing sinus rhythm with a heart rate of 71 bpm, QRS axis at +30°, absence of LV hypertrophy, absence of ischemia, no signs of ventricular pre-excitation

ANSWERS TO:

Question 1: D. Atrial Tachycardia.

Question 2:

A. **Yes. The earliest local bipolar electrogram precedes the onset of the P wave on the surface ECG by 28 ms.**

B. **Yes. The local unipolar electrogram has a "QS" aspect.**

C. **Yes. The activation map is in favor of a focal atrial tachycardia originating in this region.**

5.3   Commentary

This case illustrates a RF ablation procedure of a focal atrial tachycardia with an origin at the level of the inferolateral part of the tricuspid annulus in a 51-year-old male patient. Several observations can be made about the present case.

Atrial tachycardias represent about 10% of supraventricuar tachycardias. They are the third cause of supraventricular tachycardias in patients with structurally normal hearts, after AVNRT and AVRT. Their mechanism can be re-entry, enhanced automaticity, and triggered activity. They can also be classified into focal atrial tachycardias and macro-reentry atrial tachycardias. Focal atrial tachycardias can originate both in the right and the left atrium. In the right atrium, the most common origins are the crista terminalis, the coronary sinus ostium, the tricuspid annulus, the right atrial appendage, and the inter-atrial septum. In the left atrium, the most common origins are the pulmonary veins ostia, the left atrial appendage, and the mitral annulus [1, 2]. They can be paroxysmal, persistent or incessant, causing tachycardia-related cardiomyopathy [3]. In terms of symptoms, the spectrum varies from asymptomatic to congestive heart failure symptoms, with palpitations being the most common complaint.

Establishing the diagnosis of paroxysmal SVT (or VT) relies on the ability to record an ECG during the episode. Since a 12-lead ECG recorder is usually not available at the moment of the tachycardia onset for patients with rare episodes of tachycardia, event recorders such as smartphones, smartwatches, and one or even 6-lead ECG personal recorders are becoming increasingly available [4–7]. The present case illustrates the utility of such a smart device, which easily established the diagnosis of paroxysmal SVT. The gold-standard exam for establishing the correct diagnosis remains the electrophysiological study.

The definitive treatment is ablation of the ectopic focus. Non-fluoroscopic mapping systems can be of real help in precisely identifying the origin of the tachycardia and in reducing the fluoroscopy time and dose. In case of inadvertent catheter movement, repositioning it at the site of interest is usually not a problem. The optimal ablation criteria for focal atrial tachycardia arising from the tricuspid annulus are represented by a bipolar local atrial electrogram preceding the surface P wave by at least 20–27 ms; and a "QS" aspect of the unipolar local electrogram [2, 8]. In their study of focal atrial tachycardias arising from the tricuspid annulus, Morton et al. [9] found that most of them originate in the inferior part of the annulus (7 of 9 cases). The mean tachycardia cycle length was 371 ± 66 ms. The mean local activation time compared to the P wave onset on the 12-lead ECG was -43 ± 11 ms. The P wave morphology on the 12-lead was characterized by a positive aspect in lead aVL, negative in lead III and V1 and negative or biphasic with an initial negative component in V2 to V6. RF ablation was successful in all patients. One patient presented a recurrence, which was treated successfully with catheter ablation.

When ablating focal atrial tachycardias originating at the level of the lateral tricuspid annulus, catheter stability is usually an issue. A steerable long sheath such as Agilis (Abbott®), Chanel (Boston Scientific®), Direx (Boston Scientific®), or SureFlex (Baylis®) can offer the necessary support in order to maintain good catheter contact throughout the ablation delivery. Up to July 2020, when using the CARTO system and Smarttouch SF ablation catheters, there is no official target value for the ablation index. We used an empirical value of 450, extrapolating from our team's experience when performing PVI.

Another potential issue related to ablation of focal atrial tachycardias originating at the level of the lateral or inferolateral part of the tricuspid annulus is as illustrated in Figs. 5.6, 5.7, 5.9 and 5.11 is

the close proximity of the right coronary artery. High power ablation in this area can sometimes be complicated by right coronary artery injury [10].

Recurrences after a successful ablation are rare, between 5% and 10% [11].

Learning Point

- Focal atrial tachycardias originating from the right atrium can arise from the tricuspid annulus.
- Catheter stability can be an issue while performing ablation at the lateral part of the annulus.
- A long steerable sheath can provide the additional support necessary for performing a successful ablation.

References

1. Balla C, Foresti S, Ali H, Sorgente A, Egidy Assenza G, De Ambroggi G, et al. Long-term follow-up after radiofrequency ablation of ectopic atrial tachycardia in young patients. J Arrhythm. 2019;35(2):290–5.
2. Huo Y, Braunschweig F, Gaspar T, Richter S, Schonbauer R, Sommer P, et al. Diagnosis of atrial tachycardias originating from the lower right atrium: importance of P-wave morphology in the precordial leads V3-V6. Europace. 2013;15(4):570–7.
3. Medi C, Kalman JM, Haqqani H, Vohra JK, Morton JB, Sparks PB, et al. Tachycardia-mediated cardiomyopathy secondary to focal atrial tachycardia: long-term outcome after catheter ablation. J Am Coll Cardiol. 2009;53(19):1791–7.
4. Burke J, Haigney MCP, Borne R, Krantz MJ. Smartwatch detection of ventricular tachycardia: case series. HeartRhythm Case Rep. 2020;6(10):800–4.
5. Goldstein LN, Wells M. Smart watch-detected tachycardia: a case of atrial flutter. Oxf Med Case Reports. 2019;2019(12):495–7.
6. Ringwald M, Crich A, Beysard N. Smart watch recording of ventricular tachycardia: Case study. Am J Emerg Med. 2020;38(4):849e3–5.
7. Anjewierden S, Humpherys J, LaPage MJ, Asaki SY, Aziz PF. Detection of tachyarrhythmias in a large cohort of infants using direct-to-consumer heart rate monitoring. J Pediatr. 2021;232:147–53.
8. Okuyama Y, Mizuno H, Oka T, Komatsu S, Hirayama A, Kodama K. Atrial tachycardia originating at the tricuspid annulus. Heart Vessel. 2007;22(1):55–8.

9. Morton JB, Sanders P, Das A, Vohra JK, Sparks PB, Kalman JM. Focal atrial tachycardia arising from the tricuspid annulus: electrophysiologic and electrocardiographic characteristics. J Cardiovasc Electrophysiol. 2001;12(6):653–9.

10. Al Aloul B, Sigurdsson G, Adabag S, Li JM, Dykoski R, Tholakanahalli VN. Atrial flutter ablation and risk of right coronary artery injury. J Clin Med Res. 2015;7(4):270–3.

11. Morris GM, Segan L, Wong G, Wynn G, Watts T, Heck P, et al. Atrial tachycardia arising from the crista terminalis, detailed electrophysiological features and long-term ablation outcomes. JACC Clin Electrophysiol. 2019;5(4):448–58.

Case 6

Ronan Le Bouar, Frédéric Halbwachs,
Matthieu George, Lucien Leopold Diene,
and Nicolas Bourrelly

6

6.1 Case Presentation

A 37-year-old male patient with no significant past medical history was addressed to the Cardiology Department for asthenia that had progressively appeared during the past 3 weeks prior to his presentation to the hospital. He had no significant past medical history. He presented no chest pain, dyspnea, palpitations or syncope. He had no family history of sudden cardiac death. He was on no chronic medication. His only cardiovascular risk factor was represented by active smoking, estimated at 15 packs-year.

At physical examination, his blood pressure was 112/63 mmHg, HR 120 bpm, SpO$_2$ 97% breathing room air, $H = 175$ cm, $W = 72$ kg, BMI $= 23.51$ kg/m^2, heart sounds were rapid and regular, there were no audible murmurs, lung auscultation was clear, there were no signs of right heart failure.

His CHA$_2$DS$_2$-VASc score was 0, his HAS-BLED score was 0. His ECG at presentation is showed in Fig. 6.1.

Transthoracic echocardiography revealed a non-dilated LV with a normal systolic function, LV EF% of 59%, with a mildly dilated right and left atrium (Fig. 6.2). It also showed a normal diastolic function, absence of LV hypertrophy, a non-dilated right ventricle, absence of pulmonary hypertension, sPAP of 25 mmHg, absence of pericardial effusion, a non-dilated aorta.

His biological workup showed a Hb level of 15.1 g/dl, leucocytes 7.56 × 10^9/L, platelets 280 × 10^9/L, CRP <3 mg/L, BUN 7.0 mmol/L, creatinine 53 μmol/L, glycemia 5.7 mmol/L, Na+ 144 mmol/L, K+ 4.3 mmol/L, cTnI < 0.015 ng/ml, NT pro-BNP 430 pg/ml, TSH 0.88 IU/L, ALAT 18 IU/l, ASAT 16 IU/L.

Given the aspect of the 12-lead ECG at admittance and of that from Fig. 6.3, a 24-hour Holter ECG was performed. The result is presented in Fig. 6.4.

> **Question 1: What does the ECG in Fig. 6.1 show?**
> A. Atypical "fast-slow"AVNRT.
> B. Atypical "slow-slow".
> C. ORT using a decrementally conducting accessory pathway (Coumel tachycardia).
> D. Atrial tachycardia.
> E. ORT using nodo-ventricular fibers.

R. Le Bouar (✉) · L. L. Diene · N. Bourrelly
Cardiology Department, "Emile Muller" Hospital,
Mulhouse, France
e-mail: LEBOUARR@ghrmsa.fr

F. Halbwachs · M. George
Biosense Webster, Mulhouse, France

© The Author(s), under exclusive license to Springer Nature Switzerland AG 2022
L. Muresan (ed.), *Clinical Cases in Cardiac Electrophysiology: Supraventricular Arrhythmias*,
https://doi.org/10.1007/978-3-031-07357-1_6

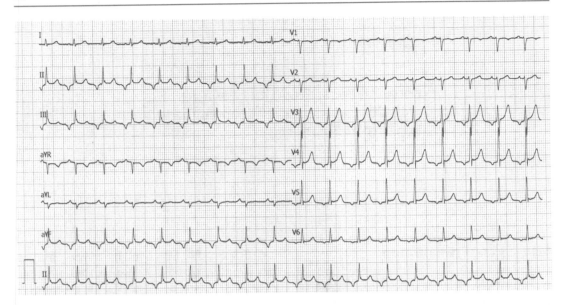

Fig. 6.1 A 12-lead ECG at admittance to the Cardiology Department showing a narrow QRS complex tachycardia with a long RP interval, with a heart rate of 120 bpm

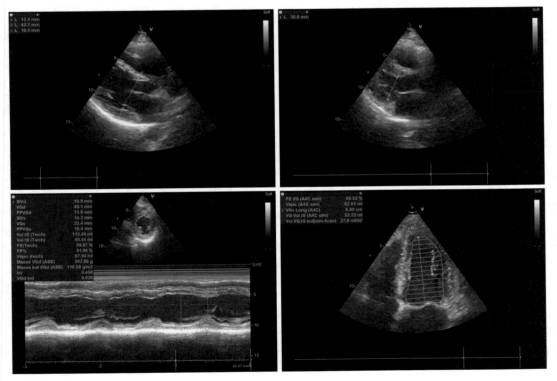

Fig. 6.2 *Left upper panel*: Transthoracic echocardiography image in parasternal long axis view showing a non-dilated LV, with an ESD of 42 mm. *Right upper panel*: parasternal long axis view showing a LV ESD of 28 mm, with an ESD of 42 mm *Left middle panel*: M-mode echocardiography in parasternal short axis showing a non-dilated LV with a preserved EF of 59%. *Right middle panel*: Apical 4 chamber view showing a LVEF of 54%. *Left lower panel*: Parasternal long axis view showing a non-dilated LA, with a diameter of 35 mm. *Right lower panel*: Apical 4 chamber view showing a slightly dilated left atrium, with a diameter of 21 cm²

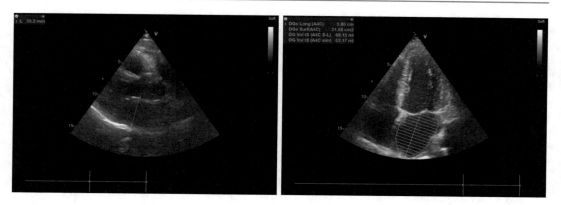

Fig. 6.2 (continued)

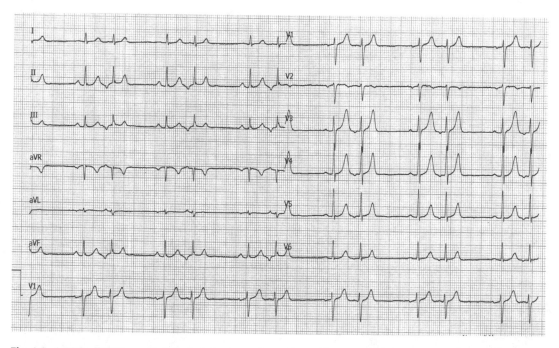

Fig. 6.3 A 12-lead ECG recorded after admittance to the Cardiology Department showing a regularly irregular rhythm: a sinus P wave followed by a narrow QRS complex, with a normal PR interval, followed by a P wave that is negative in the inferior leads with a consecutive narrow QRS complex

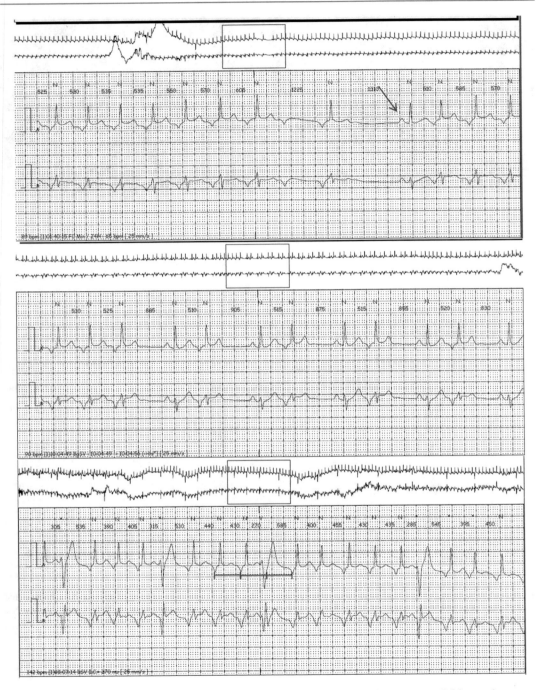

Fig. 6.4 A 24-hour Holter ECG monitoring showing in *the upper panel* the end of a long RP narrow QRS complex tachycardia episode, followed by one sinus P wave (red arrow) and immediate resumption of tachycardia. *The middle panel* shows the end of a tachycardia episode with conversion to sinus rhythm. Following this, there is an alternance between sinus P waves (red *) and negative P waves, each followed by a narrow RQS complex, aspect similar with the ECG presented in Fig. 6.3. The lower panel shows the presence of isolated wide QRS complexes (likely PVCs) during an episode of the same long RP narrow QRS complex tachycardia, without resetting the tachycardia

Question 2: What does the ECG in Fig. 6.3 show?

A. Sinus rhythm with PAC (atrial bigeminy).

B. Sinus rhythm with atrial echos (reentry using a slow AV nodal pathway).

C. Sinus rhythm with atrial echos using a decrementally conducting accessory pathway (Coumel tachycardia).

D. Sinus rhythm with "double fire" phenomenon.

E. None of the above.

Based on the ECG recorded at admittance to the hospital and on the result of the 24-hour Holter ECG, the diagnosis of incessant atrial tachycardia was established. Given the fact that long-term antiarrhythmic treatment was not desired by the patient, a catheter ablation procedure was offered and subsequently performed.

6.2   Electrophysiological Study and RF Catheter Ablation Procedure

The electrophysiological study was performed under local anesthesia and conscious sedation, without any fluoroscopic guidance, with the help of the CARTO ® 3 electro-anatomic mapping System (Biosense Webster, Johnson & Johnson).

The 12-lead ECG recorded at the beginning of the electrophysiological study is presented in Fig. 6.5.

Vascular access was obtained using the modified Seldinger technique, under Doppler ultrasound guidance. A Biosense Webster non-irrigated 4 mm tip Navistar catheter with double curve D/F was introduced in a 9F 20 cm vascular sheath at the level of the right common femoral vein and gently advanced at the level of the right common iliac vein, under constant impedance surveillance on the RF generator. The presence of the roving/ablation catheter at the level of the femoral, iliac vein, and IVC generated an impedance between 140 and 170 Ω. The entrance of the catheter in a collateral vein was rapidly accompanied by a rise in the local impedance of up to 350 Ω, and this determined retraction of the catheter in a previous position. The catheter was then gently oriented in a different manner, in such a way that its advancement determined a relatively constant impedance. The CARTO® 3 electroanatomic mapping system was used to create an anatomical map of the right common iliac vein and of the IVC, up to the point where the catheter entered the right atrium and atrial electrograms were recorded by the distal electrode of the roving/ablation catheter. Next, an anatomical map of the right atrium was created during sinus rhythm, with emphasis on the superior vena cava, the coronary sinus, the tricuspid valve, with the identification of the bundle of His and the coronary sinus ostium. The right atrium was not dilated, with a volume of 75 ml.

Next, a 6F quadripolar steerable catheter (Dynamic Extrem, Microport®) was introduced in a 6F 20 cm vascular sheath and was subsequently advanced via the right common femoral vein with the help of the CARTO system and the previously created map of the right common iliac veins and the IVC up to the coronary sinus, with the distal poles at the level of the mid portion of the great cardiac vein. A second 6F quadripolar steerable catheter (Dynamic Extrem, Microport®) was introduced in a 6F 20 cm vascular sheath and was subsequently advanced via the right common femoral vein up to the bundle of His. The roving/ablation catheter was placed inside the right ventricle.

Atrial and ventricular pacing were carried out at twice the diastolic threshold using the EP-4™ Cardiac Stimulator (Abbott®) system. Surface ECG and intracavitary ECGs were recorded by the *WorkMate* Claris™ System (Abbott®).

The AH and the HV intervals during tachycardia were of 89 ms and 53 ms (Fig. 6.6).

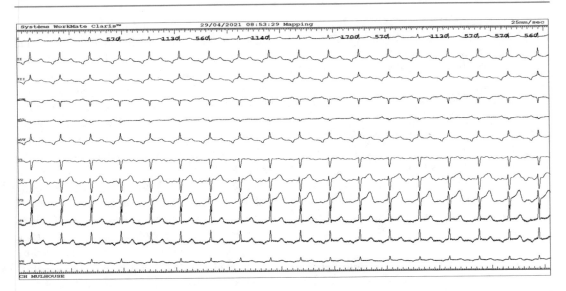

Fig. 6.5 A 12-lead ECG at the beginning of the electrophysiological study showing the presence of the patient's clinical narrow QRS complex tachycardia

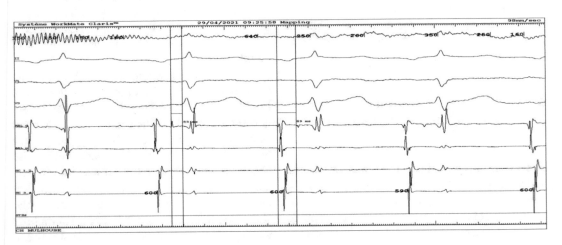

Fig. 6.6 Surface ECG leads I, II, V1 and V3 together with intracavitary leads recorded from the bipolar electrodes of the roving/ablation catheter (ABL d and ABL p) positioned at the level of the bundle of His and from the CS catheter (CS 1–2 and 3–4) showing the AH and HV intervals during tachycardia, of 89 ms and 53 ms, respectively

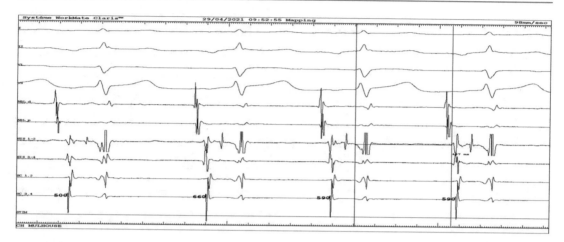

Fig. 6.7 Surface ECG leads I, II, V1 and V3 together with intracavitary leads recorded from the bipolar electrodes of the roving/ablation catheter (ABL d and ABL p) positioned at the level of the low lateral right atrial wall, the bipolar electrodes of the His catheter (His 1–2 and His 3–4) and from the CS catheter (CS 1–2 and 3–4) showing VA interval at the level of the His catheter during tachycardia, of 437 ms

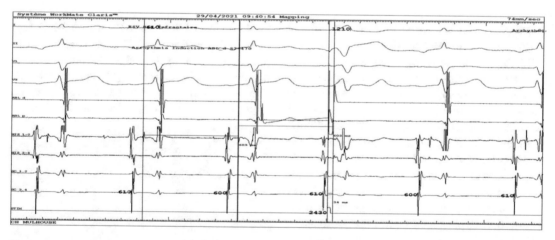

Fig. 6.8 Surface ECG leads I, II, V1 and V3 together with intracavitary leads recorded from the bipolar electrodes of the roving/ablation catheter (ABL d and ABL p) positioned at the level of the right interventricular septum and from the CS catheter (CS 1–2 and 3–4) showing the effect of a His-refractory PVC on the next activation sequence and timing as well as on the tachycardia cycle length

The VA interval during tachycardia, recorded at the level of the His catheter was 437 ms (Fig. 6.7).

The effect of a His-refractory PVC on the tachycardia cycle length and on the following atrial activation is presented in Fig. 6.8.

A short ventricular burst pacing sequence during tachycardia was performed and is presented in Fig. 6.9.

Question 3: Based on the ECGs in Figs. 6.8 and 6.9, what is the diagnosis of the patient's tachycardia?

A. Atypical "fast-slow" AVNRT.

B. Atypical "slow-slow".

C. ORT using a decrementally conducting accessory pathway (Coumel tachycardia).

D. Atrial tachycardia.

E. ORT using nodo-ventricular fibers.

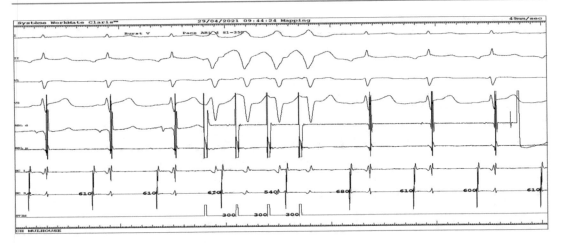

Fig. 6.9 Surface ECG leads I, II, V1 and V3 together with intracavitary leads recorded from the bipolar electrodes of the roving/ablation catheter (ABL d and ABL p) positioned at the level of the right interventricular septum and from the CS catheter (CS 1–2 and 3–4) showing a short burst of 4 ventricular beats, performed during tachycardia

Figure 6.8 shows the absence of influence of a His-refractory PVC on the TCL and on the following atrial activation sequence and timing. This does not exclude the presence of an accessory pathway, but it is not in favor of the existence of one either. Figure 6.9 shows V-A dissociation during a short sequence of burst ventricular pacing, with continuation of the tachycardia at the atrial level, best seen at the level of the coronary sinus catheter. This excludes the presence of an accessory pathway and is in favor of an atrial tachycardia. Of note, in Fig. 6.4, upper panel shows the presence of a "P-P-QRS" sequence just before termination of the tachycardia, which excludes an ORT and is also in favor of an atrial tachycardia.

The bipolar voltage map of the right atrium is shown in Figs. 6.10, 6.11, and 6.12.

Given the fact that the morphology of the P wave during tachycardia was negative in the inferior leads, positive in leads I, aVL, an origin in the inferior part of the right atrium was suspected. Mapping was therefore commenced in the right atrium.

The activation map of the right atrium is presented in Figs. 6.13 and 6.14. This confirmed the diagnosis of atrial tachycardia. The earliest local atrial activation was identified at the level of the tricuspid annulus at 6 o'clock position, where the local A preceded the surface P wave on the 12-lead ECG by 21 ms (Fig. 6.15). The local unipolar electrogram recorded by the distal electrode of the roving/ablation catheter had a "QS" aspect at this site. The activation map showed a depolarization sequence compatible with a focal mechanism.

> **Question 4: Is this a good ablation site?**
> A. Yes. The earliest local bipolar electrogram precedes the onset of the P wave on the surface ECG by 21 ms.
> B. Yes. The local unipolar electrogram has a "QS" aspect.
> C. Yes. The activation map is in favor of a focal atrial tachycardia originating in this region.
> D. No. This is an atrial tachycardia probably originating in the left atrium.
> E. No. No atrial tachycardia can originate in this region.

RF energy was applied in this region with rapid termination of the tachycardia and resumption of sinus rhythm (Fig. 6.16). Target power was 30 W and target ablation index 450. The activation map of the right atrium during tachycardia with superposed RF ablation lesions is shown in Figs. 6.17 and 6.18.

Fig. 6.10 CARTO image in LAO view showing the bipolar voltage map of the right atrium recorded during atrial tachycardia. Local voltage >0.5 mV compatible with healthy myocardial tissue is represented in violet, voltage <0.2 mV compatible with scar is represented in red, voltage between 0.2 mV and 0.5 mV is compatible with borderline tissue. The orange dots represent the bundle of His. Of note, the right atrium is not dilated, with a volume of 73 ml

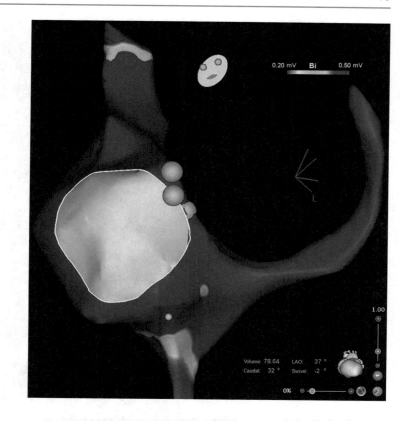

Fig. 6.11 CARTO image in postero-septal view showing the bipolar voltage map of the right atrium recorded during atrial tachycardia. Local voltage >0.5 mV compatible with healthy myocardial tissue is represented in violet, voltage <0.2 mV compatible with scar is represented in red, voltage between 0.2 mV and 0.5 mV is compatible with borderline tissue. The orange dots represent the bundle of His. Of note, the right atrium is not dilated, with a volume of 73 ml

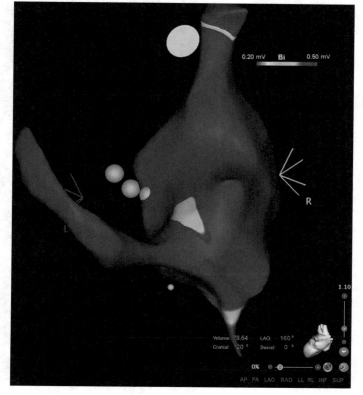

Fig. 6.12 CARTO image in inferior view showing the bipolar voltage map of the right atrium recorded during atrial tachycardia. Local voltage >0.5 mV compatible with healthy myocardial tissue is represented in violet, voltage <0.2 mV compatible with scar is represented in red, voltage between 0.2 mV and 0.5 mV is compatible with borderline tissue. The orange dots represent the bundle of His. Of note, the right atrium is not dilated, with a volume of 73 ml

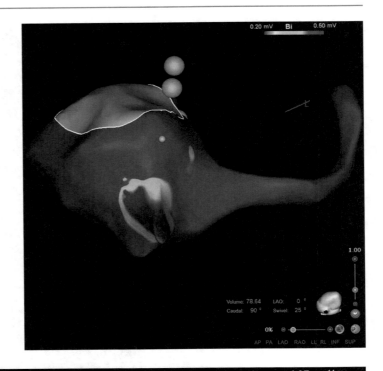

Fig. 6.13 CARTO image in LAO view showing the activation map of the right atrium during the tachycardia, showing a depolarization sequence starting in the inferior part of the tricuspid annulus (red area), from where the depolarization wavefront travels in a centrifugal manner to the rest of the atrial tissue (red → orange → yellow → green → blue → violet). The described mechanism is compatible with a focal atrial tachycardia. The red dot represents the site with the earliest activation during tachycardia. The right corner of the image shows the temporal relationship between the earliest recorded atrial electrogram recorded by the roving/ablation catheter (MAP 1–2) and the atrial electrogram recorded by the proximal pair of the coronary sinus electrodes (REF 3, 4)

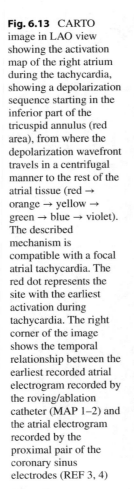

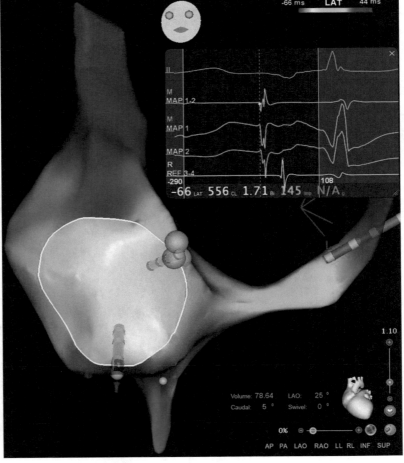

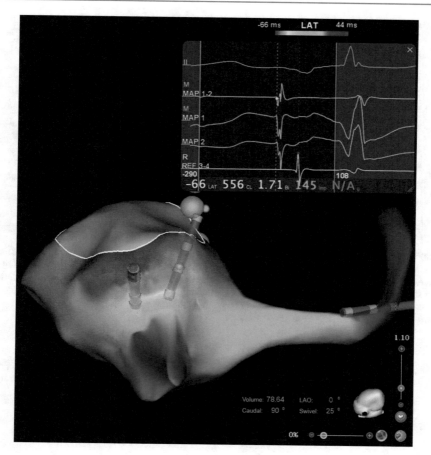

Fig. 6.14 CARTO image in inferior view showing the activation map of the right atrium during the tachycardia, showing a depolarization sequence starting in the inferior part of the tricuspid annulus (red area), from where the depolarization wavefront travels in a centrifugal manner to the rest of the atrial tissue (red → orange → yellow → green → blue → violet). The described mechanism is compatible with a focal atrial tachycardia. The red dot represents the site with the earliest activation during tachycardia. The right corner of the image shows the temporal relationship between the earliest recorded atrial electrogram recorded by the roving/ablation catheter (MAP 1–2) and the atrial electrogram recorded by the proximal pair of the coronary sinus electrodes (REF 3, 4)

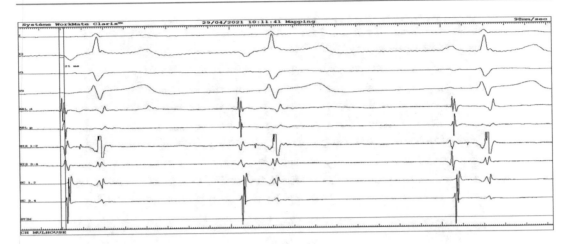

Fig. 6.15 Surface ECG leads I, II, V1, and V3 together with intracavitary leads recorded from the bipolar electrodes of the roving/ablation catheter (ABL d and ABL p) positioned at the level of the earliest atrial activation site, the bipolar electrodes of the His catheter (His 1–2 and His 3–4) and from the CS catheter (CS 1–2 and 3–4) showing the temporal relationship between the earliest recorded atrial electrogram recorded by the roving / ablation catheter (Abl d) situated at the level of the inferior tricuspid annulus and the onset of the P wave on the surface ECG, preceding it by 21 ms

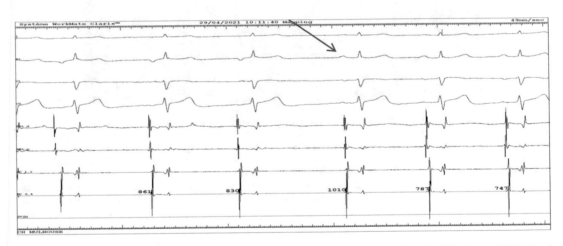

Fig. 6.16 Surface ECG leads I, II, V1, and V3 together with intracavitary leads recorded from the bipolar electrodes of the roving/ablation catheter (ABL d and ABL p) positioned at the level of the earliest atrial activation site in the right atrium, and from the CS catheter (CS 1–2 and 3–4) showing termination of the tachycardia and resumption of sinus rhythm (red arrow)

Fig. 6.17 CARTO
image in LAO view
showing the activation
map of the right atrium
during the tachycardia
with superposed RF
ablation lesions at the
successful ablation site
(red dots)

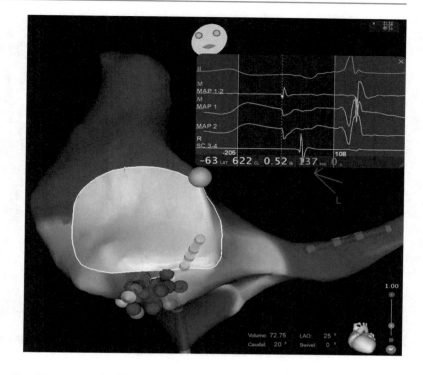

Fig. 6.18 CARTO
image in inferior view
showing the activation
map of the right atrium
during the tachycardia
with superposed RF
ablation lesions at the
successful ablation site
(red dots). The right
corner of the image
shows the temporal
relationship between the
earliest recorded atrial
electrogram recorded by
the roving/ablation
catheter (MAP 1–2) and
the atrial electrogram
recorded by the
proximal pair of the
coronary sinus
electrodes (REF 3, 4)

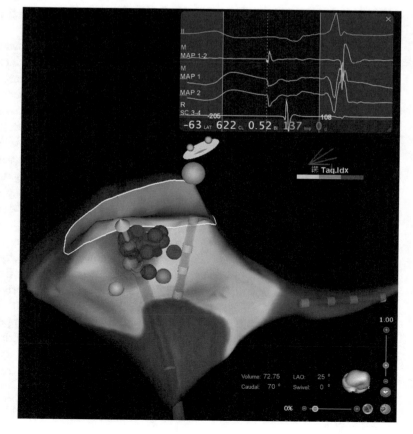

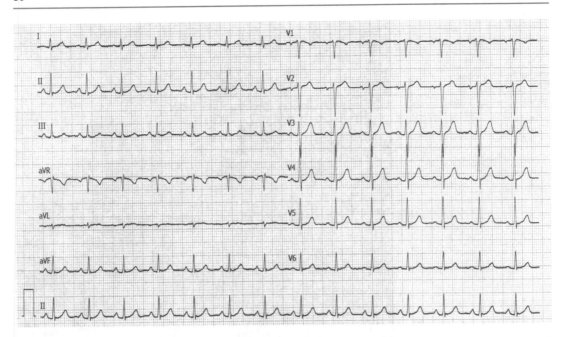

Fig. 6.19 A 12-lead ECG recorded after the ablation procedure showing sinus rhythm with a heart rate of 84 bpm, QRS axis at +60°, absence of LV hypertrophy, absence of ischemia

There was no complication related to the procedure.

The 12-lead ECG recorded after catheter ablation is shown in Fig. 6.19.

The patient was discharged from the hospital 24 h later.

ANSWERS TO:

Question 1: D. Atrial Tachycardia.

Question 2: A. Sinus rhythm with PAC (atrial bigeminy)

Question 3: D. Atrial Tachycardia.

Question 4:

    A. **Yes. The earliest local bipolar electrogram precedes the onset of the P wave on the surface ECG by 21 ms.**

    B. **Yes. The local unipolar electrogram has a "QS" aspect.**

    C. **Yes. The activation map is in favor of a focal atrial tachycardia originating in this region.**

6.3 Commentary

The present case illustrates a RF catheter ablation procedure for an incessant atrial tachycardia originating in the inferior part of the tricuspid annulus in a 37-year-old male patient with no structural heart disease. Several observations can be made about the present case.

Atrial tachycardia represents between 10% and 15% of all supraventricular tachycardias [1], the other types being represented by AVNRT and AVRT. They can appear in patients with or without structural heart disease. Their mechanism can be reentry, enhanced automatism or trigger activity. They can be macro-reentrant or focal. Focal atrial tachycardias can originate both in the right and the left atrium. In the right atrium, the most common origins are the crista terminalis, the coronary sinus ostium, the tricuspid annulus, the right atrial appendage, and the inter-atrial septum. In the left atrium, the most common origins are the pulmonary veins ostia, the left atrial appendage, and the mitral annulus [2, 3]. They can be paroxysmal, persistent, or incessant, causing tachycardia-related cardiomyopathy [4]. In terms of symptoms, the spectrum varies from asymptomatic to congestive heart failure symptoms, with palpitations being the most common complaint.

Focal atrial tachycardias arising from the tricuspid annulus have been described before [3, 5, 6]. In their study of focal atrial tachycardias arising from the tricuspid annulus, Morton et al. [5] found that most of them originate in the inferior part of the annulus (7 of 9 cases). The mean tachycardia cycle length was 371 ± 66 ms. The mean local activation time compared to the P wave onset on the 12-lead ECG was −43 ± 11 ms. The P wave morphology on the 12-lead was characterized by a positive aspect in lead aVL, negative in lead III and V1 and negative or biphasic with an initial negative component in V2 to V6. RF ablation was successful in all patients. One patient presented a recurrence, which was treated successfully with catheter ablation. The optimal ablation criteria for focal atrial tachycardia arising from the tricuspid annulus are represented by a bipolar local atrial electrogram preceding the surface P wave by at least 20–27 ms; and a "QS" aspect of the unipolar local electrogram [3, 6].

In the above-presented patient, the activation map of the right atrium performed with the CARTO system during atrial tachycardia identified the origin of the atrial tachycardia at the level of the tricuspid annulus, at 6 o'clock position in LAO 30° projection. The tachycardia cycle length was 580–590 ms, longer than that usually reported by Morton et al. [5]. The local activation time compared to the P wave onset on the 12-lead ECG was 21 ms, shorter than that reported by Morton et al. However, this was enough for a successful RF lesion. As previously described by the same group of authors, the morphology of the p wave on the 12-lead ECG was positive in lead aVL, negative in lead III, negative in V3–V6 (Fig. 6.1). However, lead V1 and lead V2 show positive P waves in lead V1 and V2, unlike the aspect described by Morton, of negative P waves in lead V1 and biphasic with an initial negative component in V2.

The CARTO system was very useful in guiding the ablation procedure. The activation map of the right atrium during tachycardia precisely localized the origin of the tachycardia. It allowed the application of several lesions at the site of the earliest atrial activation during tachycardia in order to render it non-inducible. Another important advantage of the CARTO system is that it allowed the performance of a zero-fluoroscopy procedure. No X-ray was used in this patient for the electrophysiological study and for the ablation procedure, with the technique described in the "Electrophysiological Study and RF Catheter Ablation" section. Performing ablation with zero fluoroscopy is becoming possible for several arrhythmias, notably typical atrial flutter, atrial tachycardia, AVNRT, AVRT, PVCs, and most forms of VTs [7–24].

> **Learning Point**
> - Focal atrial tachycardia can be incessant and if left untreated can give rise to tachycardia-induced cardiomyopathy.
> - Focal atrial tachycardia originating from the right atrium can arise from the tricuspid annulus.
> - A 3D electro-anatomical mapping system is a very useful tool for localizing the origin of the tachycardia and for guiding the ablation procedure.
> - Zero-fluoroscopy ablation is possible for the treatment of focal atrial tachycardias arising from the right atrium.

References

1. Steinbeck G, Hoffmann E. 'True' atrial tachycardia. Eur Heart J. 1998;19 Suppl E:E10–2. E48–9
2. Balla C, Foresti S, Ali H, Sorgente A, Egidy Assenza G, De Ambroggi G, et al. Long-term follow-up after radiofrequency ablation of ectopic atrial tachycardia in young patients. J Arrhythm. 2019;35(2):290–5.
3. Huo Y, Braunschweig F, Gaspar T, Richter S, Schonbauer R, Sommer P, et al. Diagnosis of atrial tachycardias originating from the lower right atrium: importance of P-wave morphology in the precordial leads V3-V6. Europace. 2013;15(4):570–7.

4. Medi C, Kalman JM, Haqqani H, Vohra JK, Morton JB, Sparks PB, et al. Tachycardia-mediated cardiomyopathy secondary to focal atrial tachycardia: long-term outcome after catheter ablation. J Am Coll Cardiol. 2009;53(19):1791–7.

5. Morton JB, Sanders P, Das A, Vohra JK, Sparks PB, Kalman JM. Focal atrial tachycardia arising from the tricuspid annulus: electrophysiologic and electrocardiographic characteristics. J Cardiovasc Electrophysiol. 2001;12(6):653–9.

6. Okuyama Y, Mizuno H, Oka T, Komatsu S, Hirayama A, Kodama K. Atrial tachycardia originating at the tricuspid annulus. Heart Vessel. 2007;22(1):55–8.

7. Ramos-Maqueda J, Alvarez M, Cabrera-Ramos M, Perin F, Rodriguez-Vazquez Del Rey MDM, Jimenez-Jaimez J, et al. Results of catheter ablation with zero or near zero fluoroscopy in pediatric patients with supraventricular tachyarrhythmias. Rev Esp Cardiol. 2021;75(2):166–73.

8. Lahiri A, Srinath SC, Chase D, Roshan J. Zero fluoroscopy radiofrequency ablation for Typical Atrioventricular Nodal Reentrant Tachycardia (AVNRT). Indian Pacing Electrophysiol J. 2017;17(6):180–2.

9. Yang L, Sun G, Chen X, Chen G, Yang S, Guo P, et al. Meta-analysis of zero or near-zero fluoroscopy use during ablation of cardiac arrhythmias. Am J Cardiol. 2016;118(10):1511–8.

10. Chen G, Sun G, Xu R, Chen X, Yang L, Bai Y, et al. Zero-fluoroscopy catheter ablation of severe drug-resistant arrhythmia guided by Ensite NavX system during pregnancy: Two case reports and literature review. Medicine. 2016;95(32):e4487.

11. Clark BC, Sumihara K, McCarter R, Berul CI, Moak JP. Getting to zero: impact of electroanatomical mapping on fluoroscopy use in pediatric catheter ablation. J Interv Cardiac Electrophysiol. 2016;46(2):183–9.

12. Drago F, Grifoni G, Remoli R, Russo MS, Righi D, Pazzano V, et al. Radiofrequency catheter ablation of left-sided accessory pathways in children using a new fluoroscopy integrated 3D-mapping system. Europace. 2017;19(7):1198–203.

13. Kerst G, Parade U, Weig HJ, Hofbeck M, Gawaz M, Schreieck J. A novel technique for zero-fluoroscopy catheter ablation used to manage Wolff-Parkinson-White syndrome with a left-sided accessory pathway. Pediatr Cardiol. 2012;33(5):820–3.

14. Knecht S, Sticherling C, Reichlin T, Pavlovic N, Muhl A, Schaer B, et al. Effective reduction of fluoroscopy duration by using an advanced electroanatomic-mapping system and a standardized procedural pro-tocol for ablation of atrial fibrillation: 'the unleaded study'. Europace. 2015;17(11):1694–9.

15. Luani B, Zrenner B, Basho M, Genz C, Rauwolf T, Tanev I, et al. Zero-fluoroscopy cryothermal ablation of atrioventricular nodal re-entry tachycardia guided by endovascular and endocardial catheter visualization using intracardiac echocardiography (Ice&ICE Trial). J Cardiovasc Electrophysiol. 2018;29(1):160–6.

16. Macias R, Uribe I, Tercedor L, Jimenez-Jaimez J, Barrio T, Alvarez M. A zero-fluoroscopy approach to cavotricuspid isthmus catheter ablation: comparative analysis of two electroanatomical mapping systems. Pacing Clin Electrophysiol. 2014;37(8):1029–37.

17. Plank F, Stowasser B, Till D, Schgor W, Dichtl W, Hintringer F, et al. Reduction of fluoroscopy dose for cardiac electrophysiology procedures: A feasibility and safety study. Eur J Radiol. 2019;110:105–11.

18. Proietti R, Abadir S, Bernier ML, Essebag V. Ablation of an atriofascicular accessory pathway with a zero-fluoroscopy procedure. J Arrhythm. 2015;31(5):323–5.

19. Prolic Kalinsek T, Jan M, Rupar K, Razen L, Antolic B, Zizek D. Zero-fluoroscopy catheter ablation of concealed left accessory pathway in a pregnant woman. Europace. 2017;19(8):1384.

20. Scaglione M, Ebrille E, Caponi D, Siboldi A, Bertero G, Di Donna P, et al. Zero-fluoroscopy ablation of accessory pathways in children and adolescents: CARTO3 electroanatomic mapping combined with RF and cryoenergy. Pacing Clin Electrophysiol. 2015;38(6):675–81.

21. Seizer P, Bucher V, Frische C, Heinzmann D, Gramlich M, Muller I, et al. Efficacy and safety of zero-fluoroscopy ablation for supraventricular tachycardias. Use of optional contact force measurement for zero-fluoroscopy ablation in a clinical routine setting. Herz. 2016;41(3):241–5.

22. Wang Y, Chen GZ, Yao Y, Bai Y, Chu HM, Ma KZ, et al. Ablation of idiopathic ventricular arrhythmia using zero-fluoroscopy approach with equivalent efficacy and less fatigue: a multicenter comparative study. Medicine. 2017;96(6):e6080.

23. Yamagata K, Aldhoon B, Kautzner J. Reduction of fluoroscopy time and radiation dosage during catheter ablation for atrial fibrillation. Arrhythmia Electrophysiol Rev. 2016;5(2):144–9.

24. Zhu TY, Liu SR, Chen YY, Xie LZ, He LW, Meng SR, et al. [Zero-fluoroscopy catheter ablation for idiopathic premature ventricular contractions from the aortic sinus cusp]. Nan Fang Yi Ke Da Xue Xue Bao. 2016;36(8):1105–9.

Case 7

7

Lucian Muresan, Ronan Le Bouar,
Frédéric Halbwachs, Maxime Tissier,
and Crina Muresan

7.1 Case Presentation

A 62-year-old male patient with a past medical history of AVNRT and focal atrial tachycardia originating in the right atrium, both treated with a RF catheter ablation procedure in another center at the age of 54 years, with a single episode of atrial fibrillation and atypical atrial flutter initiated during the electrophysiological study (nonclinical, therefore considered of unknown significance), first degree AV block and intermittent nocturnal type 1 s degree AV block, polymorphic isolated PVC, was addressed to the Cardiology Department for repeated episodes of intermittent palpitations accompanied by dyspnea, that had been present since 6 months after the ablation procedure. There was no notion of syncope in his past medical history, there was no family history of sudden cardiac death. His cardiovascular risk factors were represented by arterial hypertension and age >55 years. His medication at home consisted of apixaban

2×5 mg/day, bisoprolol 5 mg/day, and telmisartan 40 mg/day.

At physical examination, his blood pressure was 136/94 mmHg, HR 64 bpm, SpO_2 99% breathing room air, $H = 187$ cm, $W = 96$ kg, BMI = 27.45 kg/m^2, heart sounds were regular, there were no audible murmurs, lung auscultation was clear, there were no signs of right heart failure.

His CHA_2DS_2-VASc score was 1, his HAS-BLED score was 0.

His ECG at presentation is showed in Fig. 7.1. An ECG recorded by his treating cardiologist 1 month prior to his presentation to the hospital, during an episode of palpitations is presented in Fig. 7.2.

His biological workup showed a Hb level of 13.8 g/dl, leucocytes 6.22×10^9/L, platelets 314×10^9/L, CRP < 3 mg/L, BUN 4.5 mmol/L, creatinine 86 µmol/L, glycemia 4.9 mmol/L, HbA1c 6.2%, Na+ 141 mmol/L, K+ 3.7 mmol/L, total proteins 85 g/L, TSH 3.64 IU/L, total cholesterol 174 mg/dl, HDL 46 mg/dl, LDL 115 mg/dl, triglycerides 81 mg/dl.

A 24-hour Holter ECG confirmed the presence of nocturnal intermittent type 1 s degree AV block (Fig. 7.3).

Transthoracic echocardiography revealed a non-dilated LV (53/35 mm) with a preserved

L. Muresan (✉) · R. Le Bouar · C. Muresan
Cardiology Department, "Emile Muller" Hospital,
Mulhouse, France
e-mail: LEBOUARR@ghrmsa.fr

F. Halbwachs · M. Tissier
Biosense Webster, Mulhouse, France

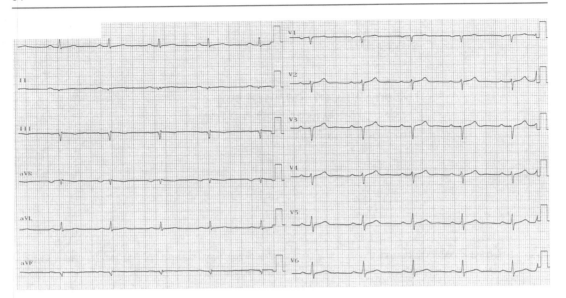

Fig. 7.1 A 12-lead ECG at admittance to the Cardiology Department showing sinus rhythm with a heart rate of 62 bpm, QRS axis at −30°, absence of LV hypertrophy, grade I AVB (PR = 212 ms), Q waves in leads III and aVF

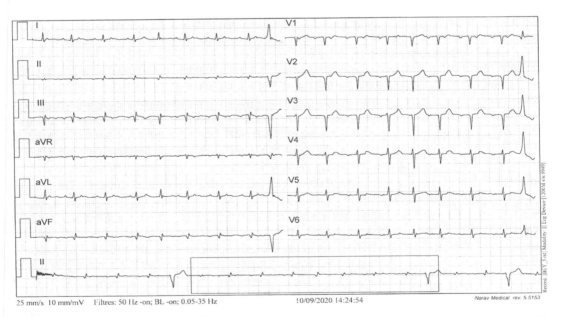

Fig. 7.2 A 12-lead ECG recorded during an episode of palpitations showing a narrow QRS complex tachycardia with a heart rate of 110 bpm, QRS axis at −15°, absence of LV hypertrophy, absence of ischemia, 1 isolated PVC

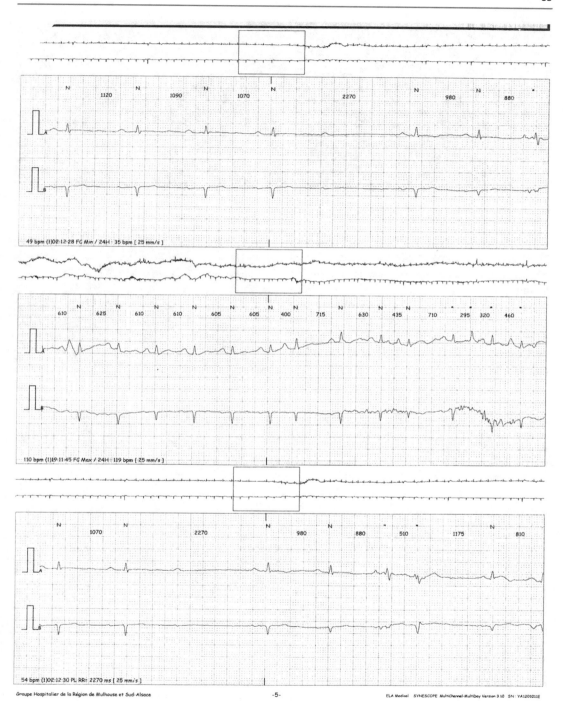

Fig. 7.3 A 24-hour Holter ECG showing the presence of second-degree AV block type 1 Luciani—Wenckebach

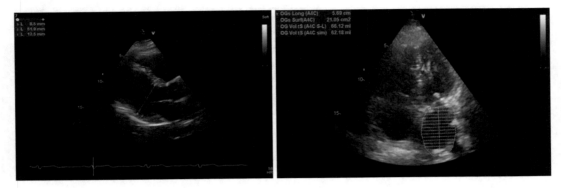

Fig. 7.4 Transthoracic echocardiography

LV EF% of 62%, type 1 diastolic dysfunction, absence of LV hypertrophy, a mildly dilated left atrium with a surface of 22 cm², normal LV filling pressure (E/e' of 7) (Fig. 7.4), non-dilated right atrium and ventricle, mild tricuspid regurgitation, absence of pulmonary hypertension, a non-dilated IVC, absence of pericardial effusion, a mildly dilated ascending aorta of 42 mm.

Question 1: What is the nature of the tachycardia presented in Fig. 7.2?
A. AVNRT
B. AVRT
C. Focal atrial tachycardia
D. Typical atrial flutter
E. Atypical atrial flutter

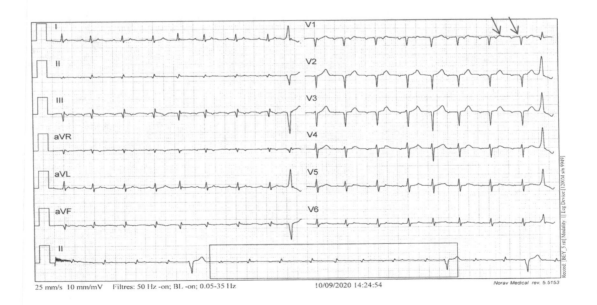

25 mm/s 10 mm/mV   Filtres: 50 Hz -on; BL -on; 0.05-35 Hz   10/09/2020 14:24:54   Norav Medical rev. 5.5153

Figure 7.2 **explained.** The ECG shows an atrial tachycardia with variable AV conduction, with a ventricular rate of 110 bpm, QRS axis at −15°, absence of LV hypertrophy, absence of ischemia, one isolated PVC. The red arrows point to the P waves, best visible in lead V1.

Given the symptomatic nature of the tachycardia from Fig. 7.2, after obtaining informed consent, an electrophysiological study was scheduled and subsequently performed.

7.2   Electrophysiological Study and RF Catheter Ablation Procedure

The electrophysiological study was performed under local anesthesia and conscious sedation, without any fluoroscopic guidance, with the help of the CARTO ® 3 electro-anatomic mapping System (Biosense Webster, Johnson & Johnson).

The 12-lead ECG recorded at the beginning of the electrophysiological study is presented in Fig. 7.5.

Vascular access was obtained using the modified Seldinger technique, under Doppler ultrasound guidance. A Biosense Webster non-irrigated 4 mm tip Navistar catheter with D curve was introduced in a 9F 20 cm vascular sheath at the level of the right common femoral vein and gen-

tly advanced at the level of the right common iliac vein, under constant impedance surveillance on the RF generator. The presence of the roving/ablation catheter at the level of the femoral, iliac vein, and IVC generated an impedance between 140 and 170 Ω. The entrance of the catheter in a collateral vein was rapidly accompanied by a rise in the local impedance of up to 350 Ω, and this determined retraction of the catheter in a previous position. The catheter was then gently oriented in a different manner, in such a way that its advancement determined a relatively constant impedance. The CARTO ® 3 electro-anatomic mapping system was used to create an anatomical map of the right common iliac vein and of the IVC, up to the point where the catheter entered the right atrium and atrial electrograms were recorded by the distal electrode of the roving/ablation catheter. Next, an anatomical map of the right atrium was created during sinus rhythm, with emphasis on the superior vena cava, the coronary sinus, the tricuspid valve, with the identification of the bundle of His and the coronary sinus ostium. The right atrium was not dilated, with a volume of 81 ml.

The AH and the HV interval were of 91 ms and 54 ms (Fig. 7.6).

Next, a 6F quadripolar steerable catheter (Dynamic Extrem, Microport®) was introduced in a 7F 20 cm vascular sheath and was subse-

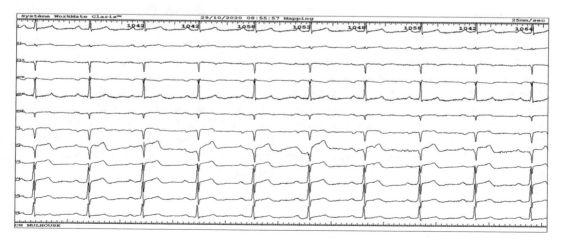

Fig. 7.5 A 12-lead ECG recorded at the beginning of the ablation procedure, showing sinus rhythm with a heart rate of 57 bpm, QRS axis at −30°, absence of LV hypertrophy, absence of ischemia

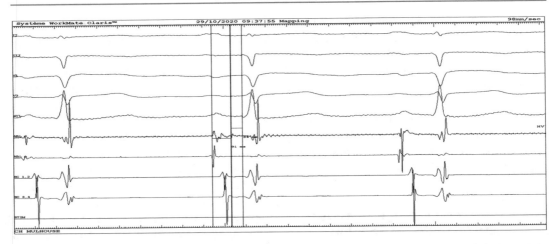

Fig. 7.6 Surface ECG leads II, III, V1, V3, and aVL, together with intracavitary leads recorded from the distal and the proximal bipolar electrodes of the roving/ablation catheter (ABL d and ABL p) and from the bipolar elec-trodes of the distal and the proximal electrodes of the coronary sinus catheter (SC 1,2 and SC 3,4) showing baseline AH and HV intervals, measuring 91 ms and 54 ms, respectively

quently advanced via the right common femoral vein with the help of the CARTO system and the previously created map of the right common iliac veins and the IVC up to the coronary sinus, with the distal poles at the level of the mid portion of the great cardiac vein. Atrial and ventricular pacing were carried out at twice the diastolic threshold using the EP-4™ Cardiac Stimulator (Abbott®) system. Surface ECG and intracavitary ECGs were recorded by the *WorkMate* Claris™ System (Abbott®).

The anterior Wenckebach point was 520 ms. Retrograde conduction was present, concentric, decremental. Parahisian pacing demonstrated an "AV nodal" response, showing no retrograde conduction over an accessory pathway.

Programmed atrial stimulation (S1 = 600 ms, S2 = 380 ms S3 = 330 ms) after isoprenaline infusion initiated of the narrow QRS complex tachycardia presented in Fig. 7.7, with a variable cycle length of 350–390 ms, which reproduced the patient's symptoms.

The 12-lead ECG during tachycardia is shown in Fig. 7.8.

A decision to ablate the atrial tachycardia was taken.

A bipolar voltage map of the RA was first created, which showed the presence of 3 areas of low-voltage/borderline voltage extending from the superior vena cava to the tricuspid annulus, at 12 o'clock position in LAO 45° (Fig. 7.9). At this level, fragmented atrial potentials and low-amplitude double potentials could be recorded.

Next, programmed atrial stimulation was repeated, and the atrial tachycardia was reinduced. An activation mapping of the right atrium was then performed during atrial tachycardia. The earliest local atrial activation was identified at the level of the tricuspid annulus at 12 o'clock position, where the local A preceded the surface P wave on the 12 lead ECG by 30 ms (Figs. 7.10 and 7.11). The local unipolar electrogram recorded by the distal electrode of the roving/ablation catheter had a "QS" aspect at this site (Fig. 7.11). The activation map showed a depolarization sequence compatible with a focal mechanism.

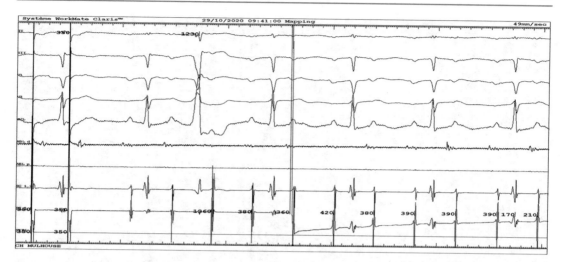

Fig. 7.7 Surface ECG leads II, III, V1, V3, and aVL, together with intracavitary leads recorded from the distal and the proximal bipolar electrodes of the roving/ablation catheter (ABL d and ABL p) and from the bipolar electrodes of the distal and the proximal electrodes of the coronary sinus catheter (SC 1,2 and SC 3,4) showing the initiation of an atrial tachycardia with a cycle length of 390 ms, with 2:1 AV conduction during burst atrial pacing with a fixed coupling interval of 350 ms. Of note, the morphology of the P wave is positive-negative in inferior leads and in lead V1, positive in lead aVL, suggesting an origin in the right atrium

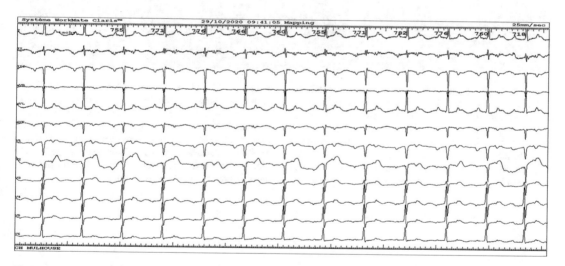

Fig. 7.8 A 12-lead ECG showing atrial tachycardia with 2:1 AV conduction, with a heart rate of 79 bpm. The morphology of the P wave is positive-negative in inferior leads and in lead V1, positive in lead I and aVL, suggesting an origin in the right atrium

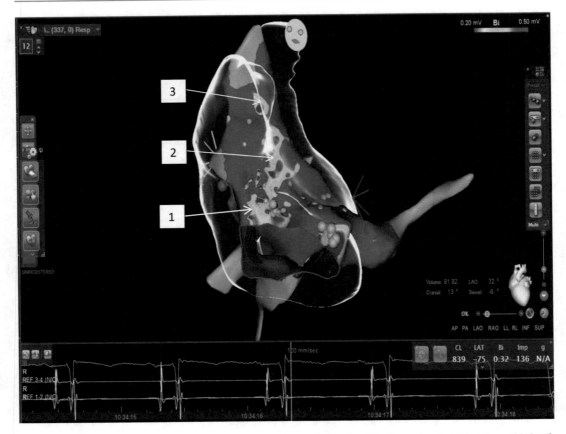

Fig. 7.9 CARTO image in LAO showing the bipolar voltage map of the right atrium during sinus rhythm. Local voltage >0.5 mV compatible with healthy myocardial tissue is represented in violet, voltage <0.2 mV compatible with scar is represented in red, voltage between 0.2 mV and 0.5 mV is compatible with borderline tissue. Of note, there are 3 areas of low-voltage/borderline voltage extending from the superior vena cava to the tricuspid annulus, at 12 o'clock position in LAO 45°. At this level, fragmented atrial potentials and low-amplitude double potentials could be recorded. The orange dots represent the bundle of His. Of note, the right atrium is not dilated, with a volume of 81 ml. Superposed in glass-gray there is the 3D reconstruction of the CT angiography performed prior to the ablation procedure, for facilitating the real-time anatomical map creation purpose

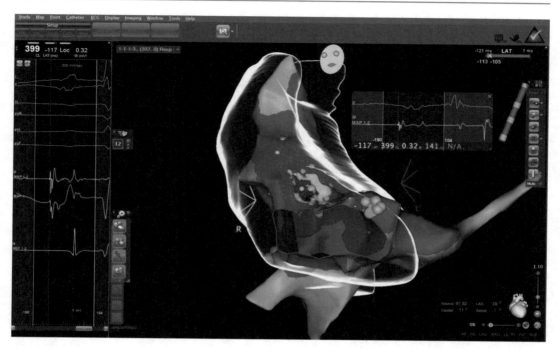

Fig. 7.10 CARTO image in LAO showing the activation map of the right atrium during atrial tachycardia. This is compatible with a focal atrial tachycardia originating close to the mitral annulus, at 12 o'clock position in LAO 45°. Of note, the earliest local atrial electrogram precedes the surface P wave by 30 ms. Double potentials can be recorded in this area, possibly as a result of the previous ablation procedure. Of note, this area corresponds to the area of low-amplitude potentials on the bipolar voltage map from Fig. 7.9

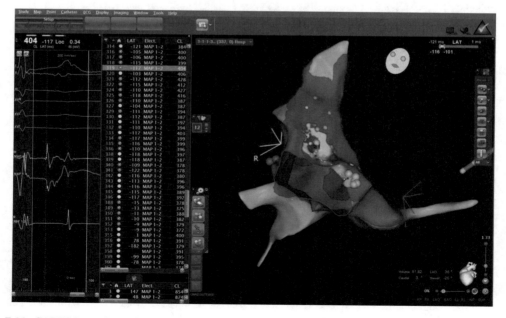

Fig. 7.11 CARTO image in LAO showing the activation map of the right atrium during atrial tachycardia. This is compatible with a focal atrial tachycardia originating close to the mitral annulus, at 12 o'clock position in LAO 45°. Of note, the earliest local atrial electrogram precedes the surface P wave by 30 ms. Double potentials can be recorded in this area, possibly as a result of the previous ablation procedure. The local unipolar electrogram has a "QS" aspect, confirming the origin of the tachycardia at this site. Of note, this area corresponds to the area of low-amplitude potentials on the bipolar voltage map from Fig. 7.9

RF energy was applied at this site, but with significant catheter instability, with short applications of less than 10 s and suboptimal catheter contact.

Question 2: What would be the next step in the management of this patient at this point of the procedure?

A. Continue applying RF energy until the tachycardia becomes non-inducible
B. Use a deflectable long sheath in order to increase catheter stability at the ablation site
C. Switch to cryoablation, given the good contact of the cryo catheter with the tissue at very low temperatures
D. Perform a superior approach of the right atrium, such as the eight internal jugular vein
E. Exchange the ablation catheter for a SmartTouch SF ablation catheter with a larger curve (F or G).

The option chosen at this point of the procedure was to use an Aglis (Abbott©) deflectable vascular sheath, that was inserted via the right common femoral vein, in order to improve contact at the target ablation site. RF energy was subsequently applied at the earliest depolarization site during tachycardia, with interruption of the tachycardia, but with constant re-induction during programmed atrial stimulation, likely due to a poor catheter contact at the ablation site.

Considering the other existing options (exchanging the RF ablation catheter for a cryo-ablation catheter or switching to a larger curve SmartTouch SF ablation catheter, or performing RF ablation via a superior approach), the right internal jugular vein approach was considered the next best step in the management of the patient. This was achieved under Doppler guidance, using the modified Seldinger technique. An 8F 20 cm vascular sheath was inserted in the right internal jugular vein and the ablation catheter was advanced at the level of the superior vena cava, and then the right atrium (Fig. 7.12).

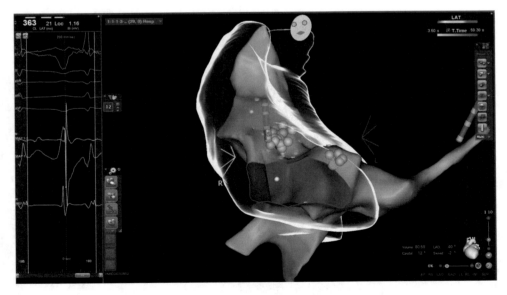

Fig. 7.12 CARTO image in LAO showing the anatomical map of the right atrium with superposed RF ablation lesions at the site of the earliest local atrial activation during atrial tachycardia. Of note, the ablation catheter is introduced in the right atrium via the right internal jugular vein and enters the right atrium through the superior vena cava. This was due to the fact that the common approach via the right common femoral vein did not assure enough catheter stability at this site, even after the insertion of a deflectable Agilis (Abbott©) sheath. Superposed in glass-blue, there is the 3D reconstruction of the CT angiography performed prior to the ablation procedure, for facilitating the real-time anatomical map creation

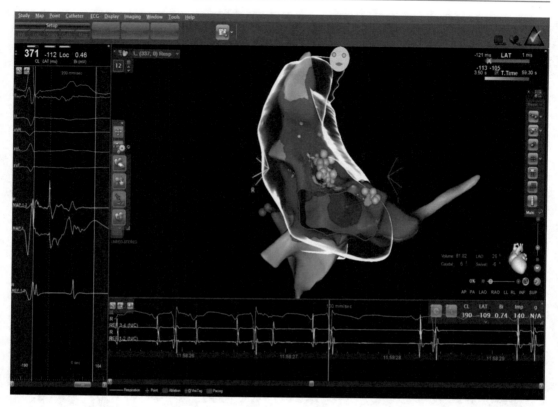

Fig. 7.13 CARTO image in LAO 26° cranial 6° showing the activation map of the right atrium during atrial tachycardia with superposed RF ablation lesions (white and pink dots) at the site of the earliest activation site during tachycardia. The orange dots represent the bundle of His.

Superposed in glass-blue, there is the 3D reconstruction of the CT angiography performed prior to the ablation procedure, for facilitating the real-time anatomical map creation purpose. In the lower part of the picture, termination of the atrial tachycardia can be seen

RF ablation was performed with power titration from 20 W to 30 Watts, with maximum application duration for each RF delivery of 60 seconds. The tachycardia was terminated during RF application (Figs. 7.13 and 7.14).

The RA bipolar voltage map with superposed RF ablation lesions is presented in Fig. 7.15.

Programmed atrial stimulation was performed at the end of the ablation of the atrial tachycardia, with induction of the tachycardia from Fig. 7.16. The 12-lead aspect of the tachycardia is shown in Fig. 7.17.

The termination of the tachycardia after a burst of atrial pacing is shown in Fig. 7.18.

> **Question 3: What is the nature of the tachycardia from Figs. 7.16 and 7.17?**
> A. This is the same atrial tachycardia from Figs. 7.7 and 7.8
> B. Atypical (fast - slow) AVNRT
> C. Typical AVNRT with 2:1 conduction block to the ventricle.ORT using a concealed left lateral accessory pathway
> D. Focal junctional tachycardia

This tachycardia was also symptomatic and sustained. It had a fixed 1:1 AV relationship. Given the

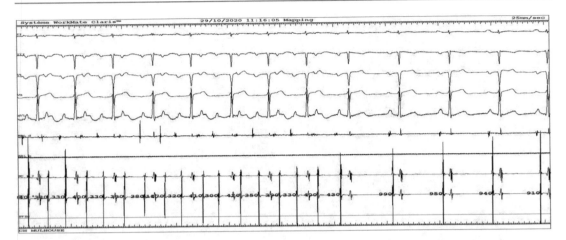

Fig. 7.14 Surface ECG leads II, III, V1, V3, and aVL, together with intracavitary leads recorded from the distal and the proximal bipolar electrodes of the roving/ablation catheter (ABL d and ABL p) and from the bipolar electrodes of the distal and the proximal electrodes of the coronary sinus catheter (SC 1,2 and SC 3,4) showing the termination of the atrial tachycardia during RF ablation

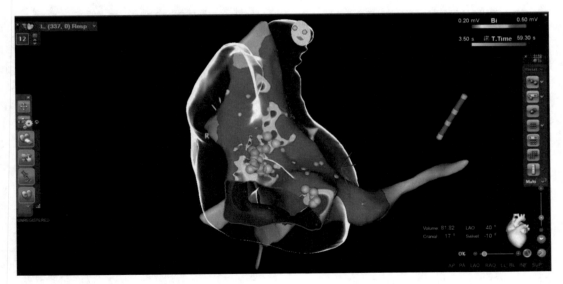

Fig. 7.15 CARTO image in LAO 40° cranial 17° showing the bipolar voltage map of the right atrium during sinus rhythm with superposed RF ablation lesions (white and pink dots) at the site of the earliest activation site during tachycardia. The orange dots represent the bundle of
His. Superposed in glass-blue, there is the 3D reconstruction of the CT angiography performed prior to the ablation procedure, for facilitating the real-time anatomical map creation

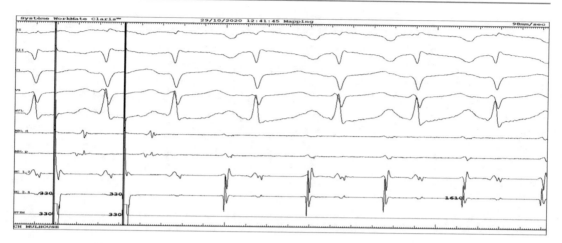

Fig. 7.16 Surface ECG leads II, III, V1, V3, and aVL, together with intracavitary leads recorded from the distal and the proximal bipolar electrodes of the roving/ablation catheter (ABL d and ABL p) and from the bipolar electrodes of the distal and the proximal electrodes of the coronary sinus catheter (SC 1,2 and SC 3,4) showing the initiation of a narrow QRS complex tachycardia with 1:1 AV conduction and a cycle length of 370 ms

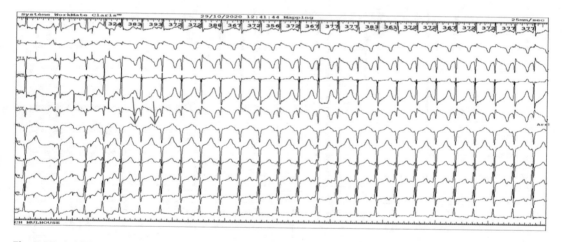

Fig. 7.17 A 12-lead ECG showing the aspect of the narrow QRS complex tachycardia from Fig. 7.16. The red arrows point to the P waves, best visible in lead V1

diagnostic maneuvers performed during the EP study (the presence of concentric retrograde conduction during V pacing in sinus rhythm, the nodal response to parahisian pacing), an ORT was considered highly unlikely. The differential diagnosis of this tachycardia included atypical AVNRT and AT. Figure 7.18 shows continuation of the tachycardia after the end of burst atrial pacing and its spontaneous termination with the sequence A-V. This makes the diagnosis of atrial tachycardia highly unlikely. Also, at the end of V pacing during

tachycardia, the response was V-A-V (not shown), supporting the diagnosis of atypical AVNRT.

The existence of a slow AV nodal pathway was subsequently demonstrated during programmed atrial stimulation, by showing the existence of an antegrade "jump" from the fast AV nodal pathway to a slow AV nodal pathway (a sudden prolongation of the AH interval by 129 ms for a 10 ms decrement in the S2-S3 interval) (Fig. 7.19).

Continuation of programmed atrial stimulation initiated a narrow QRS complex tachycardia

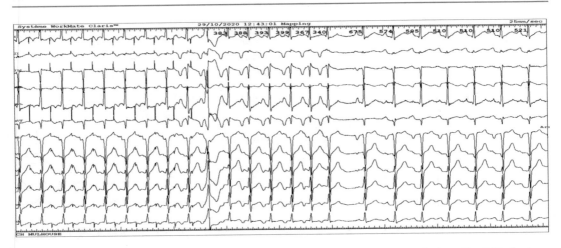

Fig. 7.18 A 12-lead ECG showing the termination of the narrow QRS complex tachycardia from Fig. 7.17 after burst atrial pacing with a fixed coupling interval of 350 ms

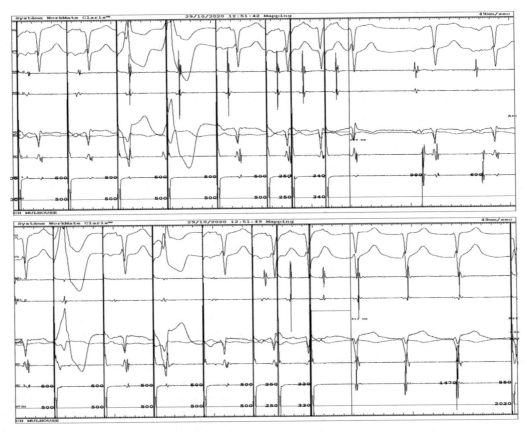

Fig. 7.19 Surface ECG leads II, III, V1, V3, and aVL, together with intracavitary leads recorded from the distal and the proximal bipolar electrodes of the roving/ablation catheter (ABL d and ABL p) and from the bipolar electrodes of the distal and the proximal electrodes of the coronary sinus catheter (SC 1,2 and SC 3,4) showing a sudden prolongation of the AV interval with 129 ms for a 10 ms decrement in the S1S2 coupling interval (from S1 = 500 ms, S2 = 350 ms, S3 = 340 ms to S1 = 500 ms, S2 = 350 ms, S3 = 330 ms), demonstrating the existence of a slow AV nodal pathway. Of note, 3 atrial echo beats can be seen. The VA interval is short of 8 ms at the level of the CS catheter

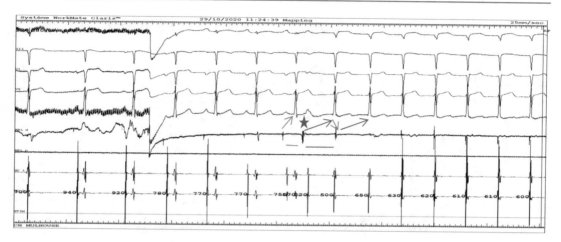

Fig. 7.20 Surface ECG leads II, III, V1, V3, and aVL, together with intracavitary leads recorded from the distal and the proximal bipolar electrodes of the roving/ablation catheter (ABL d and ABL p) and from the bipolar electrodes of the distal and the proximal electrodes of the coronary sinus catheter (SC 1,2 and SC 3,4) showing the spontaneous initiation of a narrow QRS complex tachycardia with 1:1 AV conduction, with a VA interval of 8 ms measured at the level of the CS catheter. The tachycardia initiates after a sudden prolongation of the AV interval, consistent with a "jump" from the fast AV nodal pathway to the slow AV nodal pathway. The blue arrow indicates conduction over the fast pathway, the red arrow conduction over the slow AV nodal pathway. The blue line indicates conduction over the fast pathway and the red line the first conduction over the slow AV nodal pathway, the red star indicates the atrial beat that initiates AVNRT

with 1:1 AV relationship, with a VA interval of 8 ms, compatible with typical "slow-fast" AVNRT (Figs. 7.20 and 7.21).

> **Question 4: Given the patient's personal history of intermittent grade 1 AV block and intermittent type 1 s degree AV block recorded by the 24-hour Holter ECG, the recurrence of AVNRT after the first catheter ablation procedure, what would be your approach for his typical and atypical AVNRT?**
>
> A. Medical treatment with beta blockers should be the first choice.
> B. Add Flecainide on top of beta blockers.
> C. Perform cryoablation of the slow pathway.
> D. Perform radiofrequency ablation of the slow pathway.
> E. Perform RF ablation using the right internal jugular vein approach.

Given the normal AH value during sinus rhythm at the beginning of the EP study, the ablation of the slow AV nodal pathway was decided.

RF ablation was carried out during sinus rhythm in a temperature-controlled manner, with titration of RF energy from 10 W to 30 W. Junctional beats were observed starting from 15 W when ablating the postero-septal region of the triangle of Koch, just anterior to the coronary sinus ostium (Fig. 7.22).

The local signal recorded by the ablation catheter at the successful ablation site and the deployed RF ablation lesions are presented in Fig. 7.23.

The distance between the His bundle and the successful ablation site was less than 8 mm (Fig. 7.24).

The AH interval at the end of RF ablation was 79 ms (Fig. 7.25).

Programmed atrial stimulation performed after the ablation of the slow AV nodal pathway, before and after isoprenaline administration showed absence of induction of AVNRT, absence

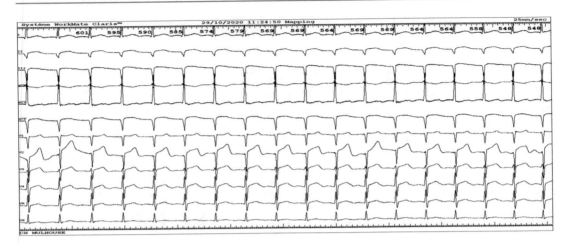

Fig. 7.21 A 12-lead ECG showing the aspect of the narrow QRS tachycardia from Fig. 7.20

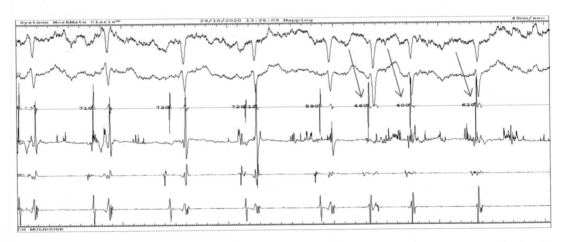

Fig. 7.22 Surface leads V1 and V3 together with intracavitary leads recorded from the proximal poles of the CS catheter (SC 3–4), from the distal and the proximal bipolar electrodes of the roving/ablation catheter (ABL d and ABL p) and from the bipolar electrodes of the distal electrodes of the coronary sinus catheter (SC 1,2) showing the presence of junctional beats during RF ablation of the slow AV nodal pathway (red arrows), indicating a good ablation site

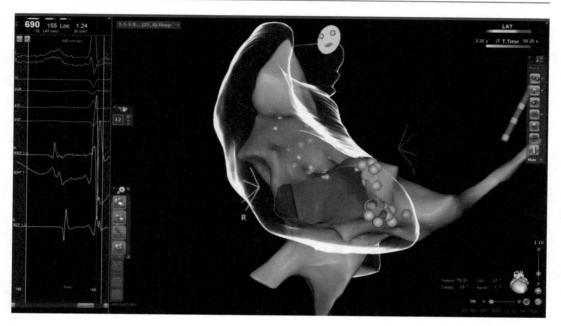

Fig. 7.23 CARTO image in LAO showing the anatomical map of the right atrium with superposed RF ablation lesions (pink and red dots) at the level of the slow pathway insertion (right lower exit). The yellow dots represent the bundle of His. The left side of the image shows the signal recorded by the ablation catheter at this site

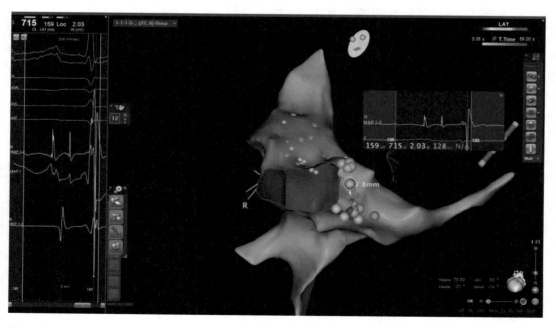

Fig. 7.24 CARTO image in LAO showing the anatomical map of the right atrium with superposed RF ablation lesions (pink and red dots) at the level of the slow pathway insertion (right lower exit). The yellow dots represent the bundle of His. The roving/ablation catheter is placed at the level of the His bundle. Note the close proximity of the His bundle to the successful ablation site (less than 8 mm)

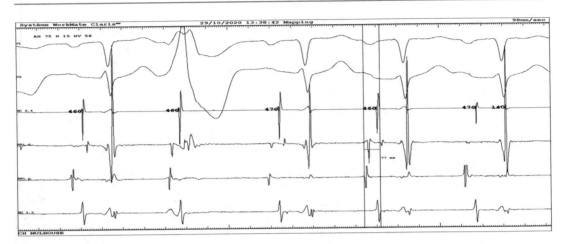

Fig. 7.25 Surface leads V1 and V3 together with intracavitary leads recorded from the proximal poles of the CS catheter (SC 3–4), from the distal and the proximal bipolar electrodes of the roving/ablation catheter (ABL d and ABL p) and from the bipolar electrodes of the distal electrodes of the coronary sinus catheter (SC 1,2) showing the AH interval at the end of the ablation procedure, measuring 79 ms (no AH prolongation as a result of the ablation, despite the close anatomical proximity of the His bundle to the successful ablation site)

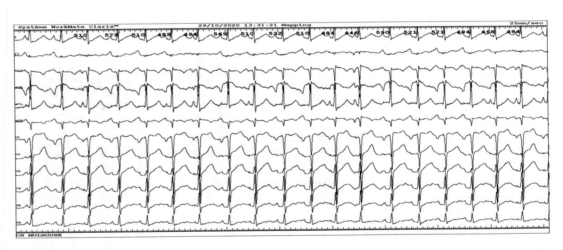

Fig. 7.26 A 12-lead ECG at the end of the ablation procedure showing sinus tachycardia (due to Isoprenaline administration during the control programmed atrial stimulation)

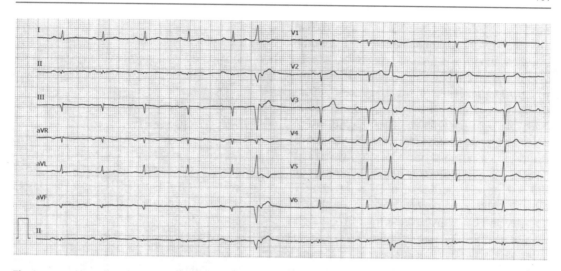

Fig. 7.27 A 12-lead ECG recorded at after the ablation procedure showing sinus rhythm with a heart rate of 75 bpm, QRS axis at −30°, absence of LV hypertrophy, absence of ischemia, 2 isolated PVC, PR interval of 190 ms

of atrial echos and absence of a conduction "jump," confirming the elimination of the slow AV nodal pathway.

There were no complications related to the procedure. The ECG recorded at the end of the ablation procedure is presented in Fig. 7.26.

The 12-lead ECG recorded after the ablation procedure is shown in Fig. 7.27.

ANSWERS TO:
Question 1: C. Focal atrial tachycardia.
Question 2: D. Perform a superior approach of the right atrium, such as the eight internal jugular vein.
Question 3: B. Atypical (fat - slow) AVNRT.
Question 4: D. Perform RF ablation of the slow AV nodal pathway.

7.3 Commentary

The present case illustrates a catheter ablation procedure of a focal atrial tachycardia originating close to the tricuspid annulus and of a typical and atypical AVNRT in a 62-year-old male patient without structural heart disease. Several aspects merit further discussion.

The tricuspid annulus is one of the possible origins of focal atrial tachycardias arising from the right atrium, along with the crista terminalis, the right atrial appendage, and the coronary sinus ostium [1–5]. In their experience, Morton et al. [3] found 13% of their patients with right atrial tachycardias to have an origin at the tricuspid annulus level. Most of these (7 of 9 patients) had an origin in the inferior part of the tricuspid annulus, compared to only 2 patients who had an origin at the superior part of the annulus. The mean tachycardia cycle length of the atrial tachycardias in their study was 371 ± 66 ms, which is very similar to the cycle length of the tachycardia present in the above-described case. The success rate of the ablation procedure was high, and the recurrence rate is low (1 of 9 patients), and the patient who presented the recurrence was successfully treated with a second ablation procedure. Of note, this was also the case for the above-presented patient since he had undergone catheter ablation for his atrial tachycardia several years prior in another center.

Ablating focal atrial tachycardias originating from the tricuspid annulus at 12 o'clock position in LAO 45° projection can sometimes be technically challenging, since a good contact between the ablation catheter and the tricuspid annulus is difficult to obtain, due to catheter instability.

Possible solutions include using a long deflectable sheath for catheter stabilization [6], switching to a superior approach (via the subclavian vein or the internal jugular vein) [7] or switching to cryoablation (since the cryo catheter adheres to the myocardial tissue during ablation) [8]. Each of these possible solutions has its advantages and its downsides. As shown in the above-presented case, the Agilis (Abbott®) deflectable sheath, although extremely helpful in other cases, did not provide sufficient support in order to allow a stable good contact between the ablation catheter and the tachycardia origin. Switching to a right internal jugular vein approach was the solution in this case since the superior approach of the tricuspid annulus allowed sufficient contact between the ablation catheter and the tachycardia origin in order to perform a successful ablation. This approach has already been described as successfully used in SVT ablation in children [9], typical atrial flutter [10], atrial fibrillation in patients with interrupted inferior vena cava [11] and performing transseptal puncture for atrial fibrillation ablation or left atrial appendage closure [11].

Regarding AVNRT, coexistence of typical and atypical AVNRT in the same patient is rare, as demonstrated by Katritsis et al., who identified 20 patients out of 1299 (1.5%) to have both types of AVNRT [12]. Ablation of both types of AVNRT is usually performed at the right extension of the AV node, in the lower part of Koch's triangle [13]. Success rate is high, and recurrence rate is low.

The procedure was performed without any fluoroscopic guidance. As described in the "Electrophysiological Study and RF Catheter Ablation Procedure "section of the case report, the CARTO system can provide sufficient information for catheter positioning and RF ablation in order to completely avoid utilization of fluoroscopy. Experience with AVNRT ablation guided by an electroanatomical mapping system [14] or by remote magnetic navigation [15] is increasing.

Learning Point

- Typical (slow-fast) and atypical (fast-slow or slow-slow) AVNRT can coexist in the same patient.
- AVNRT and focal atrial tachycardia can coexist in the same patient.
- When ablating focal atrial tachycardias originating from the tricuspid annulus at 12 o'clock position in LAO 45° projection, catheter stability is usually an issue. Utilizing a long deflectable sheath or switching to a superior approach (via the subclavian vein or the internal jugular vein) can provide the desired catheter stability in order to perform a successful ablation.
- Catheter ablation of AVNRT and of SVT can be safely accomplished with the use of an electroanatomical mapping system, without the use of fluoroscopy.

References

1. Femenia F, Arce M, Arrieta M, Baranchuk A. [Incessant focal atrial tachycardia arising from the right appendage: risk of tachycardia mediated cardiomyopathy. Role of the radiofrequency ablation]. Arch Argent Pediatr. 2011;109(2):e33–e38.
2. Kistler PM, Fynn SP, Haqqani H, Stevenson IH, Vohra JK, Morton JB, et al. Focal atrial tachycardia from the ostium of the coronary sinus: electrocardiographic and electrophysiological characterization and radiofrequency ablation. J Am Coll Cardiol. 2005;45(9):1488–93.
3. Morton JB, Sanders P, Das A, Vohra JK, Sparks PB, Kalman JM. Focal atrial tachycardia arising from the tricuspid annulus: electrophysiologic and electrocardiographic characteristics. J Cardiovasc Electrophysiol. 2001;12(6):653–9.
4. Uhm JS, Shim J, Wi J, Mun HS, Pak HN, Lee MH, et al. An electrocardiography algorithm combined with clinical features could localize the origins of focal atrial tachycardias in adjacent structures. Europace. 2014;16(7):1061–8.
5. Zhang T, Li XB, Wang YL, Yin JX, Zhang P, Zhang HC, et al. Focal atrial tachycardia arising from the right atrial appendage: electrophysiologic and elec-

trocardiographic characteristics and catheter ablation. Int J Clin Pract. 2009;63(3):417–24.

6. Piorkowski C, Eitel C, Rolf S, Bode K, Sommer P, Gaspar T, et al. Steerable versus nonsteerable sheath technology in atrial fibrillation ablation: a prospective, randomized study. Circ Arrhythm Electrophysiol. 2011;4(2):157–65.

7. Miranda R, Simpson CS, Nolan RL, Diez JC, Michael KA, Redfearn DP, et al. Superior approach for radiofrequency ablation of atrio-ventricular nodal reentrant tachycardia in a patient with anomalous inferior vena cava and azygos continuation. Europace. 2010;12(6):908–9.

8. Bastani H, Insulander P, Schwieler J, Tabrizi F, Braunschweig F, Kenneback G, et al. Safety and efficacy of cryoablation of atrial tachycardia with high risk of ablation-related injuries. Europace. 2009;11(5):625–9.

9. Ergul Y, Ozgur S, Sahin GT, Kafali HC, Celebi SB, Bay B, et al. The transjugular approach: an alternative route to improve ablation success in right anteriorly and anterolaterally-located supraventricular tachycardia substrates in children. Pediatr Cardiol. 2019;40(3):477–82.

10. Tung R, Shivkumar K, Mandapati R. Ablation of post transplant atrial flutter and pseudo-fibrillation using magnetic navigation via a superior approach. Indian Pacing Electrophysiol J. 2012;12(5):229–32.

11. Hanley A, Bode WD, Heist EK, Leyton-Mange J, Chatterjee N, Chokshi M, et al. Management of patients with interrupted inferior vena cava requiring electrophysiology procedures. J Cardiovasc Electrophysiol. 2020;31(5):1083–90.

12. Katritsis DG, Marine JE, Latchamsetty R, Zografos T, Tanawuttiwat T, Sheldon SH, et al. Coexistent types of atrioventricular nodal re-entrant tachycardia: implications for the tachycardia circuit. Circ Arrhythm Electrophysiol. 2015;8(5):1189–93.

13. Katritsis DG, Marine JE, Contreras FM, Fujii A, Latchamsetty R, Siontis KC, et al. Catheter Ablation of Atypical Atrioventricular Nodal Reentrant Tachycardia. Circulation. 2016;134(21):1655–63.

14. Earley MJ, Showkathali R, Alzetani M, Kistler PM, Gupta D, Abrams DJ, et al. Radiofrequency ablation of arrhythmias guided by non-fluoroscopic catheter location: a prospective randomized trial. Eur Heart J. 2006;27(10):1223–9.

15. Bhaskaran A, Albarri M, Ross N, Al Raisi S, Samanta R, Roode L, et al. Slow pathway radiofrequency ablation using magnetic navigation: a description of technique and retrospective case analysis. Heart Lung Circ. 2017;26(12):1297–302.

Case 8

Frédéric Halbwachs, Ronan Le Bouar, David Kenizou, and Yasmine Doghmi

8

8.1 Case Presentation

A 45-year-old female patient with a long history of undocumented palpitations (2–3 episodes/year since the age or 24 years, with a duration of several minutes, with sudden onset and spontaneous termination) presents herself to the Emergency Department complaining of rapid palpitations with a sudden onset and regular rhythm accompanied by dyspnea, that had started 20 min before her presentation at the hospital. She had no personal history of heart disease or syncope, no family history of sudden cardiac death. A cardiovascular exam performed several years prior (ECG, transthoracic echocardiography, 24-hour Holter ECG) was normal. Her cardiovascular risk factors were represented by smoking (15 packs-year) and grade 1 overweight. She was on no chronic medication. At physical exam, her blood pressure was 100/65 mmHg, heart rate of 150 bpm, SpO_2 98% breathing room air, $H = 1.74$ m, $W = 88$ kg, BMI = 29.06 kg/m^2, heart sounds were rapid, there was no audible heart murmur, there were no signs of heart failure, pulmonary auscultation was normal. Her ECG is presented in Fig. 8.1.

The tachycardia presented in Fig. 8.1 terminated spontaneously while in the Emergency Department and the patient was addressed to the Cardiology Department.

An ECG was recorded after the termination of the tachycardia (Fig. 8.2).

Transthoracic echocardiography was performed, which showed a non-dilated left ventricle, absence of LV hypertrophy, with a preserved LV EF% of 77% (Fig. 8.3). It also showed normal diastolic function, mild mitral regurgitation, non-dilated left atrium, right atrium and right ventricle, trivial tricuspid regurgitation, absence of pulmonary hypertension, absence of pericardial effusion.

Her biological workup showed a Hb level of 14.7 g/dl, leucocytes 8.0×10^9/L, platelets 360×10^9/L, CRP 5 mg/L, BUN 3.2 mmol/L, creatinine75 µmol/L, glycemia 4.7 mmol/L, Na+ 138 mmol/L, K+ 4.2 mmol/L, NT pro-BNP 412 pg/ml, TSH 1.51 IU/L, total cholesterol 201 mg/dl, HDL 73 mg/dl, LDL 113 mg/dl, and triglycerides 96 mg/dl.

F. Halbwachs (✉)
Biosense Webster, Mulhouse, France

R. Le Bouar · D. Kenizou · Y. Doghmi
Cardiology Department, "Emile Muller" Hospital, Mulhouse, France

© The Author(s), under exclusive license to Springer Nature Switzerland AG 2022
L. Muresan (ed.), *Clinical Cases in Cardiac Electrophysiology: Supraventricular Arrhythmias*,
https://doi.org/10.1007/978-3-031-07357-1_8

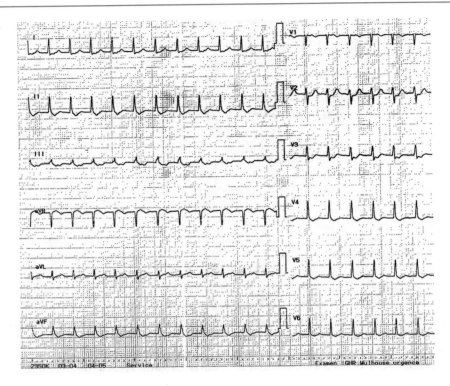

Fig. 8.1 Narrow QRS complex tachycardia with a heart rate of 150 bpm, QRS axis at +60°, absence of LV hypertrophy, flattened T waves in V3–V6, negative in II, III, and aVF

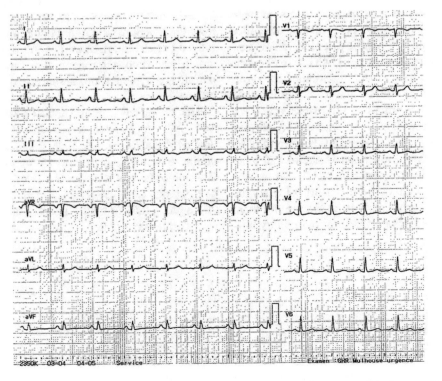

Fig. 8.2 A 12-lead ECG showing sinus rhythm with a heart rate of 90 bpm, QRS axis at +60°, absence of LV hypertrophy, absence of ischemia, PR interval of 160 ms

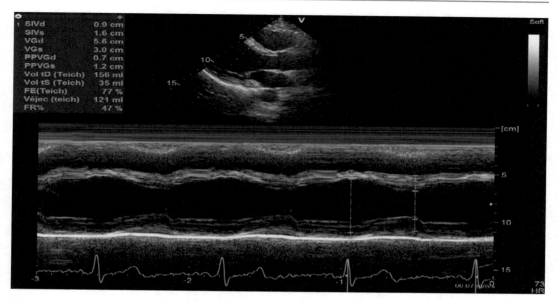

Fig. 8.3 M mode echocardiographic image showing a non-dilated LV with a preserved LVEF of 77%, absence of LV hypertrophy

Her chest X-ray is presented in Fig. 8.4.

Question 1: What is the nature of the tachycardia presented in Fig. 8.1?
A. Sinus tachycardia.
B. Atrial tachycardia.
C. Typical slow-fast AVNRT.
D. Slow-slow AVNRT.
E. AVRT.

Below is a more detailed analysis of the ECG presented in Fig. 8.1.

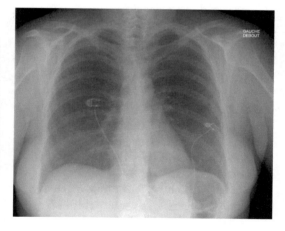

Fig. 8.4 Chest X-ray in postero-anterior view showing a non-enlarged cardiac silhouette, absence of pleural effusion, image compatible with a normal chest X-ray

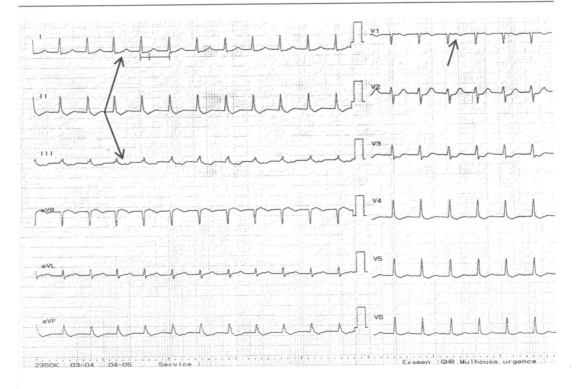

Figure 8.1 (**explained**). Narrow QRS complex tachycardia with a heart rate of 150 bpm, QRS axis at +60°, the morphology of the QRS complex being identical to the QRS in sinus rhythm. P waves are visible in lead I, III, and V1 at the end of the QRS complex (red arrows), with a RP interval < PR interval (blue lines, lead I), but greater than 80 ms. The differential diagnosis comprises atypical AVNRT, orthodromic AVRT, and atrial tachycardia.

In order to establish the correct diagnosis, an electrophysiological study was performed.

8.2 Electrophysiological Study and RF Catheter Ablation Procedure

The electrophysiological study was performed under local anesthesia and conscious sedation. Vascular access was obtained using the modified Seldinger technique, under Doppler ultrasound guidance. A 6F quadripolar steerable catheter (Dynamic Extrem, Microport®) was introduced

in a 9F 20 cm vascular sheath and was subsequently advanced via the right common femoral vein up to the bundle of His. A 6F decapolar steerable catheter (Inquiry, Abbott®) was introduced in a 6F 20 cm vascular sheath and placed via the right common femoral vein in the coronary sinus, with the distal poles at the level of the lateral mitral annulus. A bipolar non-steerable catheter (Viking, Boston Scientific®) was introduced in a 6F 20 cm vascular sheath and was subsequently advanced via the right common femoral vein up to the right ventricular apex. Atrial and ventricular pacing were carried out at twice the diastolic threshold using the EP-4™ Cardiac Stimulator (Abbott®) system. Surface ECG and intra-cavitary ECGs were recorded by the *WorkMate* Claris™ System (Abbott®). Radiofrequency ablation was delivered using a Biosense Webster® SmartTouch SF open-irrigated 3.5 mm tip with D curve. The CARTO ® 3 electro-anatomic mapping System (Biosense Webster, Johnson & Johnson) was used to guide mapping and ablation. Baseline AH was 79 ms, the HV interval was 45 ms. Anterior Wenckebach

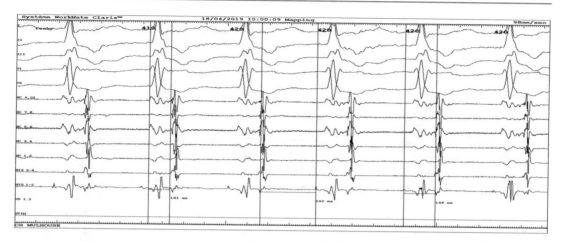

Fig. 8.5 Surface ECG leads I, II, III, V1, and V6 together with intracavitary leads recorded from the bipolar electrodes of the coronary sinus catheter (SC 9,10 to SC 1,2) and the His catheter (His 3–4 and His 1–2) at 200 mm/s showing the VA interval of 101 ms, AH interval of 242 ms, and the HA interval of 148 ms during tachycardia

point was 400 ms. Retrograde conduction was present, concentric, decremental.

Programmed atrial stimulation demonstrated the existence of 2 slow AV nodal pathways (2 "jumps"). Continuation of programmed atrial stimulation resulted in initiation of a narrow QRS complex tachycardia, with the earliest retrograde atrial depolarization situated at the level of the ostium of the coronary sinus. The AH interval during tachycardia at the level of the His catheter was 262 ms. The HA interval was 148 ms (Fig. 8.5).

At the end of ventricular pacing at a fixed coupling interval of 390 ms, the return sequence was V-A-V. A single ventricular extrastimulus during His refractoriness did not advance the tachycardia. PPI at the apex of the right ventricle – TCL = 130 ms. SA – VA during tachycardia was >85 ms.

The fact that at the end of ventricular pacing at a fixed coupling interval of 390 ms, the return sequence was V-A-V, excluded an atrial tachycardia. The fact that a single ventricular extrastimulus during His refractoriness did not advance the tachycardia was not in favor of an ORT, even though this did not exclude it. The PPI at the apex of the right ventricle—TCL greater than 120 ms and the SA—VA during tachycardia >85 ms were in favor of AVNRT. The AH of 262 ms and the HA of 148 ms were in favor of a "slow-slow" AVNRT.

Programmed atrial stimulation also initiated the tachycardia in Fig. 8.6.

At the end of ventricular pacing at a fixed coupling interval of 340 ms, the return sequence was V-A-V. A single ventricular extrastimulus during His refractoriness did not advance the tachycardia. PPI at the apex of the right ventricle—TCL = 150 ms. SA—VA during tachycardia was >85 ms.

Question 2: What is the tachycardia presented in Fig. 8.5?
A. Typical "slow-fast" AVNRT.
B. Atypical "fast-slow" AVNRT.
C. Atypical "slow-slow" AVNRT.
D. ORT using a concealed parahisian accessory pathway.
E. Focal atrial tachycardia originating in the interatrial septum area.

Question 3: What is the tachycardia presented in Fig. 8.6?
A. Typical "slow-fast" AVNRT.
B. Atypical "fast-slow" AVNRT.
C. Atypical "slow-slow" AVNRT.
D. ORT using a concealed parahisian accessory pathway.
E. Focal atrial tachycardia originating in the interatrial septum area.

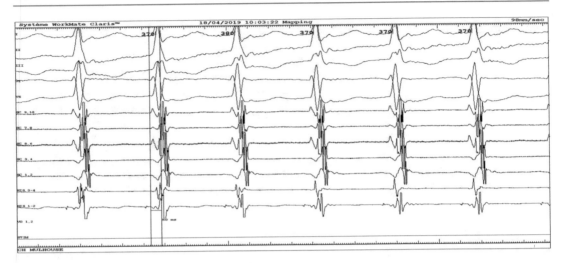

Fig. 8.6 Surface ECG leads I, II, III, V1, and V6 together with intracavitary leads recorded from the bipolar electrodes of the coronary sinus catheter (SC 9,10 to SC 1,2) and the His catheter (His 3–4 and His 1–2) at 200 mm/s showing the VA interval during the second narrow QRS complex tachycardia, of 50 ms

The fact that at the end of ventricular pacing at a fixed coupling interval of 340 ms, the return sequence was V-A-V, excluded an atrial tachycardia. The fact that a single ventricular extrastimulus during His refractoriness did not advance the tachycardia was not in favor of an ORT, even though this did not exclude it. The PPI at the apex of the right ventricle—TCL greater than 120 ms and the SA—VA during tachycardia >85 ms were in favor of AVNRT. The AV of 250 ms and the VA of 50 ms were in favor of a typical "slow-fast" AVNRT.

Question 4: What would be the best ablation strategy in this patient?
A. Ablate the slow pathway of the AV node during sinus rhythm.
B. Ablate the slow pathway of the AV node during "slow-slow" AVNRT.
C. Ablate the slow pathway of the AV node during "slow-fast" AVNRT.
D. Ablate the fast pathway of the AV node during sinus rhythm.
E. Identify the slow-pathway insertion during "slow-slow" AVNRT using activation mapping and ablate it during sinus rhythm.

A decision to ablate the slow pathway of the AV node was taken.

The SmartTouch SF roving/ablation catheter was introduced in the 9F sheath and advanced at the level of the right atrium.

An anatomical map of the left atrium was first created, showing a volume of 90 ml. Activation mapping of the atrial myocardium around the tricuspid valve was then performed, with emphasis on the retrograde atrial activation during "slow-slow" AVNRT. The earliest local atrial activation was confirmed at the level of the coronary sinus ostium, where the shortest VA interval during tachycardia was 52 ms (Fig. 8.7).

RF ablation was carried out during sinus rhythm in a temperature-controlled manner, with titration of RF energy from 10 W to 30 W (Figs. 8.8 and 8.9). Active junctional rhythm was observed starting from 15 W when ablating the postero-septal region of the triangle of Koch, just anterior to the coronary sinus ostium (Fig. 8.10).

Programmed atrial stimulation performed after the ablation of the slow AV nodal pathway, before and after isoprenaline administration showed absence of induction of AVNRT, absence of atrial echos, and absence of a conduction "jump," confirming the elimination of the slow AV nodal pathway.

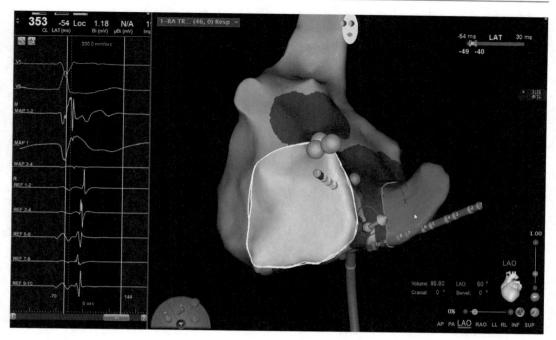

Fig. 8.7 CARTO image in LAO 60° of the right atrium showing the activation map during the tachycardia. The tricuspid valve is represented by the white circle, the coronary sinus is represented in blue, containing a decapolar diagnostic catheter, the His bundle is represented by the yellow dots. The earliest endocardial atrial activation is recorded by the roving/ablation catheter in the triangle of Koch, in an area (red color) slightly below the ostium of the coronary sinus, away from the earliest atrial activation recorded during SVT 1 (orange dot). The left side of the image shows surface ECG leads together with the atrial activation recorded by the coronary sinus catheter (REF 1, 2 to REF 9, 10) and the roving/ablation catheter (MAP 1–2)

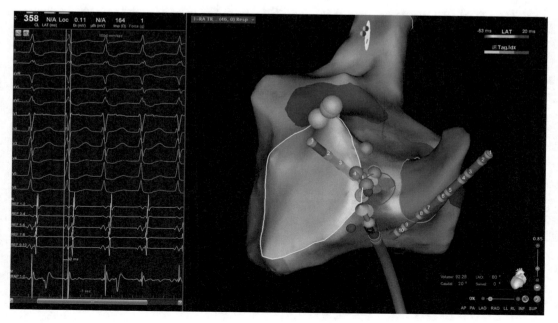

Fig. 8.8 CARTO image of the right atrium, same view as in Fig. 8.5. The shortest VA interval is recorded by the roving/ablation catheter at the ostium of the CS, measuring 52 ms (left side of the image)

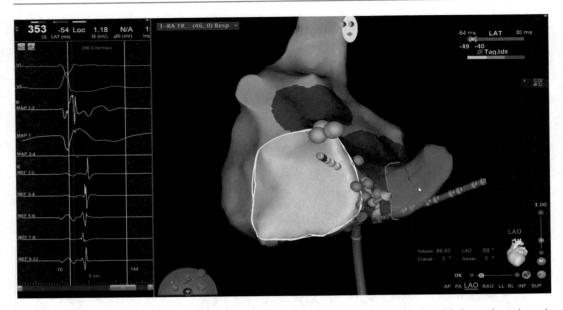

Fig. 8.9 CARTO image of the right atrium, same view as in Figs. 8.7 and 8.8. The roving/ablation catheter is positioned at the level of the slow-pathway insertion in the triangle of Koch. Pink dots represent ablation lesions

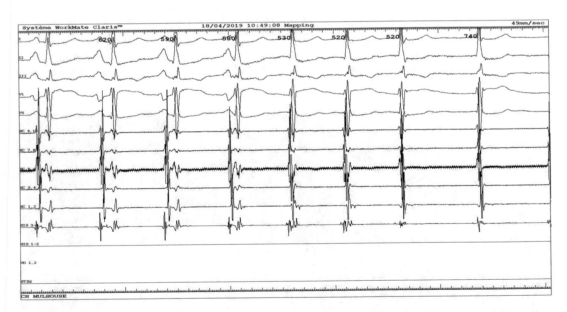

Fig. 8.10 Surface ECG leads I, II, III, V1, and V6 together with intracavitary leads recorded from the bipolar electrodes of the coronary sinus catheter (SC 9,10 to SC 1,2) and the His catheter (His 3–4 and His 1–2) at 200 mm/s showing the presence of active junctional rhythm during RF ablation of the slow AV nodal pathway

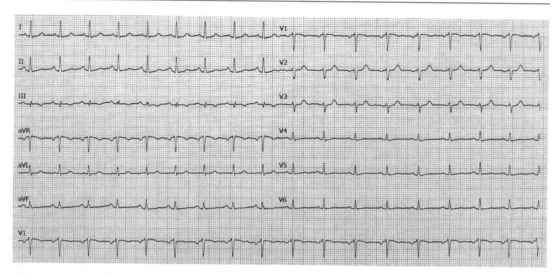

Fig. 8.11 A 12-lead ECG after RF ablation of the slow AV nodal pathway, showing sinus rhythm with a heart rate of 100 bpm, ARS axis at +30°, absence of ischemia, PR interval of 150 ms

There were no complications related to the procedure.

The 12-lead ECG recorded after the ablation procedure is shown in Fig. 8.11.

The patient was discharged from the hospital 24 h later on no antiarrhythmic treatment.

ANSWERS TO:
Question 1: D. Slow-slow AVNRT.
Question 2: C. Atypical "slow-slow" AVNRT.
Question 3: A. Typical "slow-fast" AVNRT.
Question 4: E. Identify the slow-pathway insertion during "slow-slow" AVNRT using activation mapping and ablate it during sinus rhythm.

8.3   Commentary

This case illustrates a RF ablation procedure of the slow AV nodal pathway for typical "slow-fast" and atypical "fast-slow" AVNRT in a 45-year-old female patient with no structural heart disease. Several observations merit further comments.

This specific case was chosen for presentation in order to illustrate the fact that typical "slow-fast" and atypical "fast-slow" AVNRT can coexist in the same patient. For "slow-fast" AVNRT, the anterior limb of the tachycardia is represented by the slow AV nodal pathway, and the retrograde limb is represented by the fast AV nodal pathway. For "fast-slow" AVNRT, the antegrade limb is represented by the fast AV nodal pathway, and the retrograde limb is represented by the slow AV nodal pathway. Of note, several slow pathways can coexist in the same patient, giving rise to the "slow-slow" type of AVNRT, where both the antegrade limb and the retrograde limb of the tachycardia are represented by a slow AV nodal pathway [1]. Whatever the type of AVNRT, the treatment is almost always the same: slow AV nodal pathway ablation. The only exception might be, according to some authors, in patients presenting with first degree AV block during sinus rhythm, who have an altered conduction over the fast pathway of the AV node, in which fast AV nodal pathway might be targeted for ablation [2].

Dual AV nodal pathways can be demonstrated in 10% to 35% of individuals in the general population [3]. However, only a minority of patients who have dual AV nodal physiology will develop AVNRT.

As elegantly demonstrated by Jackmann et al. [4], the slow pathway of the AV node has 4 extensions, which can all, in theory, be targeted for ablation of AVNRT. These are (1) **the right inferior extension**, situated in the triangle of Koch, anterior to the coronary sinus ostium and inferior to the tendon of Todaro, which is almost always the first target for slow-pathway ablation; (2) **the left inferior-lateral extension**, situated at the lateral and inferior part of the mitral annulus, at 5 o'clock position when viewing the mitral annulus in LAO 45°. This may be targeted for slow-pathway ablation if ablation of the right inferior extension fails, this being the successful ablation site in 25% of cases of failed AVNRT ablations; (3) **the left inferior extension**, situated on the left and inferior side of the interatrial septum, corresponding to the 7 o'clock position when viewing the mitral annulus in LAO 45°. This can also be targeted for slow-pathway ablation in the case of prior failed ablations of the right inferior extension; and (4) **the antero-superior extension**, which is situated in the right atrium, in the antero-septal region, which is not usually targeted for slow-pathway ablation.

Ablation of typical "slow-fast" AVNRT is generally performed during sinus rhythm. This is especially because of the fact that mapping during tachycardia identifies the earliest retrograde atrial depolarization, which uses the fast AV nodal pathway, which is not the target for ablation. The slow pathway is identified by carefully mapping its insertion at the level of the triangle of Koch, in a small area between the ostium of the coronary sinus, the tendon of Todaro and the tricuspid valve, where a sharp local signal, as originally described by Jackmann et al. [5] or a "dome-type" local signal, as originally described by Haissaguerre et al. [6] of the slow AV nodal pathway can be recorded.

Ablation of the "fast-slow" or "slow-slow" AVNRT can be performed either in sinus rhythm, similar to "slow-fast" AVNRT or during tachycardia. This is due to the fact that the retrograde activation of the atrium uses the slow AV nodal pathway, which is the target for ablation. In our case, mapping of fast-slow AVNRT was performed during "slow-slow" AVNRT, identifying the earliest retrograde atrial activation and therefore the right interior extension of the slow AV nodal pathway; RF ablation was carried out during sinus rhythm, and active junction rhythm was obtained at the site corresponding to the earliest retrograde atrial depolarization during "slow-slow" AVNRT.

One of the best indicators of efficient slow-pathway ablation for slow-fast AVNRT is the appearance of active junctional rhythm [7, 8]. Cases of successful slow-pathway ablation without obtaining active junctional rhythm have also been described [9]. In the case of slow-pathway ablation for slow-slow AVNRT, some authors observed V-A dissociation during RF energy application, which might not require immediate interruption of the RF application, indicating success of the ablation of the retrograde slow pathway [10]. The solution for verifying integrity of conduction over the fast AV nodal pathway is pacing the atrium and surveying conduction over the fast pathway (the AH interval should not augment during RF application, and AV block should not occur).

The end point of the AVNRT ablation procedure is non-inducibility of the tachycardia. Complete slow-pathway elimination is not always necessary for preventing AVNRT recurrence since modulation of the slow AV nodal pathway with a significant prolongation of its refractory period is sometimes sufficient [11]. Some authors accept as an ablation end point persistence of a "jump" from the fast to the slow pathway with maximum 1 atrial "echo" [12].

The success rate of the slow-pathway ablation procedure can be as high as 98% [4]. In experienced hands, recurrences are rare, about 2–5%. Complications are also rare, the main being vascular complications (1–2%) and complete AV block (0.5–1%), in the case of inadvertent AV nodal ablation, which, if not rapidly reversible, require pacemaker implantation [13].

We used RF energy titration in this patient starting from 10 W and progressively increasing the power up to 30 W, in sites where active junction rhythm was seen. It is our experience to titrate RF energy and not to apply maximum RF energy from the beginning of each RF application, in order to avoid complete AV block in case of RF energy application close to the compact AV node. Inadvertent AV nodal ablation with low power (10–15 W) is generally reversible. Of note, junctional rhythm was observed in this patient only when the power reached 15 W. In our experience, this value is slightly higher compared to ablation of the slow AV nodal pathway using non-irrigated catheters. In our knowledge, as of July 2020, there is no standardized RF ablation parameter end point in terms of ablation index for slow-pathway ablation when using an electroanatomical mapping system. An empirically chosen value of 450 was used (the same value that our team uses for PVI).

We believe that using the CARTO system for AVNRT ablation has several advantages over the "classic" fluoroscopic-only approach: (1) a lower fluoroscopy time and dose; (2) a more accurate activation map during fast-slow or slow-slow AVNRT; (3) contact force monitoring before and during RF application (contact between the distal electrode of the ablation catheter and the myocardium). (4) assessment of the orientation of the force vector, allowing a better contact between the distal electrode of the ablation catheter and the myocardium. (5) ease of catheter repositioning in case of inadvertent catheter movement. (6) ease of applying additional RF lesions at the successful ablation site, if needed. The shortcomings of systematically using a non-fluoroscopic electroanatomical mapping system for AVNRT ablation are related to a higher cost of the procedure.

Learning Point

- Typical and atypical AVNRT can coexist in the same patient.
- Ablation of the slow AV nodal pathway is the treatment of choice for both typical and atypical (fast–slow or slow–slow) AVNRT.

References

1. Heidbuchel H, Jackman WM. Characterization of subforms of AV nodal reentrant tachycardia. Europace. 2004;6(4):316–29.
2. Tuohy S, Trulock KM, Wiggins NB, Bassiouny M, Ono M, Kiehl EL, et al. Should fast pathway ablation be reconsidered in typical atrioventricular nodal re-entrant tachycardia? J Cardiovasc Electrophysiol. 2019;30(9):1569–77.
3. Mani BC, Pavri BB. Dual atrioventricular nodal pathways physiology: a review of relevant anatomy, electrophysiology, and electrocardiographic manifestations. Indian Pacing Electrophysiol J. 2014;14(1):12–25.
4. S P. Warren Jackman's Art of War: A Sniper's Approach to Catheter Ablation; 2019.
5. Jackman WM, Beckman KJ, McClelland JH, Wang X, Friday KJ, Roman CA, et al. Treatment of supraventricular tachycardia due to atrioventricular nodal reentry by radiofrequency catheter ablation of slow-pathway conduction. N Engl J Med. 1992;327(5):313–8.
6. Haissaguerre M, Gaita F, Fischer B, Commenges D, Montserrat P, d'Ivernois C, et al. Elimination of atrioventricular nodal reentrant tachycardia using discrete slow potentials to guide application of radiofrequency energy. Circulation. 1992;85(6):2162–75.
7. Iakobishvili Z, Kusniec J, Shohat-Zabarsky R, Mazur A, Battler A, Strasberg B. Junctional rhythm quantity and duration during slow pathway radiofrequency ablation in patients with atrioventricular nodal re-entry supraventricular tachycardia. Europace. 2006;8(8):588–91.
8. Katritsis DG, Zografos T, Siontis KC, Giannopoulos G, Muthalaly RG, Liu Q, et al. Endpoints for successful slow pathway catheter ablation in typical and atypical atrioventricular nodal re-entrant tachycardia: a contemporary, multicenter study. JACC Clin Electrophysiol. 2019;5(1):113–9.
9. Hsieh MH, Chen SA, Tai CT, Yu WC, Chen YJ, Chang MS. Absence of junctional rhythm during successful slow-pathway ablation in patients with atrioventricular nodal reentrant tachycardia. Circulation. 1998;98(21):2296–300.
10. Fujiki A, Sakamoto T, Sakabe M, Tsuneda T, Sugao M, Nakatani Y, et al. Junctional rhythm associated with ventriculoatrial block during slow pathway ablation in atypical atrioventricular nodal re-entrant tachycardia. Europace. 2008;10(8):982–7.
11. Wegner FK, Bogeholz N, Leitz P, Frommeyer G, Dechering DG, Kochhauser S, et al. Occurrence of primarily noninducible atrioventricular nodal reentry tachycardia after radiofrequency delivery in the slow pathway region during empirical slow pathway modulation. Clin Cardiol. 2017;40(11):1112–5.
12. Stern JD, Rolnitzky L, Goldberg JD, Chinitz LA, Holmes DS, Bernstein NE, et al. Meta-analysis to assess the appropriate endpoint for slow pathway

ablation of atrioventricular nodal reentrant tachycardia. Pacing Clin Electrophysiol. 2011;34(3):269–77.

13. O'Hara GE, Philippon F, Champagne J, Blier L, Molin F, Cote JM, et al. Catheter ablation for cardiac arrhythmias: a 14-year experience with 5330 consecutive patients at the Quebec Heart Institute, Laval Hospital. Can J Cardiol. 2007;23 Suppl B:67B–70B.

Case 9

9

Matthieu George, Marine Kinnel,
Robert Dallemand, and Gabriel Cismaru

9.1 Case Presentation

A 56-year-old male patient with a long history of undocumented palpitations (several episodes during the past 23 years, with duration of several minutes, with sudden onset and spontaneous termination) presented himself to the Cardiology Department for a detailed cardiology workup and treatment. He had no personal history of known heart disease, no family history of sudden cardiac death. His cardiovascular risk factors were represented by age >55 years and arterial hypertension. His treatment at home consisted of a combination of verapamil 240 mg + trandolapril 2 mg, but despite this, his episodes of palpitations kept recurring.

At physical exam, his blood pressure was 130/76 mmHg, heart rate of 68 bpm, SpO$_2$ 97% breathing room air, heart sounds were regular, there was no audible heart murmur, there were no signs of heart failure, pulmonary auscultation was normal.

His ECG is presented in Fig. 9.1.

M. George (✉)
Biosense Webster, Mulhouse, France

M. Kinnel · R. Dallemand
Cardiology Department, "Emile Muller" Hospital, Mulhouse, France

G. Cismaru
Cardiology Department, Rehabilitation Hospital, Cluj-Napoca, Romania

A transthoracic echocardiography was performed, showing a non-dilated LV, absence of LV hypertrophy, with a preserved EF% of 55% (Fig. 9.2). It also showed mild diastolic dysfunction, a non-dilated left atrium (surface = 17.3 cm^2, antero-posterior diameter in parasternal long axis = 37 mm), absence of significant valve disease, a non-dilated right ventricle, trivial tricuspid regurgitation, absence of pulmonary hypertension, a non-dilated IVC, no pericardial effusion, a non-dilated aorta.

His biological workup showed a Hb level of 14.0 g/dl, leucocytes 7.8 × 10^9/L, platelets 205 × 10^9/L, CRP <3 mg/L, BUN 6.0 mmol/L, creatinine 86 μmol/L, glycemia 6.0 mmol/L, Na+ 138 mmol/L, K+ 4.9 mmol/L, and total proteins 71 g/L.

Given the presence of palpitations, an electrophysiological study was subsequently offered and performed.

9.2 Electrophysiological Study and RF Catheter Ablation Procedure

The electrophysiological study was performed under local anesthesia and conscious sedation. Vascular access was obtained using the modified Seldinger technique, under Doppler ultrasound guidance. A 6F quadripolar steerable catheter (Dynamic Extrem, Microport®) was introduced

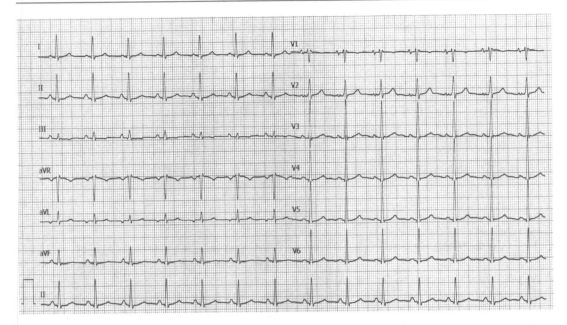

Fig. 9.1 A 12-lead ECG at admittance to the Cardiology Department showing sinus rhythm with a heart rate of 84 bpm, QRS axis at + 40°, absence of LV hypertrophy, absence of ischemia, incomplete RBBB, QTc interval of 437 ms

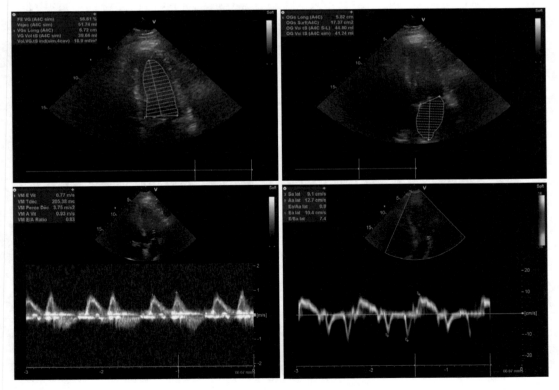

Fig. 9.2 *Left upper panel*: Transthoracic echocardiography image in apical 4 chamber view showing a preserved LV EF% of 56% (Simpson single plane method). *Right upper panel*: Apical 4 chamber view showing a non-dilated LA, with an area of 17.3 cm². *Left lower panel*: Trans-mitral flow interrogation showing the presence of mild diastolic dysfunction (*E/A* < 1). *Right lower panel*: Tissue Doppler image at the lateral level of the mitral annulus demonstrating non-increased LV filling pressure, with a ratio of *E/e'* of 7.4

in a 6F 20 cm vascular sheath and was subsequently advanced via the right common femoral vein up to the bundle of His. Another 6F quadripolar steerable catheter (Dynamic Extrem, Microport®) was introduced in a 6F 20 cm vascular sheath and placed via the right common femoral vein in the coronary sinus, with the distal poles at the level of the lateral mitral annulus. A Biosense Webster® SmartTouch SF open-irrigated 3.5 mm tip with F curve was introduced in a 8F 20 cm vascular sheath and was subsequently advanced via the right common femoral vein up to the right atrium. It was used for the creation of the anatomical maps and the activation maps of

the right and left atrium. Atrial and ventricular pacing were carried out at twice the diastolic threshold using the EP-4™ Cardiac Stimulator (Abbott®) system. Surface ECG and intracavitary ECGs were recorded by the WorkMate Claris™ System (Abbott®).

The CARTO® 3 electro-anatomic mapping System (Biosense Webster, Johnson & Johnson) was used to guide mapping and ablation of the accessory pathway.

The ECG at the beginning of the ablation procedure is presented in Fig. 9.3.

Baseline AH was 102 ms, the HV interval was 37 ms (Fig. 9.4).

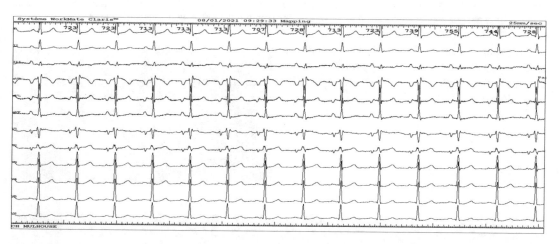

Fig. 9.3 A 12-lead ECG at the beginning of the ablation procedure showing sinus rhythm with a heart rate of 84 bpm, incomplete RBBB

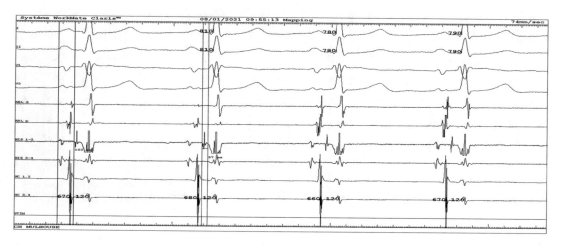

Fig. 9.4 Surface ECG leads I, II, V1, and V3, together with intracavitary leads recorded from the distal and the proximal electrodes of the roving/ablation catheter (Abl d, Abl p), His bundle catheter (His 1–2, His 3–4) and the coronary sinus catheter (SC 1–2 and 3–4), showing normal AH and HV intervals, of 102 ms, and 37 ms

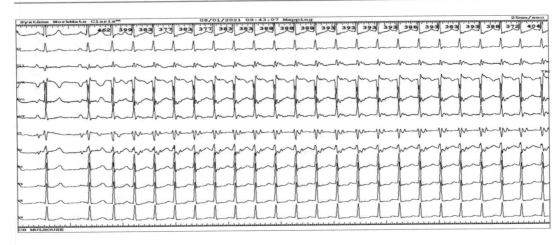

Fig. 9.5 A 12-lead ECG showing the initiation of a narrow QRS complex tachycardia, with a heart rate of 156 bpm, with the QRS morphology being identical to the one in sinus rhythm, reproducing the patient's symptoms

Programmed atrial stimulation initiated the narrow QRS complex tachycardia from Fig. 9.5. The cycle length of the tachycardia was 400 ms.

Question 1: What is the most likely diagnosis of the tachycardia from Fig. 9.5?
A. Typical "slow-fast" AVNRT
B. Atypical "slow-slow" AVNRT
C. Atypical "fast-slow"
D. Atrial tachycardia
E. AVRT

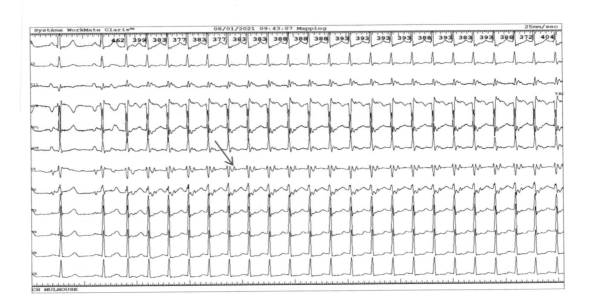

Figure 9.5 **explained**. A 12-lead ECG showing the initiation of a narrow QRS complex tachycardia, with a heart rate of 156 bpm, with the QRS morphology being identical to the one in sinus rhythm. The RP interval is shorter than the PR interval. A P wave can be seen at the end of each QRS complex (1 to 1 P wave to QRS relationship), best visible in lead V1 (red arrow), with a VA interval of more than 80 ms, making the diagnosis of typical AVNRT unlikely. The P waves are positive in lead V1, suggesting a depolarization of the atria coming from the left atrium, in favor of a left accessory pathway or a left atrial tachycardia.

The aspect of the intracavitary electrograms during the narrow QRS complex tachycardia is presented in Figs. 9.6 and 9.7. The earliest atrial activation was recorded by the distal electrodes

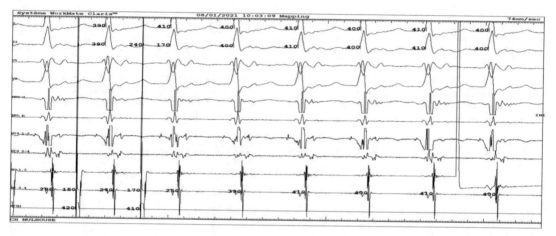

Fig. 9.6 Surface ECG leads I, II, V1, and V3, together with intracavitary leads recorded from the distal and the proximal electrodes of the roving/ablation catheter (Abl d, Abl p), His bundle catheter (His 1–2, His 3–4) and the coronary sinus catheter (SC 1–2 and 3–4), showing the initiation of the tachycardia during programmed atrial stimulation

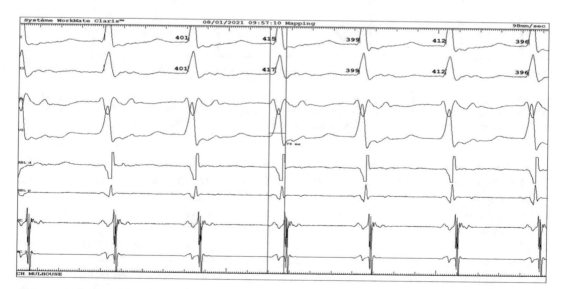

Fig. 9.7 Surface ECG leads I, II, V1, and V3, together with intracavitary leads recorded from the distal and the proximal electrodes of the roving/ablation catheter (Abl d, Abl p), His bundle catheter (His 1–2, His 3–4) and the coronary sinus catheter (SC 1–2 and 3–4), showing the shortest VA interval during tachycardia being recorded at the level of the distal pole of the CS catheter, corresponding to the lateral part of the mitral annulus. The local VA measures 80 ms

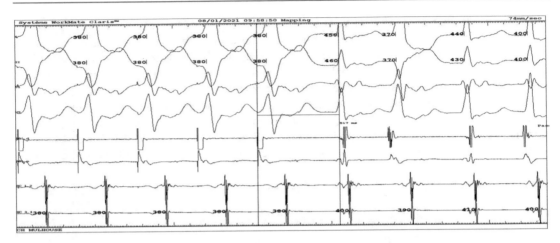

Fig. 9.8 Surface ECG leads I, II, V1, and V3, together with intracavitary leads recorded from the distal and the proximal electrodes of the roving/ablation catheter (Abl d, Abl p), His bundle catheter (His 1–2, His 3–4), and the coronary sinus catheter (SC 1–2 and 3–4), showing the response at the end of RV pacing during tachycardia (the catheter in in the RVOT). This is V-A-V. The PPI – TCL is 517 – 41 ms = 107 ms

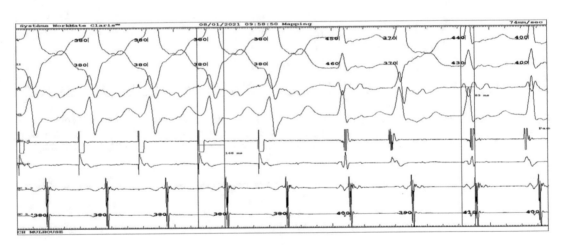

Fig. 9.9 Surface ECG leads I, II, V1, and V3, together with intracavitary leads recorded from the distal and the proximal electrodes of the roving/ablation catheter (Abl d, Abl p), His bundle catheter (His 1–2, His 3–4), and the coronary sinus catheter (SC 1–2 and 3–4), showing SA – VA = 168 – 83 = 85 ms

of the coronary sinus catheter, corresponding to the lateral region of the mitral annulus. The shortest VA interval was also recorded at this level, measuring 80 ms.

The His catheter was advanced at the level of the RVOT, and RV pacing was performed during the tachycardia. The response after the termination of ventricular pacing during tachycardia with a fixed coupling interval of 380 ms is pre-

sented in Fig. 9.8. This was V-A-V. The PPI – TCL was 107 ms. The SA – VA interval was 85 ms (Fig. 9.9).

The termination of the tachycardia is presented in Figs. 9.10 and 9.11.

The tachycardia was initiated once again with a single PVC.

The next step consisted of creation of an anatomical map of the right atrium. This was mildly

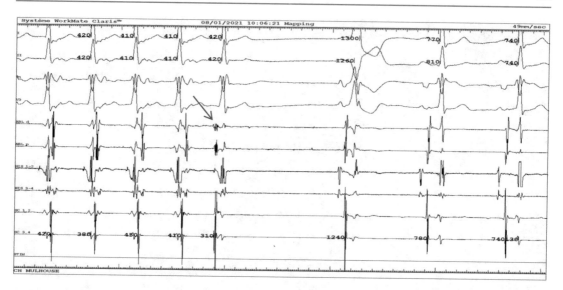

Fig. 9.10 Surface ECG leads I, II, V1, and V3, together with intracavitary leads recorded from the distal and the proximal electrodes of the roving/ablation catheter (Abl d, Abl p), His bundle catheter (His 1–2, His 3–4) and the coronary sinus catheter (SC 1–2 and 3–4), showing the termination of the tachycardia with a premature atrial beat produced by the roving/ablation catheter (red arrow) and resumption of sinus rhythm

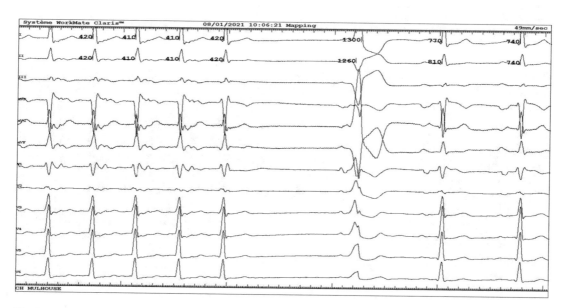

Fig. 9.11 A 12-lead ECG showing termination of an episode of tachycardia (the same as in Fig. 9.10)

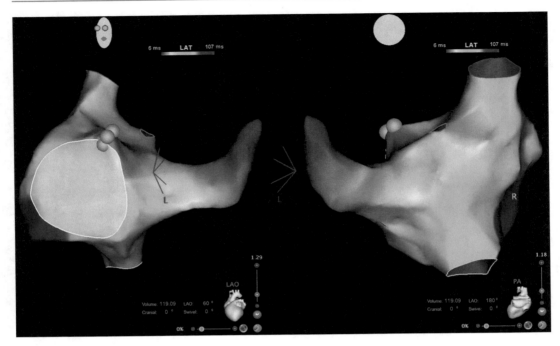

Fig. 9.12 CARTO image in LAO 60° (left panel) and posterior view (right panel) showing the activation map of the right atrium during tachycardia, with the earliest local atrial activation being recorded in the distal part of the coronary sinus (red color). The right atrium is mildly dilated, with a volume of 120 ml

dilated, with a volume of 130 ml. Next, an activation map of the right atrium was created during the tachycardia (Fig. 9.12).

Question 2: What is the most likely diagnosis of the tachycardia?
A. Typical "slow-fast" AVNRT
B. Atypical "slow-slow" AVNRT
C. Atypical "fast-slow"
D. Atrial tachycardia
E. AVRT

Question 3: What is the next best step at this point of the procedure?
A. Ablate inside the coronary sinus in the region of the earliest atrial activation.
B. Perform activation mapping of the left atrium using a retrograde aortic approach.
C. Perform activation mapping of the left atrium using an anterograde transseptal approach.
D. Remap the right atrium.
E. None of the above.

The response at the end of ventricular pacing during tachycardia is V-A-V, which excludes the diagnosis of atrial tachycardia. The PPI – TCL interval of 107 ms and the SA – VA interval of 85 ms are arguments in favor of the presence of an orthodromic AVRT.

Given the ECG aspect of the tachycardia, the diagnostic maneuvers, and the activation map of the right atrium during the tachycardia, the diagnosis was an orthodromic AVRT using a concealed accessory pathway.

Question 4: Where is the accessory pathway situated?
A.   Right antero-septal.
B.   Right postero-septal.
C.   Left postero-septal.
D.   Left antero-lateral.
E.   Right lateral.

Given the atrial depolarization sequence and the activation map of the tachycardia in Fig. 9.12, the location of the accessory pathway is left lateral. Mapping of the left atrium was decided at this point of the procedure using an antegrade approach of the mitral valve.

Access to the mitral valve was therefore obtained using an antegrade approach. A single transseptal puncture was performed under fluoroscopic guidance using an 8.5F 67 cm Swartz SL0™ transseptal sheath (Abbott®) and a BRK ™ XS 71 cm needle (Abbott®).

After the transseptal puncture, anticoagulation was obtained with unfractionated Heparin 70 IU/kg given as bolus, followed by continuous infusion of 12 IU/kg/h, with a target ACT of 300 seconds.

Once the access to the left atrium was granted, the SmartTouch SF roving/ablation catheter was introduced in the SL0 transseptal sheath.

An anatomical map of the left atrium was first created. The left atrium was not dilated, with a volume of 76 ml. Activation mapping of the atrial myocardium around the mitral valve was then performed during orthodromic tachycardia, with

emphasis on the retrograde atrial activation (Figs. 9.13 and 9.14). The earliest local atrial activation was recorded in the lateral region of the annulus, corresponding to the 1'clock position, where the local atrial electrogram preceded the atrial electrogram recorded by the distal poles of the coronary sinus by 30 ms. At this level, the local V and A electrograms were fused (Fig. 9.15).

Target ablation parameters were a power of 30 W, with an ablation index of 450.

Application of RF energy at the site of the earliest local ventricular activation, where the sharp local potential was recorded eliminated the conduction over the accessory pathway (Figs. 9.16 and 9.17).

Figures 9.18 and 9.19 present the activation map of the LA during the tachycardia with superposed RF ablation lesions at the successful ablation site. Figure 9.18 also presents the local signal at the successful ablation site

An activation site of the left atrium was subsequently created. This is presented in Fig. 9.20. Figure 9.21 presents the retrograde conduction properties post-ablation.

There was no complication related to the procedure.

The 12-lead ECG recorded at the end of the catheter ablation procedure is presented in Fig. 9.22.

The 12-lead ECG recorded after the catheter ablation procedure is presented in Fig. 9.23.

The patient was discharged from the hospital 24 h later, on no antiarrhythmic medication.

ANSWERS TO:
Question 1: E. AVRT.
Question 2: E. AVRT.
Question 3: both are correct
B. **Perform activation mapping of the left atrium using a retrograde aortic approach**
C. **Perform activation mapping of the left atrium using an anterograde transseptal approach**
Question 4: D. Left antero-lateral.

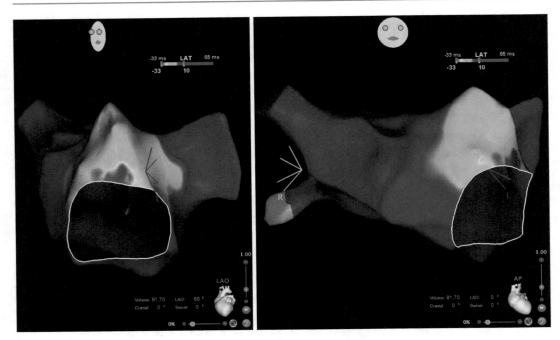

Fig. 9.13 CARTO image in LAO 60° (*left panel*) and antero-posterior view (*right panel*) showing the activation map of the left atrium during tachycardia. The earliest atrial activation sequence is recorded at the level of the antero-lateral part of the mitral annulus, corresponding to the 1 o'clock in the LAO 60° projection (M1). From this point, the depolarization spreads in a radial manner. Of note, the left atrium is not dilated, with a volume of 76 ml

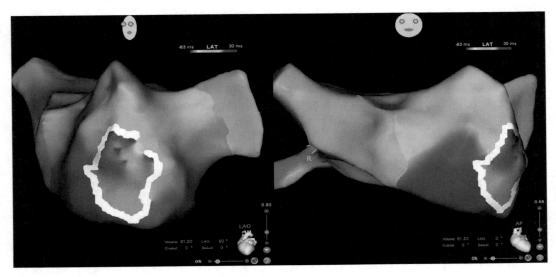

Fig. 9.14 CARTO image in LAO 60° (*left panel*) and antero-posterior view (*right panel*) showing the activation map of the left atrium during tachycardia. This was created by first recording the activation wavefront on the ventricular side of the annulus, around the mitral annulus (red color) and then progressively withdrawing the roving/ablation catheter in the left atrium and recording the activation wavefront around the mitral annulus on its atrial side. The white circular incomplete line represents areas with local VA interval greater than 60 ms. The site corresponding to the 1 o'clock position in LAO 60° (M1) at the level of the mitral annulus represents the site with the shortest VA interval, indicating the location of the accessory pathway. Of note, this site corresponds to the earliest retrograde atrial activation indicated by the activation map from Fig. 9.13

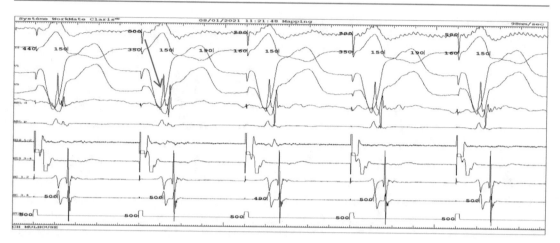

Fig. 9.15 Surface ECG leads I, II, V1, and V3, together with intracavitary leads recorded from the distal and the proximal electrodes of the roving/ablation catheter (Abl d, Abl p), His bundle catheter (His 1–2, His 3–4) and the coronary sinus catheter (SC 1–2 and 3–4), showing the shortest VA interval (red arrow) recorded by the roving/ablation catheter (Abl d) at the level of the earliest atrial activation site, corresponding to the antero-lateral part of the mitral annulus

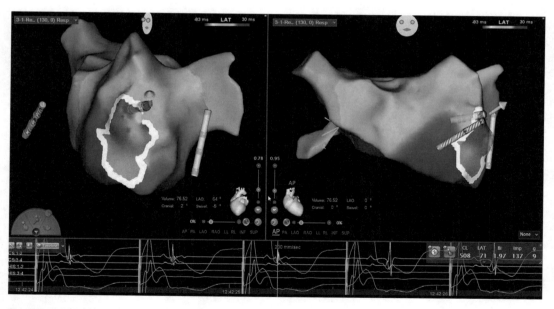

Fig. 9.16 CARTO image in LAO 60° (*left panel*) and antero-posterior view (*right panel*) showing the activation map of the left atrium during tachycardia. The roving/ablation catheter is positioned at the level of the earliest atrial activation site. Application of RF energy at this level promptly interrupted the conduction over the accessory pathway. This can be seen in the lower part of the image, showing the retrograde conduction during RV pacing. After the fourth spike, a sudden increase in the local VA interval can be seen, explained by the sudden change of the retrograde conduction from the accessory pathway to the fast AV nodal pathway

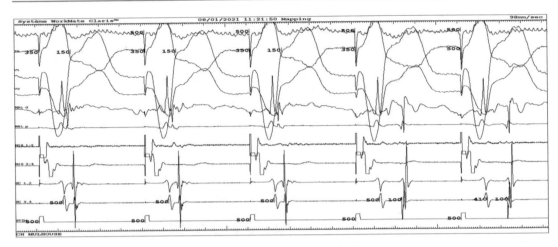

Fig. 9.17 Surface ECG leads I, II, V1, and V3, together with intracavitary leads recorded from the distal and the proximal electrodes of the roving/ablation catheter (Abl d, Abl p), His bundle catheter (His 1–2, His 3–4), and the coronary sinus catheter (SC 1–2 and 3–4), showing the interruption of conduction over the accessory pathway during RF ablation at the level of the antero-lateral part of the mitral annulus and a switch in the retrograde conduction from the accessory pathway to the fast AV nodal pathway

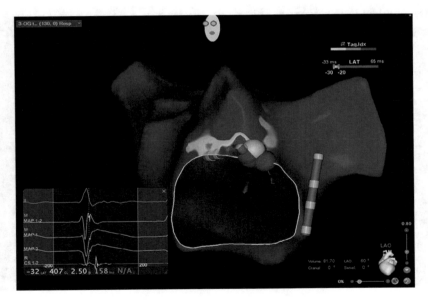

Fig. 9.18 CARTO image in LAO 60° showing the activation map of the left atrium during tachycardia with the earliest retrograde activation sequence situated at the antero-lateral part of the mitral annulus with superposed RF ablation lesions. The local signal recorded by the roving/ablation catheter is presented in the left part of the image (MAP 1–2), together with electrograms recorded by surface lead II and the distal bipolar electrodes of the coronary sinus catheter (CS 1–2)

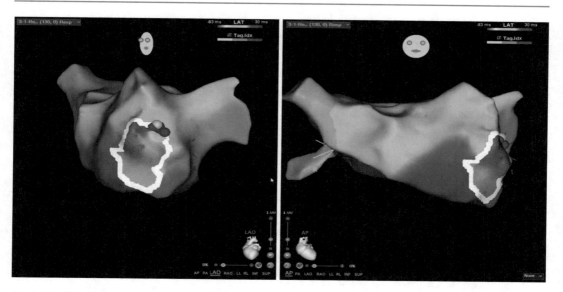

Fig. 9.19 CARTO image in LAO 60° (*left panel*) and antero-posterior view (*right panel*) showing the activation map of the left atrium during tachycardia superposed RF ablation lesions at the level of the accessory pathway

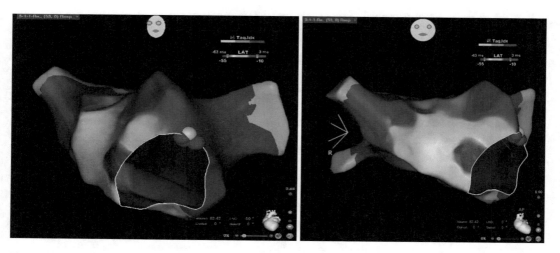

Fig. 9.20 CARTO image in LAO 60° (*left panel*) and antero-posterior view (*right panel*) showing the activation map of the left atrium recorded during RV pacing, after the RF ablation of the accessory pathway, showing a different retrograde atrial depolarization pattern, with the earliest retrograde atrial activation region at the level of the inter-atrial septum. This corresponds to the retrograde activation over the fast AV nodal pathway

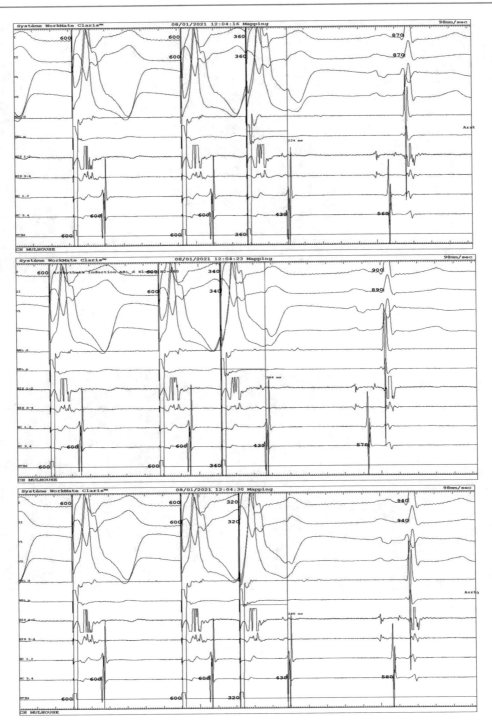

Fig. 9.21 Surface ECG leads I, II, V1, and V3, together with intracavitary leads recorded from the distal and the proximal electrodes of the roving/ablation catheter (Abl d, Abl p), His bundle catheter (His 1–2, His 3–4), and the coronary sinus catheter (SC 1–2 and 3–4), showing the decremental properties of the retrograde conduction after RF ablation of the accessory pathway (progressive increase in the VA interval from 224 ms to 246 ms and to 265 ms by decreasing the coupling interval between the ventricular extra-stimuli from 360 ms to 340 ms to 320 ms). This is an argument confirming the absence of conduction over the accessory pathway

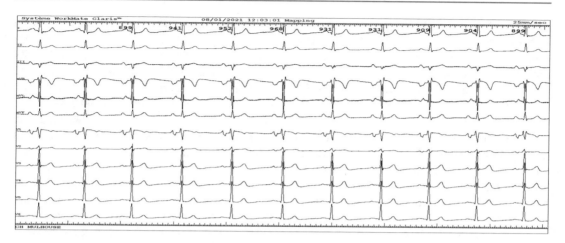

Fig. 9.22 A 12-lead ECG recorded at the end of the ablation procedure, showing sinus rhythm with a heart rate of 67 bpm

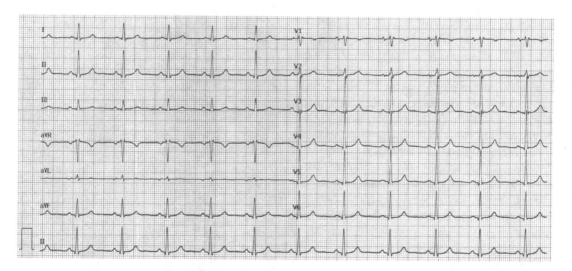

Fig. 9.23 A 12-lead ECG recorded after the ablation procedure, showing sinus rhythm with a heart rate of 68 bpm

9.3 Commentary

The present case illustrates an RF ablation procedure of a concealed antero-left lateral accessory pathway in a patient with symptomatic orthodromic reciprocating tachycardia, using an antegrade (transseptal) approach of the mitral valve. Several observations can be made about the present case.

The interpretation of a 12-lead ECG in a young patient complaining of palpitations suggesting a paroxysmal tachycardia should be done patiently and systematically. One should look for signs of ventricular pre-excitation: short PR interval, the presence of delta waves, which can be very subtle and an enlarged QRS duration; ST segment elevation with a negative T wave in lead V1 in favor of a Brugada type 1 or type 2 pattern should be sought; epsilon waves should be looked for, especially in lead V1, suggesting arrhythmogenic cardiomyopathy; the QT interval should be systematically measured, looking for long or short QT syndrome; and last but not least, signs of ischemia such as pathologic q waves, T wave inversion, ST segment elevation, or ST segment depression.

Orthodromic reciprocating tachycardia is the most common form of arrhythmia in patients with WPW syndrome accounting for more than 90% of arrhythmias [1], followed by pre-excited atrial fibrillation and antidromic tachycardia, the latter occurring in 3–8% of WPW patients [2]. It is the second most common type of SVT in patients without WPW syndrome, after AVNRT. The treatment of choice is catheter ablation of the accessory pathway. For a left lateral accessory pathway, this can be accomplished either by an antegrade (transeptal) approach of the mitral valve or by a retrograde transaortic approach. Both techniques have a similar success rate when magnetically guided ablation is used [3]. Otherwise, the antegrade approach has a slightly higher (but significantly) success rate compared to the transaortic approach: 98% vs. 94%. The retrograde approach is associated with a slightly higher incidence of vascular complications. There is no significant difference in the procedure time and the fluoroscopy time between the 2 approaches. Recurrences after a successful procedure are rare and do not significantly differ between the 2 approaches [4].

Ablation of a concealed accessory pathway can be performed during ventricular pacing or during AV reentry tachycardia. The most common problem associated with ablation of the accessory pathway during tachycardia is catheter movement immediately after the termination of the tachycardia. This is due to a first prolonged diastole after interruption of the tachycardia circuit and a subsequent "vigorous" systole, which determines a slight catheter movement. However, with the use of an electroanatomically mapping system, this problem can be overcome, since

recording of the ablation catheter position at the successful site is done automatically and its repositioning to the successful ablation site is usually not a problem. Another advantage of using an electroanatomically mapping system and an ablation catheter equipped with a contact force sensor electrode for accessory pathway ablation is the possibility to assure a proper contact of the distal electrode of the ablation catheter and the myocardial tissue before RF delivery. Recurrences are associated with a poor contact of the ablation catheter with the myocardial tissue. The orientation of the force vector of the ablation catheter is another important detail in assuring a successful catheter ablation.

> **Learning Point**
> - Orthodromic reciprocating tachycardia is the second most common type of SVT in patients with structurally normal heart.
> - The most common location of a concealed accessory pathway is the left lateral location.
> - Ablation of the accessory pathway can be accomplished either by an anterograde (transseptal) approach of the mitral valve or a retrograde (transaortic) approach.
> - The use of an electroanatomical mapping system is a very valuable tool in guiding the ablation procedure.

References

1. Page RL, Joglar JA, Caldwell MA, et al. 2015 ACC/AHA/HRS Guideline for the Management of Adult Patients With Supraventricular Tachycardia: A Report of the American College of Cardiology/American Heart Association Task Force on Clinical Practice Guidelines and the Heart Rhythm Society. J Am Coll Cardiol. 2016;67:e27–e115.

2. Brugada J, Katritsis DG, Arbelo E, et al. 2019 ESC Guidelines for the management of patients with supraventricular tachycardia. The Task Force for the management of patients with supraventricular tachycardia of the European Society of Cardiology (ESC). Eur Heart J. 2020;41:655–720.

3. Schwagten B, Jordaens L, Rivero-Ayerza M, et al. A randomized comparison of transseptal and transaortic approaches for magnetically guided ablation of left-sided accessory pathways. Pacing Clin Electrophysiol. 2010;33:1298–303.

4. Anselmino M, Matta M, Saglietto A, et al. Transseptal or retrograde approach for transcatheter ablation of left sided accessory pathways: a systematic review and meta-analysis. Int J Cardiol. 2018;272:202–7.

Case 10

Ronan Le Bouar, Frédéric Halbwachs,
Charline Daval, and Serban Schiau

10

10.1 Case Presentation

A 28-year-old male patient with no significant past medical history presents to the Emergency Department for a first episode of palpitations with a sudden onset and irregular rhythm, which had started 30 min prior to his presentation to the hospital. He had no cardiovascular risk factors, apart from overweight. He had no personal history of syncope, no family history of sudden cardiac death. He denied consumption of alcohol of illicit drugs. He was on no chronic medication. At physical exam, his blood pressure was 122/82 mmHg, heart rate of 150 bpm, SpO_2 98% breathing room air, $H = 175$ cm, $W = 85$ kg, BMI $= 27.75$ kg/m^2, heart sounds were rapid and irregular, there was no audible heart murmur, there were no signs of heart failure, pulmonary auscultation was normal. His ECG is presented in Fig. 10.1.

His biological workup showed a Hb level of 14.9 g/dl, leucocytes 8.56×10^9/L, platelets 359×10^9/L, CRP <3 mg/K, BUN 3.4 mmol/L, creatinine 86 μmol/l, glycemia 6.8 mmol/l, Na$^+$ 142 mmol/l, K$^+$ 3.8 mmol/l, total proteins 77 g/l, D-dimers 281 ng/ml, TSH 2.6 IU/L, NT pro-BNP <30 pg/ml.

Transthoracic echocardiography showed a non-dilated LV with a preserved LV EF%, absence of LV hypertrophy, no significant valve disease, non-dilated right ventricle, absence of pericardial fluid.

Given the recent onset of atrial fibrillation, oral metoprolol 50 mg was administered, together with the flecainide 2 mg/kg intravenously. Five minutes after the end of flecainide infusion, the ECG in Fig. 10.2 was recorded. A couple of minutes later, the ECG in Fig. 10.3 was recorded.

The patient was transferred to the Cardiology Department for further diagnostic testing and treatment.

A transthoracic echocardiography was performed in sinus rhythm, showing a LV EF of 63% and a non-dilated left atrium of 15.4 cm^2 (Fig. 10.4).

> **Question 1: What is the tachycardia shown in Fig. 10.2?**
> A. AVNRT
> B. AVRT
> C. Atrial tachycardia
> D. Sinus tachycardia
> E. Fascicular ventricular tachycardia

R. Le Bouar (✉) · C. Daval · S. Schiau
Cardiology Department, "Emile Muller" Hospital,
Mulhouse, France
e-mail: LEBOUARR@ghrmsa.fr

F. Halbwachs
Biosense Webster, Mulhouse, France

© The Author(s), under exclusive license to Springer Nature Switzerland AG 2022
L. Muresan (ed.), *Clinical Cases in Cardiac Electrophysiology: Supraventricular Arrhythmias*,
https://doi.org/10.1007/978-3-031-07357-1_10

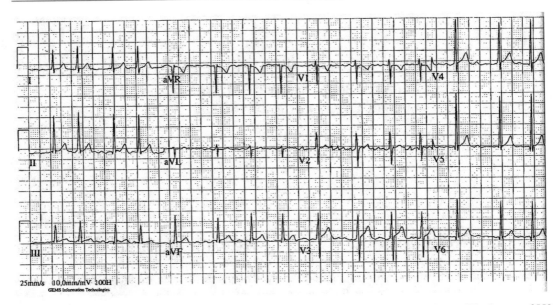

Fig. 10.1 A 12-lead ECG showing atrial fibrillation with a heart rate of 100 bpm, QRS axis at +60°, absence of LV hypertrophy, absence of ischemia

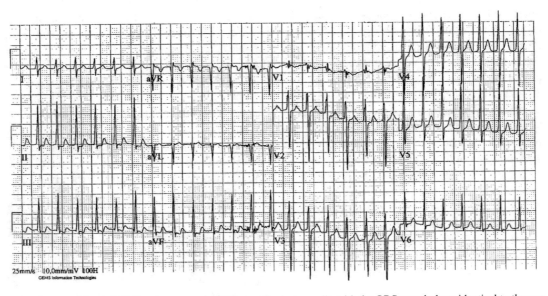

Fig. 10.2 A 12-lead ECG showing a narrow QRS complex tachycardia with the QRS morphology identical to the one in sinus rhythm, with a heart rate of 160 bpm

Figure 10.2 is explained below

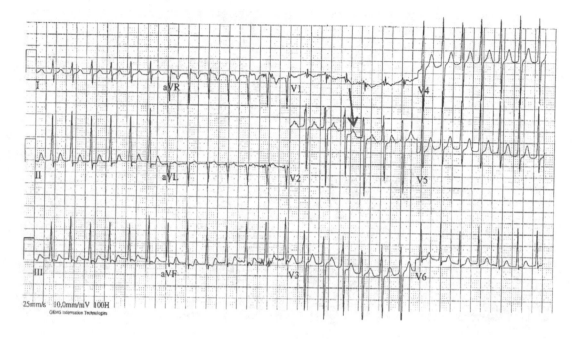

Figure 10.2 **explained.** A **12-**lead ECG showing a narrow QRS complex tachycardia with the QRS morphology identical to the one in sinus rhythm. P waves are visible superposed on the peak of the T waves, with a RP interval >80 ms, but with a PR >RP interval, suggesting a possible AVRT tachycardia using a left-sided accessory pathway

> **Question 2: What would be your ablation strategy in this case?**
> A. Pulmonary veins isolation and AVRT ablation.
> B. AVRT ablation alone.
> C. Pulmonary veins isolation alone.
> D. Antiarrhythmic therapy + anticoagulant depending on his CHA_2DS_2-VASc score.
> E. None of the above.

After obtaining informed consent, an electrophysiological study was offered and accepted by the patient.

10.2   Electrophysiological Study and RF Catheter Ablation Procedure

The electrophysiological study was performed under local anesthesia and conscious sedation. Vascular access was obtained using the modified Seldinger technique, under Doppler ultrasound guidance.

A 6F quadripolar steerable catheter (Dynamic Extrem, Microport®) was introduced in a 9F 20 cm vascular sheath and was subsequently advanced via the right common femoral vein up to the bundle of His. Another 6F decapolar steerable catheter (Inquiry, Abbott®) was introduced in a 7F 20 cm vascular sheath and placed via the

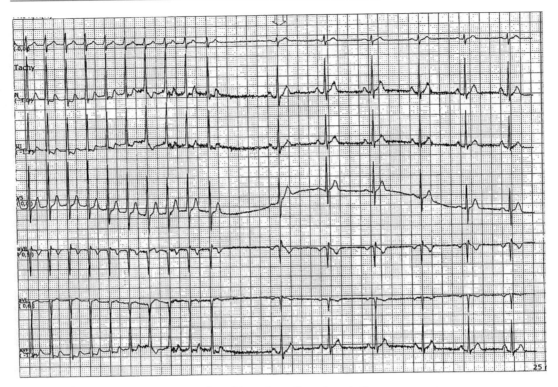

Fig. 10.3 A 7-lead ECG showing conversion of the tachycardia to sinus rhythm

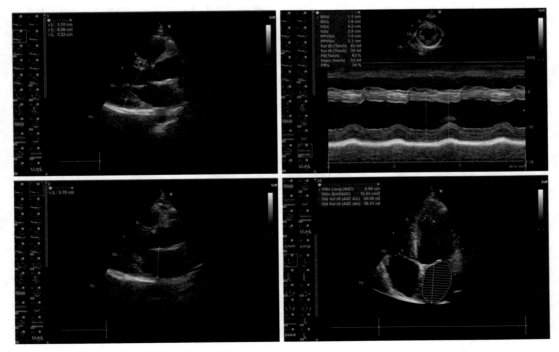

Fig. 10.4 *Left upper panel*: Transthoracic echocardiogra- phy image in parasternal long axis view showing a non- dilated LV, with an end diastolic diameter of 43 mm. *Right upper panel*: M-mode echocardiography image in para- sternal short axis showing a non-dilated LV with preserved systolic function, a LVEF% of 63% (Teicholz method). *Left lower panel*: Parasternal long axis view showing a non-dilated LA, with the AP diameter of 37.5 mm. *Right lower panel*: Apical 4 chamber view showing a non-dilated left atrium, with a surface of 15.44 mm

right common femoral vein in the coronary sinus, with the distal poles at the level of the lateral mitral annulus. A bipolar non-steerable catheter (Viking, Boston Scientific®) was introduced in a 6F 20 cm vascular sheath and was subsequently advanced via the right common femoral vein up to the right ventricular apex.

Atrial and ventricular pacing were carried out at twice the diastolic threshold using the EP-4™ Cardiac Stimulator (Abbott®) system. Surface ECG and intracavitary ECGs were recorded by the WorkMate Claris™ System (Abbott®).

Radiofrequency ablation was delivered using a Biosense Webster® SmartTouch SF open-irrigated 3.5 mm tip with D curve. The CARTO ® 3 electro-anatomic mapping System (Biosense Webster, Johnson & Johnson) was used to guide mapping and ablation of the accessory pathway.

Baseline AH was 78 ms, the HV interval was 41 ms. Anterior Wenckebach point was 240 ms. Retrograde conduction was eccentric, non-decremental.

Programmed atrial stimulation initiated a narrow QRS complex tachycardia, with a cycle length of 250 ms, with an eccentric atrial activation sequence, with the earliest atrial depolarization situated at the level of the mid electrodes of the coronary sinus catheter, corresponding to the posterior/postero-septal region of the mitral annulus (Fig. 10.5).

At the end of ventricular pacing at a fixed coupling interval of 230 ms, the return sequence was V-A-V, excluding an atrial tachycardia. A single ventricular extrastimulus during His refractoriness advanced the tachycardia with 14 ms. PPI at the apex of the right ventricle – TCL = 84 ms. SA – VA during tachycardia was <85 ms, confirming the diagnosis of AVRT using a concealed accessory pathway. Given the fact that the earliest depolarization sequence during tachycardia corresponded to the left postero-septal region, a decision to map the mitral annulus was taken.

Access to the mitral valve was obtained using an antegrade approach, via a PFO. The roving/

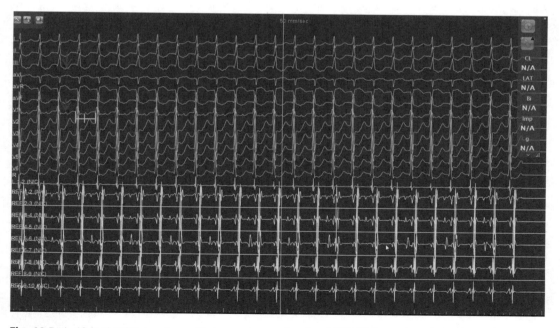

Fig. 10.5 A 12-lead ECG together with intracavitary electrograms recorded by the bipolar electrodes of the decapolar coronary sinus catheter showing a narrow QRS complex tachycardia with RP <PR (green lines under the fourth and fifth QRS complexes in lead V1), with P waves best seen in leads III and V1 (red arrow). The differential diagnosis includes atypical AVNRT, AVRT, and atrial tachycardia. Paper speed at 50 mm/s

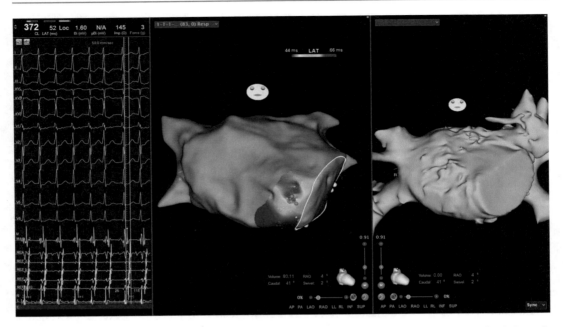

Fig. 10.6 CARTO image in RAO 4° caudal 41° showing in the middle panel the activation map of the left atrium in the peri-mitral region during ORT. The area of the earliest retrograde atrial activation is recorded in the postero-septal region (red area in the *middle panel*), where the shortest VA was recorded. *Left panel*: Surface ECG leads and intracavitary leads recorded from the distal electrode of the roving/ablation catheter (MAP 1–2) and the decapolar diagnostic catheter (REF 1, 2 → 9–10) inserted inside the coronary sinus during ORT. *Right panel*: 3D reconstruction of the CT angiographic image of the left atrium

ablation catheter was positioned inside the left atrium using an 8.5F 67cm Swartz SL0TM™ transseptal sheath (Abbott®).

After placing the roving/ablation catheter in the LA, anticoagulation was obtained with unfractionated heparin 70 IU/kg given as bolus, followed by continuous infusion of 12 IU/kg/h, with a target ACT of 300 s.

An anatomical map of the left atrium was first created. Activation mapping of the atrial myocardium around the mitral valve was then performed during orthodromic tachycardia. The earliest local atrial activation was recorded in the postero-septal region of the annulus, corresponding to the 7'clock position, where the local atrial electro-gram preceded the atrial electrogram recorded by the distal poles of the coronary sinus by 12 ms. At this level, the local V and A electrograms were fused (Figs. 10.6 and 10.7).

Application of RF energy at this level interrupted the conduction over the accessory pathway.

The successful ablation site is presented in Figs. 10.7 and 10.8.

Ventricular pacing after the RF application demonstrated absence of retrograde conduction over the accessory pathway.

There were no complications related to the ablation procedure.

The ECG after the ablation procedure is presented in Fig. 10.9.

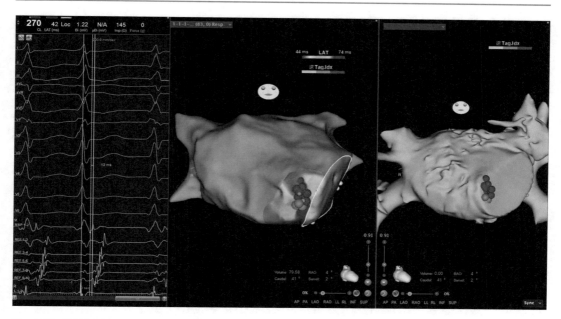

Fig. 10.7 CARTO image in RAO 4° caudal 41° (same as in Fig. 10.4) showing in the *middle panel* the activation map of the left atrium in the peri-mitral region during ORT with superposed RF ablation lesions at the site of earliest retrograde atrial activation. *Left panel*: surface ECG leads and intracavitary leads recorded from the distal electrode of the roving/ablation catheter (MAP 1–2) and the decapolar diagnostic catheter (REF 1, 2 → 9–10)

inserted inside the coronary sinus during ORT showing the earliest retrograde atrial electrogram recorded by the roving/ablation catheter, which precedes the earliest retrograde atrial electrogram from the proximal poles of the coronary sinus catheter by 12 ms. *Right panel*: 3D reconstruction of the CT angiographic image of the left atrium with superposed RF ablation lesions at the site of earliest retrograde atrial activation

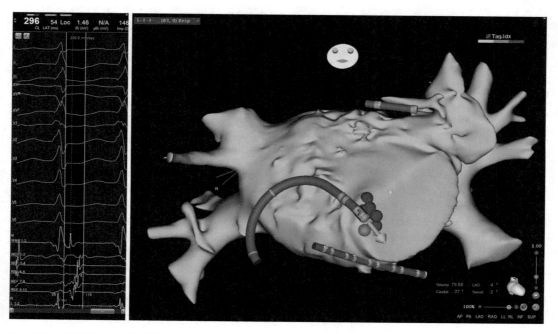

Fig. 10.8 CARTO image in LAO 4° caudal 37° showing the 3D reconstruction of the CT angiographic image of the left atrium with superposed RF ablation lesions and

the roving/ablation catheter at the site of earliest retrograde atrial activation

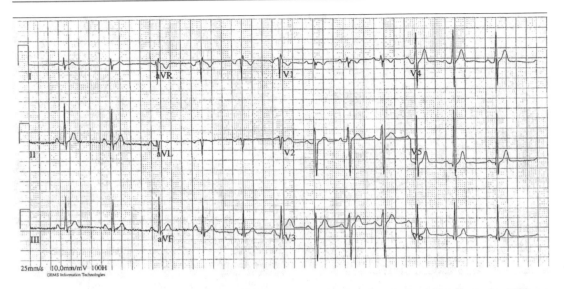

Fig. 10.9 A 12-lead ECG recorded after the RF ablation procedure showing sinus rhythm with a heart rate of 70 bpm, QRS axis at +75°, absence of LV hypertrophy, absence of ischemia, PR interval of 172 ms

The patient was discharged from the hospital 24 h later.

After 1 year of follow-up, the patient remains asymptomatic.

> **ANSWERS TO:**
> **Question 1: B. AVRT**
> **Question 2: AVRT ablation alone.**

10.3   Commentary

The present case illustrates an RF ablation procedure of a concealed left postero-septal accessory pathway using an antegrade approach of the mitral valve in a 28-year-old male patient with symptomatic ORT. Several comments can be made about the present case.

Atrial fibrillation occurs in up to 50% of patients with manifest accessory pathways [1]. It also occurs in patients with concealed accessory pathways, but with a much lower prevalence [2, 3].

A first important observation would be the fact that in young patients with atrial fibrillation, the presence of an underlying condition, such as the presence of a manifest or a concealed accessory pathway should be suspected and ruled out before establishing the need to perform pulmonary vein isolation. If present, such in the above-described case, ablation of the accessory pathway alone should be performed, and no PVI should be done, since PVI in addition to accessory pathway ablation does not reduce the recurrence rate of atrial fibrillation post-ablation [4].

AVNRT can also initiate AF in young individuals. Slow pathway ablation is the only needed treatment in such cases, and pulmonary vein isolation is generally not needed. Potential triggers of AF such as excessive alcohol consumption or illicit drugs should be searched for and if identified, eliminated.

A second observation would be that postero-septal accessory pathways are the second most frequent location of accessory pathways, after the left lateral location [5]. Among postero-septal accessory pathways, left postero-septal are more common than right postero-septal accessory pathways [6]. Ablating left postero-septal pathways can be done using an antegrade transseptal approach of the mitral valve or a retrograde transaortic approach. In the above-presented patient, the presence of a PFO favored the antegrade approach. The success rate of the ablation procedure can reach 98.5% in the hands of experienced operators [7]. Three-dimensional electroanatomic mapping systems can be of great help in mapping and ablating accessory pathways, providing important information concerning catheter stability, force and offering the possibility to reposition the ablation catheter in key sites in case of inadvertent catheter movement [8, 9].

Learning Point

- In young patients with atrial fibrillation, the presence of an accessory pathway should be ruled out before pulmonary vein isolation is offered.
- This may require performing an electrophysiological study before proposing catheter ablation of atrial fibrillation.
- This is very important to keep in mind since catheter ablation of the accessory pathway may eliminate the presence of atrial fibrillation and therefore the need to administer long-term antiarrhythmic treatment or to perform unnecessary pulmonary vein isolation.

References

1. Brugada J, Katritsis DG, Arbelo E, et al. 2019 ESC Guidelines for the management of patients with supraventricular tachycardia The Task Force for the management of patients with supraventricular tachycardia of the European Society of Cardiology (ESC). Eur Heart J. 2020;41:655–720.
2. Ma L, Li Y, Wang Y, et al. Relationship between accessory pathway location and occurrence of atrial fibrillation in patients with atrioventricular re-entrant tachycardia. Exp Clin Cardiol. 2004;9:196–9.
3. Della Bella P, Brugada P, Talajic M, et al. Atrial fibrillation in patients with an accessory pathway: importance of the conduction properties of the accessory pathway. J Am Coll Cardiol. 1991;17:1352–6.
4. Kawabata M, Goya M, Takagi T, et al. The impact of B-type natriuretic peptide levels on the suppression of accompanying atrial fibrillation in Wolff-Parkinson-White syndrome patients after accessory pathway ablation. J Cardiol. 2016;68:485–91.
5. Birati EY, Eldar M, Belhassen B. Gender differences in accessory connections location: an Israeli study. J Interv Cardiac Electrophysiol. 2012;34:227–9.
6. Wen MS, Yeh SJ, Wang CC, et al. Radiofrequency ablation therapy of the posteroseptal accessory pathway. Am Heart J. 1996;132:612–20.
7. Pappone C, Vicedomini G, Manguso F, et al. Wolff-Parkinson-White syndrome in the era of catheter ablation: insights from a registry study of 2169 patients. Circulation. 2014;130:811–9.
8. Worley SJ. Use of a real-time three-dimensional magnetic navigation system for radiofrequency ablation of accessory pathways. Pacing Clin Electrophysiol. 1998;21:1636–45.
9. Kim YH, Chen SA, Ernst S, et al. 2019 APHRS expert consensus statement on three-dimensional mapping systems for tachycardia developed in collaboration with HRS, EHRA, and LAHRS. J Arrhythm. 2020;36:215–70.

Case 11

Frédéric Halbwachs, Maxime Tissier,
Aubrietia Lawson, and Romaric Bouillard

11

11.1 Case Presentation

A 31-year-old male patient with no history of cardiovascular disease collapsed during a tennis match. His tennis partner found no perceptible pulse and started CPR. Five minutes later, paramedics arrived and confirmed cardiorespiratory arrest. They performed orotracheal intubation and connected an automatic external defibrillator, which recorded the trace from Fig. 11.1. This showed ventricular fibrillation, and the patient received 3 external shocks, after which sinus rhythm was restored (Fig. 11.2). The patient was transported to the intensive care unit of the local hospital, where he was rapidly extubated, given his stable vital signs. History taking confirmed the absence of relevant cardiovascular disease. He was on no chronic medication at home.

His only cardiovascular risk factor was represented by overweight. He had no family history of sudden cardiac death. He denied smoking, alcohol consumption, or consumption of illicit drugs.

At physical exam, his blood pressure was 130/75 mmHg, heart rate of 80 bpm, SpO$_2$ 98% breathing room air, H = 192 cm, W = 106 kg, BMI = 28.75 kg/m^2, heart sounds were rapid and regular, there was no audible heart murmur, there were no signs of heart failure, pulmonary auscultation was also normal.

His ECG recorded at admittance to the intensive care unit is presented in Fig. 11.3. Once the condition of the patient stabilized, he was transferred to the Cardiology Department for further tests and treatment.

Transthoracic echocardiography showed a non-dilated LV with a preserved LV EF% of 68%, absence of LV hypertrophy, no significant valve disease, non-dilated right ventricle, absence of pericardial fluid (Figs. 11.4, 11.5, 11.6, 11.7, and 11.8).

His biological workup showed a Hb level of 14.3 g/dl, leucocytes 8.27 × 10^9/L, platelets 237 × 10^9/L, CRP <3 mg/L, BUN 4.5 mmol/L, creatinine 78 μmol/L, glycemia 5.5 mmol/L, Na$^+$ 140 mmol/L, K$^+$ 3.9 mmol/L, total proteins 81 g/L, TSH 2.67 IU/L, NT pro-BNP 253 pg/ml.

F. Halbwachs (✉) · M. Tissier · R. Bouillard
Biosense Webster, Mulhouse, France

A. Lawson
Cardiology Department, "Emile Muller" Hospital,
Mulhouse, France

L. Muresan (ed.), *Clinical Cases in Cardiac Electrophysiology: Supraventricular Arrhythmias*,
https://doi.org/10.1007/978-3-031-07357-1_11

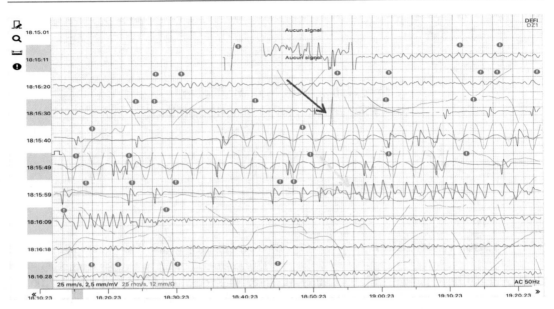

Fig. 11.1 A 1-lead ECG recorded by the automatic external defibrillator showing ventricular fibrillation successfully terminated by external electrical cardioversion (red arrow). Resumption of ventricular activity is subsequently observed, but with degeneration into a rapid and irregular ventricular rhythm, most likely ventricular fibrillation (yellow arrow)

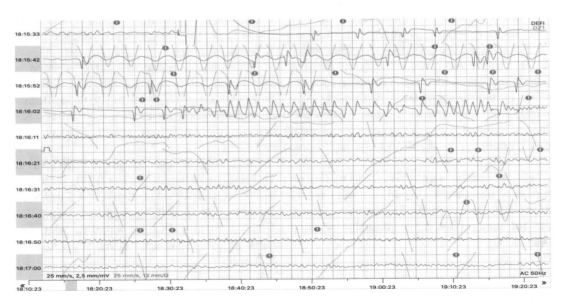

Fig. 11.2 1-lead ECG recorded by the automatic external defibrillator showing in the first part of the tracing the events described in Fig. 11.1, with subsequent ongoing ventricular fibrillation

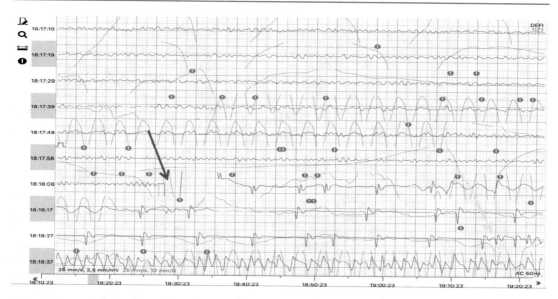

Fig. 11.3 1-lead ECG recorded by the automatic external defibrillator showing successful defibrillation (red arrow) with resumption of ventricular activity with an irregular rhythm. The yellow arrow indicates the initiation of a rapid and irregular ventricular rhythm, most likely ventricular fibrillation

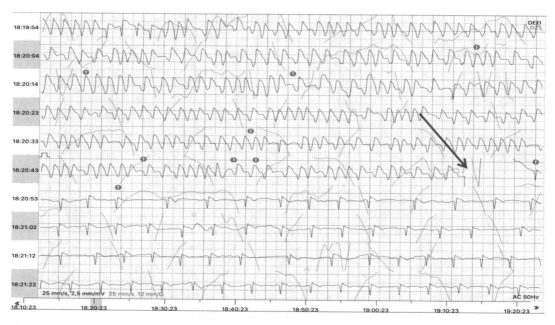

Fig. 11.4 1-lead ECG recorded by the automatic external defibrillator showing successful cardioversion of ventricular fibrillation with resumption of ventricular electrical activity

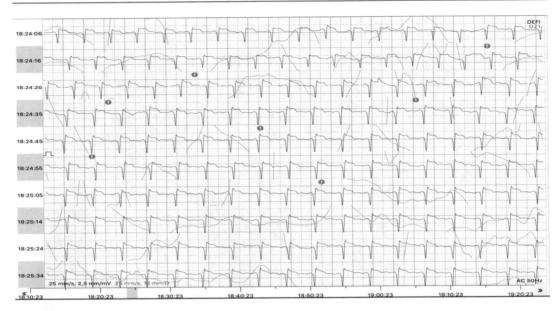

Fig. 11.5 1-lead ECG recorded by the automatic external defibrillator showing stable sinus rhythm post defibrillation

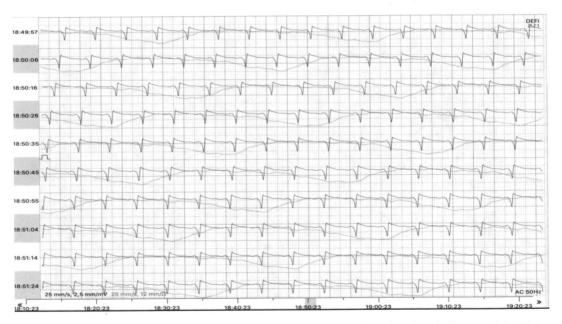

Fig. 11.6 1-lead ECG recorded by the automatic external defibrillator showing stable sinus rhythm post defibrillation

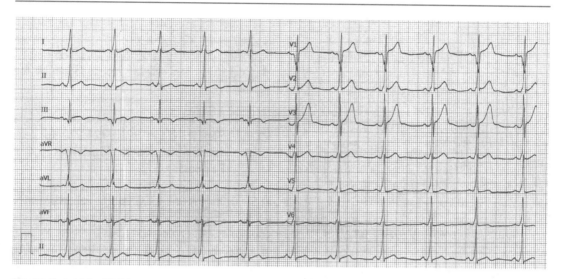

Fig. 11.7 A 12-lead ECG at recorded at admittance to the Cardiology Department

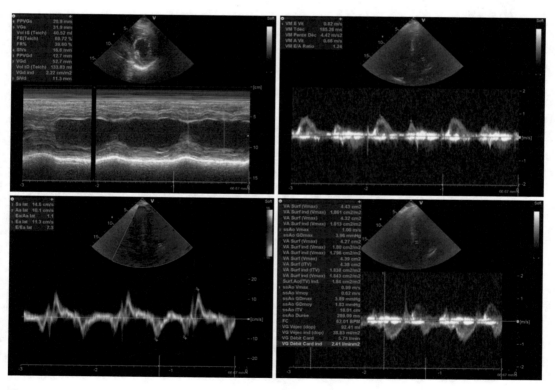

Fig. 11.8 *Left upper panel*: Transthoracic echocardiography image in apical 4 chamber view axis showing a non-dilated LV with preserved systolic function, a LVEF% of 68% (Teicholz method). *Right upper panel*: Pulsed wave Doppler interrogation of the transmitral flow showing normal diastolic function, with E >A wave. *Left lower panel*: Tissue Doppler at the level of the lateral mitral annulus showing normal LV filling pressure, with an E/e' ratio of 7.3. *Right lower panel*: Pulsed wave Doppler interrogation of the LVOT flow showing a preserved cardiac index of 2.41 l/min/m²

Question 1: Are there any clues on the 12-lead ECG in Fig. 11.7 **suggesting a specific diagnosis?**

A. No. This is a normal ECG.

B. Yes. Q waves in lead III, aVF suggesting remote inferior wall myocardial infarction.

C. Yes. Delta waves suggesting ventricular pre-excitation.

D. Yes. Negative T waves in I, aVL, suggesting LV lateral wall ischemia.

E. Yes. Incomplete RBBB suggesting arrhythmogenic cardiomyopathy.

Question 2: Where is the accessory pathway located?

A. Left lateral.

B. Left postero-septal.

C. Right postero-septal.

D. Right antero-lateral.

E. Right mid-septal.

Given the presence of resuscitated sudden cardiac death, the presence of ventricular pre-excitation on the 12-lead ECG, an electrophysiological study was offered and accepted by the patient.

11.2 Electrophysiological Study and RF Catheter Ablation Procedure

The electrophysiological study was performed under local anesthesia and conscious sedation, without any fluoroscopic guidance, with the help of the CARTO ® 3 electro-anatomic mapping System (Biosense Webster, Johnson & Johnson).

The 12-lead ECG recorded at the beginning of the electrophysiological study is presented in Fig. 11.9.

Vascular access was obtained using the modified Seldinger technique, under Doppler ultrasound guidance. A Biosense Webster non-irrigated 4 mm tip Navistar catheter with D curve was introduced in a 9F 20 cm vascular sheath at the level of the right common femoral vein and gently

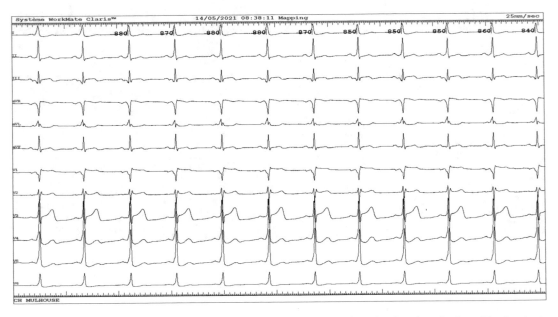

Fig. 11.9 A 12-lead ECG recorded at the beginning of the ablation procedure showing sinus rhythm with a heart rate of 70 bpm, ventricular pre-excitation

advanced at the level of the right common iliac vein, under constant impedance surveillance on the RF generator. The presence of the roving/ablation catheter at the level of the femoral, iliac vein, and IVC generated an impedance between 140 and 170 Ω. The entrance of the catheter in a collateral vein was rapidly accompanied by a rise in the local impedance of up to 350 Ω, and this determined retraction of the catheter in a previous position. The catheter was then gently oriented in a different manner, in such a way that its advancement determined a relatively constant impedance. The CARTO ® 3 electro-anatomic mapping system was used to create an anatomical map of the right common iliac vein and of the IVC, up to the point where the catheter entered the right atrium, and atrial electrograms were recorded by the distal electrode of the roving/ablation catheter. Next, an anatomical map of the right atrium was created during sinus rhythm, with emphasis on the superior vena cava, the coronary sinus, the tricuspid valve, with the identification of the bundle of His

and the coronary sinus ostium. The right atrium was mildly dilated, with a volume of 130 ml.

Measurement of basal conduction intervals is shown in Fig. 11.6. The recorded HV interval is short (<35 ms), confirming ventricular pre-excitation.

The antegrade effective refractory period of the accessory pathway was <270 ms, value which corresponded to the atrial refractory period (Fig. 11.10).

Retrograde conduction was present, concentric, non-decremental (Fig. 11.8), up to a coupling interval of 220 ms, value which represented the ventricular effective refractory period (Fig. 11.11).

Manipulation of the roving/ablation catheter in the right ventricle induced a narrow complex QRS tachycardia, with a cycle length of 340 ms. The initiation and the termination of the tachycardia are presented in Figs. 11.12 and 11.13. The tachycardia terminated spontaneously before any differential diagnosis maneuvers were per-

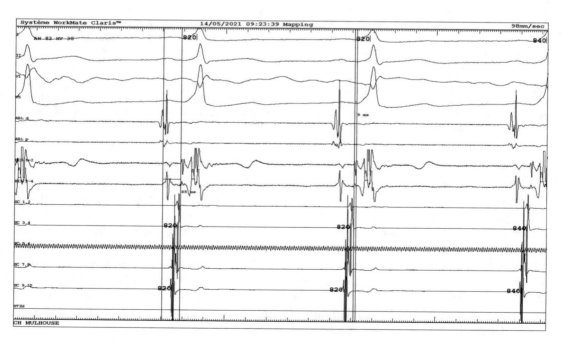

Fig. 11.10 Surface ECG leads I, II and V1, V5 together with intracavitary leads recorded from the distal and the proximal electrodes of the roving/ablation catheter (Abl d, Abl p) and from the coronary sinus catheter (SC 9–10, 7–8, 5–6, 3–4 and 1–2), showing a short HV interval, of 9 ms, confirming ventricular pre-excitation. The AH interval was 85 ms

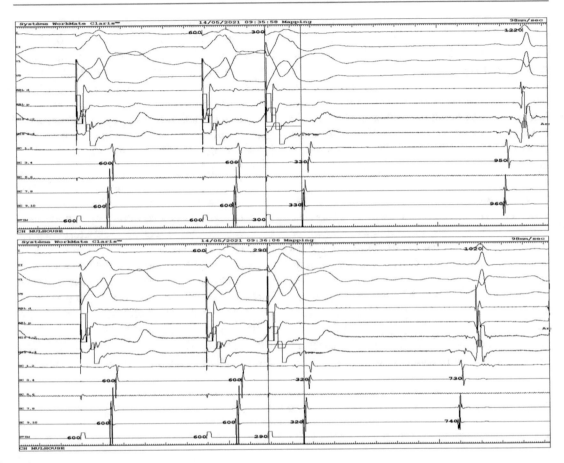

Fig. 11.11 Surface ECG leads I, II and V1, V5 together with intracavitary leads recorded from the distal and the proximal electrodes of the roving/ablation catheter (Abl d, Abl p) and from the coronary sinus catheter (SC 9–10, 7–8, 5–6, 3–4, and 1–2), showing the presence of non-decremental retrograde conduction. The VA interval measures 220 ms for a coupling interval of 300 ms (*upper panel*), the same as for a coupling interval of 290 ms (*lower panel*)

formed. This was likely ORT, but this could not be proved.

Programmed atrial stimulation with up to 3 extrastimuli, at a coupling interval of 600 ms and 400 ms did not induce any sustained arrhythmia. Programmed ventricular stimulation (S1 = 400 ms, S2 = 240 ms, S3 = 220 ms, S4 = 200 ms) induced the wide QRS complex tachycardia from Fig. 11.14, with a 1:1 AV relationship and a cycle length of 240 ms. This tachycardia was highly likely antidromic atrioventricular reentry tachycardia, but this rapidly degenerated into atrial fibrillation (Fig. 11.15), and no differential diagnosis maneuvers could be performed (Fig. 11.16).

The shortest RR interval during pre-excited atrial fibrillation was 180 ms (Fig. 11.17). Together with the effective refractory period of the accessory pathway, this proved its malignant character.

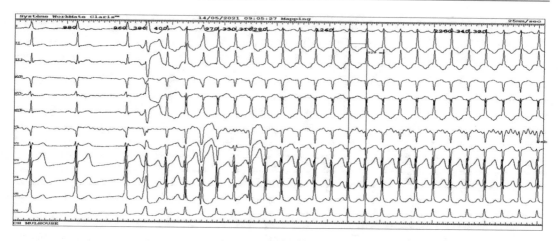

Fig. 11.12 A 12-lead ECG showing initiation of a narrow complex QRS tachycardia with a cycle length of 340 ms

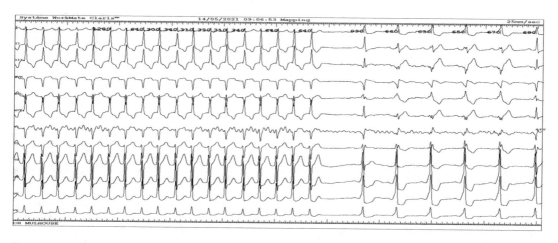

Fig. 11.13 A 12-lead ECG showing the termination of the narrow complex QRS tachycardia and restoration of sinus rhythm

Question 3: What would be your strategy at this point of the procedure?

A. Administer Flecainide 2 mg/kg iv.
B. Administer Amiodarone 300 mg in 10 min.
C. Perform electrical cardioversion.
D. Perform activation mapping of the right basal ventricle and subsequent ablation of the accessory pathway.
E. Wait 30 more minutes for the atrial fibrillation to spontaneously stop.

Administering flecainide at this point of the procedure had the risk of blocking conduction over the accessory pathway, apart from terminating atrial fibrillation. Ablation of the malignant accessory pathway would be compromised. Amiodarone is contraindicated in cases of pre-excited atrial fibrillation since it can precipitate ventricular fibrillation (see the Commentary section). Performing activation mapping during atrial fibrillation had the risk of not precisely identifying the localization of the accessory pathway, and given its likely location based on the 12-lead ECG (mid-septal), performing ablation based on this map seemed too risky.

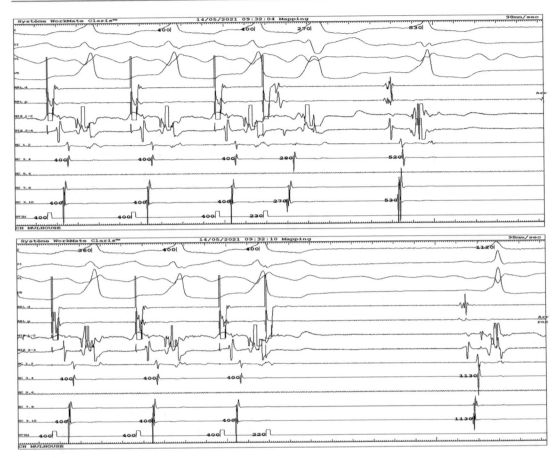

Fig. 11.14 Surface ECG leads I, II and V1, V5 together with intracavitary leads recorded from the distal and the proximal electrodes of the roving/ablation catheter (Abl d, Abl p) and from the coronary sinus catheter (SC 9–10, 7–8, 5–6, 3–4, and 1–2), showing a refractory period of the accessory pathway of less than 220 ms. Note that the extrastimulus delivered at a coupling interval of 220 ms is blocked at the level of the atrium (no atrial electrogram visible after the spike), so the refractory period of the accessory pathway is actually shorter than this value

Waiting 30 more minutes did not seem a good option, since atrial fibrillation might have continued longer than that. Electrical cardioversion was therefore performed (Fig. 11.18), after administering Propofol 1 mg/kg.

Given the malignant character of the accessory pathway and the presence of symptomatic episodes of narrow and wide QRS complex tachycardia (probably ORT and ART) and atrial fibrillation, a decision to ablate the accessory pathway was taken. The aspect during maximal pre-excitation (positive delta waves in leads I, aVL, II, aVF, V2-V6, negative delta waves in leads V1, III) suggested a right mid-septal origin.

Mapping of the tricuspid annulus was performed, using the CARTO system.

An anatomical map of the right atrium was first created. An activation map targeting the earliest local ventricular activation was subsequently created during atrial pacing, in order to obtain maximal pre-excitation, with careful analysis of the local ventricular electrograms recorded around the tricuspid annulus. The earliest local ventricular activation was recorded in the mid-septal region of the annulus, corresponding to the 3'clock position, where the local ventricular electrogram preceded the onset of the surface QRS complex by 16 ms (Figs. 11.19, 11.20, and 11.21). The unipolar electrogram recorded by the distal electrogram of the roving/ablation catheter had a "QS" aspect at this site (Figs. 11.21 and 11.22).

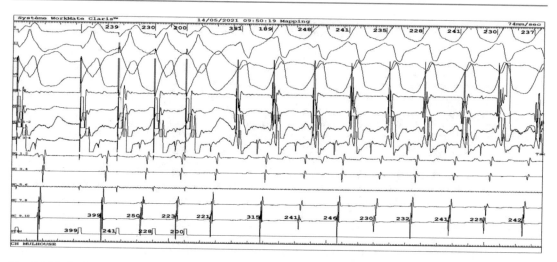

Fig. 11.15 Surface ECG leads I, II, aVF, V1, and V5 together with intracavitary leads recorded from the distal and the proximal bipolar electrodes of the roving/ablation catheter (ABL 1–2, ABL 3–4), from the distal and the proximal bipolar electrodes of the His catheter (His 1–2, His 3–4) and of the coronary sinus catheter (SC 1–2 to S-C 9–10) showing the initiation of a wide QRS complex tachycardia, corresponding to antidromic AV reentry

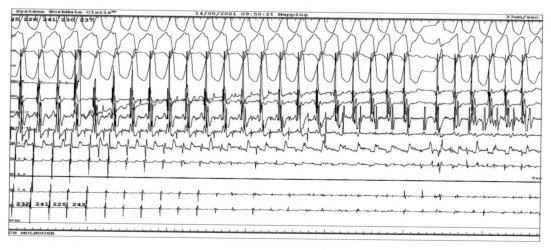

Fig. 11.16 Surface ECG leads I, II, aVF, V1, and V5 together with intracavitary leads recorded from the distal and the proximal bipolar electrodes of the roving/ablation catheter (ABL 1–2, ABL 3–4), from the distal and the proximal bipolar electrodes of the His catheter (His 1–2, His 3–4) and of the coronary sinus catheter (SC 1–2 to S-C 9–10) showing antidromic tachycardia degenerating into atrial fibrillation

Question 4: Is this a good ablation site?

A. Yes. The bipolar EGM precedes the surface ECG by 16 ms.

B. Yes. The unipolar EGM shows a "QS" aspect.

C. Yes. The local AV is short.

D. No. The surface ECG suggests a left postero-septal origin.

E. No. The local bipolar EGM is not the earliest local EGM that can be recorded in this patient.

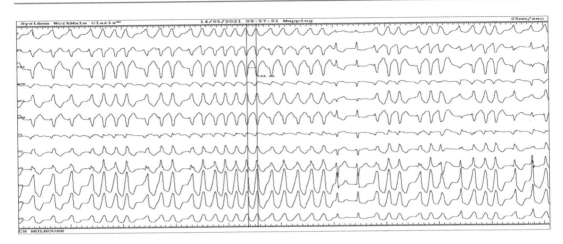

Fig. 11.17 A 12-lead ECG leads showing pre-excited atrial fibrillation with the shortest RR interval oF 186 ms, confirming the malignant character of the accessory pathway

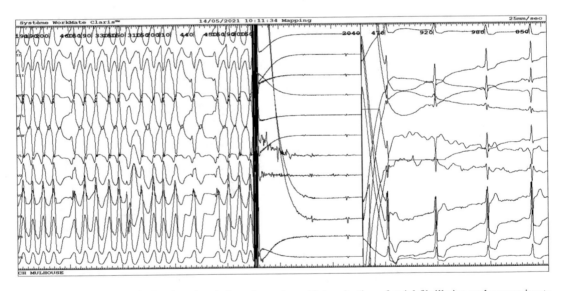

Fig. 11.18 A 12-lead ECG showing electrical cardioversion with termination of atrial fibrillation and conversion to sinus rhythm

Application of RF energy at this level interrupted the conduction over the accessory pathway 5 seconds after the initiation of RF delivery (Figs. 11.23, 11.24, and 11.25), with no recurrence of conduction over the accessory pathway. This was carried out during atrial stimulation from the CS electrodes, in order to increase the degree of pre-excitation. Target ablation parameters were a power of 30 W, with energy titration starting from 15 W.

The distance between the successful ablation site and the bundle of His was 11 mm (Fig. 11.26).

Programmed ventricular stimulation demonstrated the presence of decremental concentric retrograde conduction, compatible with conduction over the AV node (Fig. 11.27).

The AH and HV interval post ablation are presented in Fig. 11.28.

Programmed atrial stimulation before and after isoprenaline administration was negative.

Fig. 11.19 CARTO image in AP view showing the activation map of the left atrium during coronary sinus pacing. The area of the earliest antegrade ventricular activation is recorded in the mid-septal region of the tricuspid valve (red area), where the shortest AV was recorded

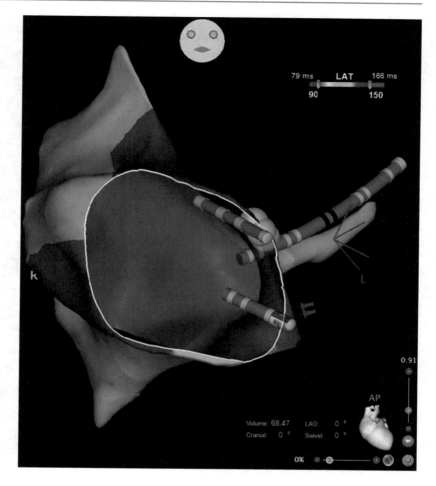

The antegrade effective refractory period of the AV node was 290 ms (Fig. 11.29).

The ECG at the end of the ablation procedure is shown in Fig. 11.30.

The ECG recorded 24 h after the ablation procedure is shown in Fig. 11.31.

The patient was discharged from the hospital 24 h later.

ANSWERS TO:
Question 1: C. Yes. Delta waves suggesting ventricular pre-excitation.
Question 2:
A. **Yes. The bipolar EGM precedes the surface ECG by 15 ms.**
B. **Yes. The unipolar EGM shows a "QS" aspect.**
C. **Yes. The local AV is short.**

Question 3: C. Perform electrical cardioversion
Question 4:
A. **Yes. The bipolar EGM precedes the surface ECG by 16 ms.**
B. **Yes. The unipolar EGM shows a "QS" aspect.**
C. **Yes. The local AV is short.**

11.3   Commentary

The present case illustrates a RF catheter ablation procedure of a malignant accessory pathway in a 31-year-old male patient with resuscitated sudden cardiac death, highly likely due to pre-excited rapid atrial fibrillation degenerating into ventric-

Fig. 11.20 CARTO image in LL view showing the activation map of the left atrium during coronary sinus pacing. The area of the earliest antegrade ventricular activation is recorded in the mid-septal region of the tricuspid valve (red area), where the shortest AV was recorded

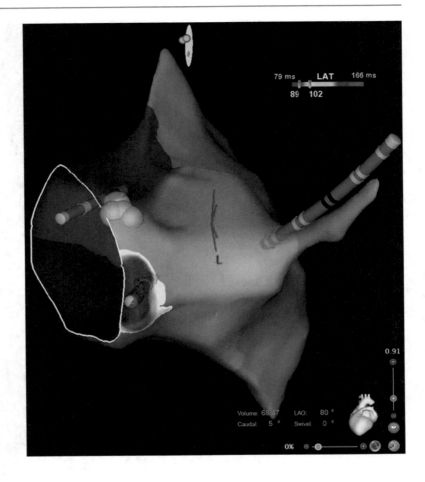

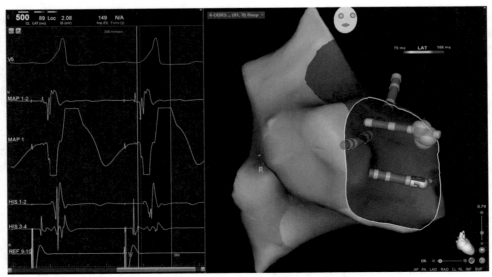

Fig. 11.21 CARTO image in RAO view showing the activation map of the left atrium during coronary sinus pacing. The area of the earliest antegrade ventricular acti-vation is recorded in the mid-septal region of the tricuspid valve (red area), where the shortest AV was recorded

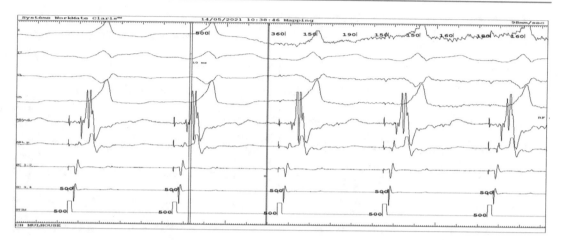

Fig. 11.22 Surface ECG leads I, II and V1, V5 together with intracavitary leads recorded from the distal and the proximal electrodes of the roving/ablation catheter (Abl d, Abl p) and from the coronary sinus catheter (SC 1–2 and 3–4), showing the earliest local ventricular electrogram, recorded in the mid-septal region of the tricuspid valve, preceding the onset of the QRS complex on the surface ECG by 16 ms. Note that at this site, the A and V electrograms recorded by the ablation catheter are fused

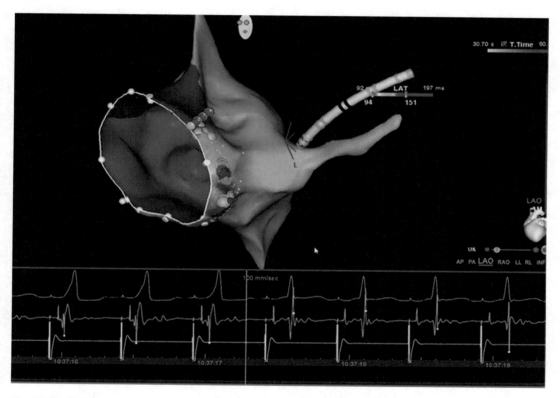

Fig. 11.23 CARTO image in LAO 60° showing the activation map of the right atrium during coronary sinus pacing. The area of the earliest antegrade ventricular activation is recorded in the antero-lateral region of the tricuspid annulus (red area), where the shortest AV was recorded. Red and pink dots represent ablation lesions. The bottom part of the image: surface ECG lead II with intracavitary leads recorded from the distal pole of the ablation catheter (MAP 1–2) and from the proximal pole of the coronary sinus catheter (REF 9, 10) during the successful RF application at the site of the earliest antegrade ventricular activation with rapid interruption of the antegrade conduction at the level of the accessory pathway (first QRS complex after the vertical red line)

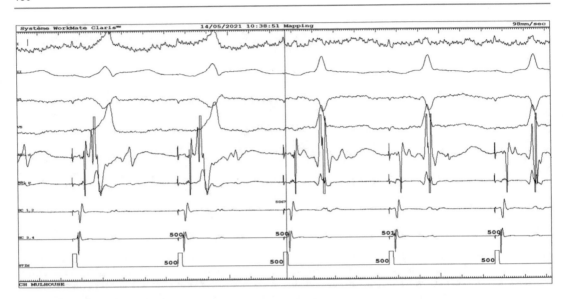

Fig. 11.24 A 12-lead ECG showing disappearance of conduction over the accessory pathway during RF application (red arrow)

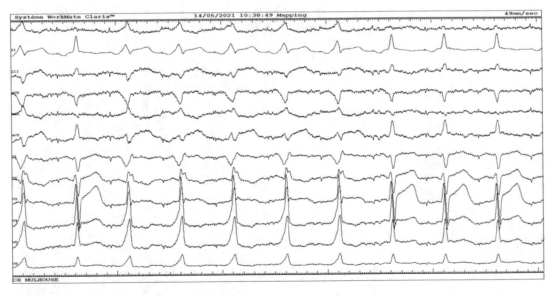

Fig. 11.25 A 12-lead ECG showing disappearance of conduction over the accessory pathway during RF application (red arrow)

ular fibrillation. Several aspects related to this case merit discussion.

Sudden cardiac death can be the first clinical manifestation of WPW syndrome. It is generally due to rapid pre-excited atrial fibrillation degenerating into ventricular fibrillation. Atrial fibrillation occurs in up to 50% of patients with

WPW syndrome [1]. In the acute setting, electrical cardioversion is the treatment of choice for pre-excited atrial fibrillation, especially when the patient is hemodynamically unstable. Intravenous flecainide is an alternative. Amiodarone is considered contraindicated in cases of pre-excited atrial fibrillation, since it

Fig. 11.26 CARTO image in LAO 60° showing the activation map of the right atrium during coronary sinus pacing. The area of the earliest antegrade ventricular activation is recorded in the antero-lateral region of the tricuspid annulus (red area), where the shortest AV was recorded. Red and pink dots represent ablation lesions. The distance between the successful ablation site and the bundle of His was 11.7 mm

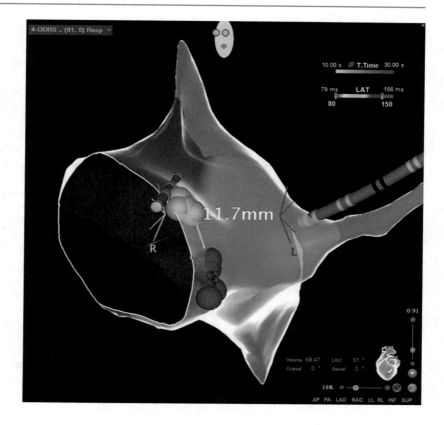

can precipitate ventricular fibrillation [2, 3]. Outside of an acute setting, the definitive treatment for atrial fibrillation in patients with WPW is catheter ablation of the accessory pathway. Interestingly, pulmonary vein isolation in addition to accessory pathway ablation is not recommended since it is not associated with a reduced AF recurrence after catheter ablation [4].

Malignant accessory pathways are characterized by a short antegrade refractory period (of less than 250 ms) and a short RR interval during pre-excited atrial fibrillation (less than 200 ms) [5–8]. The best marker of malignancy is considered the shortest pre-excited RR interval during atrial fibrillation since marked variations in the effective refractory period of the accessory pathway can exist in the same patient [9].

In the experience of Tai et al. [10], mid-septal accessory pathway can be differentiated from antero-septal and parahisian accessory pathway by taking into account several observations: (1)

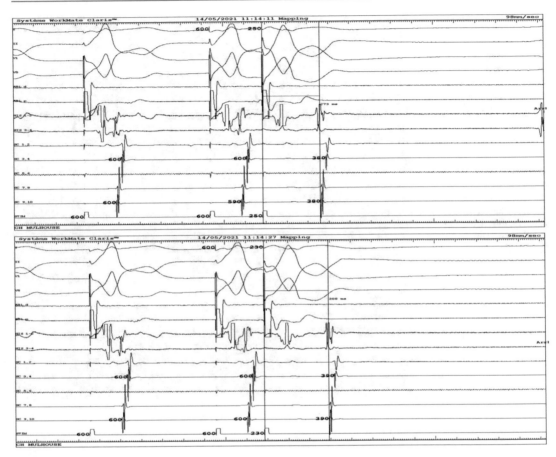

Fig. 11.27 Surface ECG leads I, II and V1, V5 together with intracavitary leads recorded from the distal and the proximal electrodes of the roving/ablation catheter (Abl d, Abl p) and from the coronary sinus catheter (SC 9–10, 7–8, 5–6, 3–4 and 1–2), showing the presence of decremental retrograde conduction, compatible with conduction over the AV node. This is different from the non-decremental conduction recorded before the ablation of the accessory pathway, which was in favor of retrograde conduction over the accessory pathway. The VA interval measures 273 ms for a coupling interval of 250 ms (*upper panel*), compared to 308 ms for a coupling interval of 230 ms (*lower panel*)

during sinus rhythm, mid-septal accessory pathway is characterized by a negative delta wave in lead III and a biphasic delta wave in lead aVF; during ORT, by a negative retrograde P wave in two inferior leads; (2) mid-septal accessory pathways have better antegrade conduction properties and a significantly higher incidence of inducible atrial fibrillation(61.5%); (3) radiofrequency catheter ablation using lower energy (20 ± 6 W) has a comparable effect to ablation using higher energy (36 ± 5 W), but without impairment of atrioventricular node conduction or development of AV block.

Another aspect worth mentioning is that this catheter ablation procedure was performed without the use of fluoroscopy. Zero-fluoroscopy catheter ablation procedures have become feasible for several types of arrhythmias and are more and more widespread [11–15]. This is usually accomplished with the use of a non-fluoroscopic three-dimensional mapping system, such as the CARTO system.

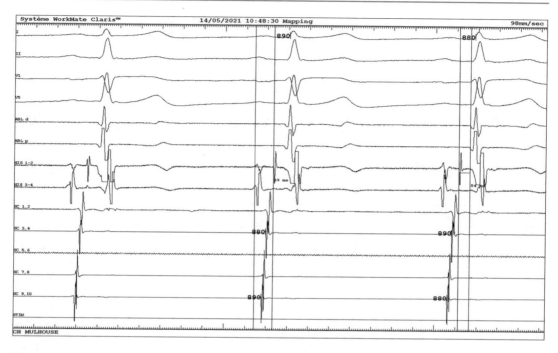

Fig. 11.28 Surface ECG leads I, II and V1, V5 together with intracavitary leads recorded from the distal and the proximal electrodes of the roving/ablation catheter (Abl d, Abl p) and from the coronary sinus catheter (SC 9–10, 7–8, 5–6, 3–4, and 1–2), showing a normal HV interval, of 54 ms, confirming ventricular pre-excitation. The AH interval was 89 ms

Learning Point
- Sudden cardiac death can be the first clinical manifestation of WPW syndrome. It is generally due to rapid pre-excited atrial fibrillation degenerating into ventricular fibrillation.
- In the acute setting, electrical cardioversion is the treatment of choice for pre-excited atrial fibrillation, especially when the patient is hemodynamically unstable. Intravenous flecainide is an alternative. Amiodarone is contraindicated in this setting since it can precipitate ventricular fibrillation.

- Malignant accessory pathways are characterized by a short antegrade refractory period (of less than 250 ms) and a short RR interval during pre-excited atrial fibrillation (less than 200 ms).
- Catheter ablation of the accessory pathway is the treatment of choice, especially for malignant accessory pathways.
- A three-dimensional electro-anatomical mapping system is very helpful in reducing the fluoroscopy time and dose throughout the procedure and accurately identifies its location.

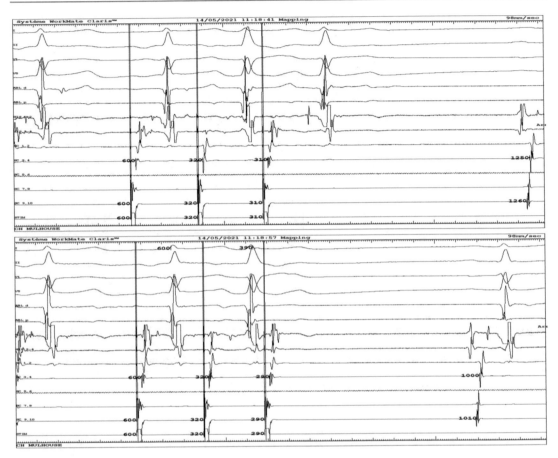

Fig. 11.29 Surface ECG leads I, II and V1, V5 together with intracavitary leads recorded from the distal and the proximal electrodes of the roving/ablation catheter (Abl d, Abl p), from the distal and the proximal electrodes of the His catheter (His 1–2 and His 3–4) and from the coronary sinus catheter (SC 9–10, 7–8, 5–6, 3–4 and 1–2), showing the antegrade effective refractory period of the AV node of 290 ms. Of note, there is no antegrade conduction over an accessory pathway (normal HV interval and absence of pre-excitation aspect on the surface ECG)

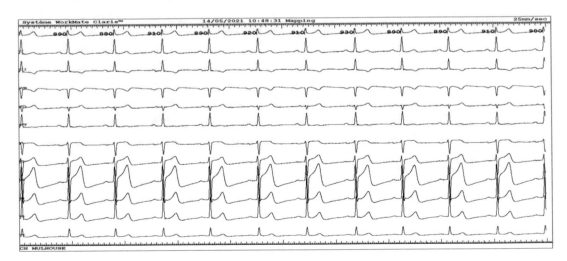

Fig. 11.30 A 12-lead ECG recorded at the end of the ablation procedure, showing sinus rhythm and absence of ventricular pre-excitation

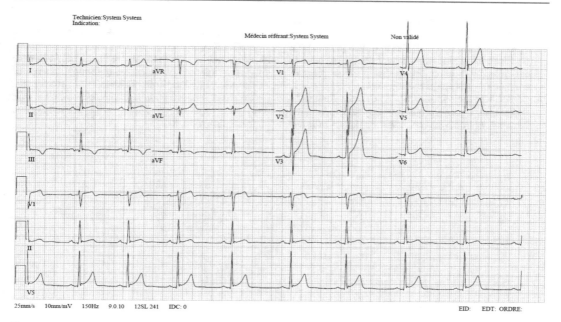

Fig. 11.31 A 12-lead ECG recorded 24 h after the ablation procedure, showing sinus rhythm with a heart rate of 75 bpm, QRS axis at +60° and absence of ventricular pre-excitation

References

1. Brugada J, Katritsis DG, Arbelo E, Arribas F, Bax JJ, Blomstrom-Lundqvist C, et al. 2019 ESC Guidelines for the management of patients with supraventricular tachycardiaThe Task Force for the management of patients with supraventricular tachycardia of the European Society of Cardiology (ESC). Eur Heart J. 2020;41(5):655–720.

2. Ren J, Yang Y, Zhu J, Wu S, Wang J, Zhang H, et al. The use of intravenous amiodarone in patients with atrial fibrillation and Wolff-Parkinson-White syndrome. Pacing Clin Electrophysiol. 2021;44(1):35–43.

3. Tijunelis MA, Herbert ME. Myth: Intravenous amiodarone is safe in patients with atrial fibrillation and Wolff-Parkinson-White syndrome in the emergency department. CJEM. 2005;7(4):262–5.

4. Kawabata M, Goya M, Takagi T, Yamashita S, Iwai S, Suzuki M, et al. The impact of B-type natriuretic peptide levels on the suppression of accompanying atrial fibrillation in Wolff-Parkinson-White syndrome patients after accessory pathway ablation. J Cardiol. 2016;68(6):485–91.

5. Pappone C, Vicedomini G, Manguso F, Baldi M, Pappone A, Petretta A, et al. Risk of malignant arrhythmias in initially symptomatic patients with Wolff-Parkinson-White syndrome: results of a pro-spective long-term electrophysiological follow-up study. Circulation. 2012;125(5):661–8.

6. Rao AL, Salerno JC, Asif IM, Drezner JA. Evaluation and management of wolff-Parkinson-white in athletes. Sports Health. 2014;6(4):326–32.

7. Valaparambil AK. Variability of accessory pathway refractory periods: what should be the criteria for ablation in asymptomatic wpw. Indian Pacing Electrophysiol J. 2012;12(3):79–81.

8. Kubus P, Vit P, Gebauer RA, Materna O, Janousek J. Electrophysiologic profile and results of invasive risk stratification in asymptomatic children and adolescents with the Wolff-Parkinson-White electrocardiographic pattern. Circ Arrhythm Electrophysiol. 2014;7(2):218–23.

9. Oliver C, Brembilla-Perrot B. Is the measurement of accessory pathway refractory period reproducible? Indian Pacing Electrophysiol J. 2012;12(3):93–101.

10. Tai CT, Chen SA, Chiang CE, Lee SH, Chang MS. Electrocardiographic and electrophysiologic characteristics of anteroseptal, midseptal, and para-hisian accessory pathways. Implication for radiofrequency catheter ablation. Chest. 1996;109(3):730–40.

11. Plank F, Stowasser B, Till D, Schgor W, Dichtl W, Hintringer F, et al. Reduction of fluoroscopy dose for cardiac electrophysiology procedures: A feasibility and safety study. Eur J Radiol. 2019;110:105–11.

12. Proietti R, Abadir S, Bernier ML, Essebag V. Ablation of an atriofascicular accessory path-

way with a zero-fluoroscopy procedure. J Arrhythm. 2015;31(5):323–5.

13. Prolic Kalinsek T, Jan M, Rupar K, Razen L, Antolic B, Zizek D. Zero-fluoroscopy catheter ablation of concealed left accessory pathway in a pregnant woman. Europace. 2017;19(8):1384.

14. Ramos-Maqueda J, Alvarez M, Cabrera-Ramos M, Perin F, Rodriguez-Vazquez Del Rey MDM, Jimenez-Jaimez J, et al. Results of catheter ablation with zero or near zero fluoroscopy in pediatric patients with supraventricular tachyarrhythmias. Rev Esp Cardiol. 2021;75(2):166–73.

15. Scaglione M, Ebrille E, Caponi D, Siboldi A, Bertero G, Di Donna P, et al. Zero-fluoroscopy ablation of accessory pathways in children and adolescents: CARTO3 electroanatomic mapping combined with rf and cryoenergy. Pacing Clin Electrophysiol. 2015;38(6):675–81.

Case 12

Ronan Le Bouar, Matthieu George, Crina Muresan,
and Emmanuelle Gain

12

12.1 Case Presentation

A 58-year-old male patient with a history of undocumented palpitations (3 episodes during the past 5 years, with duration of several minutes, with sudden onset and spontaneous termination) presents himself to the Cardiology Department for a detailed cardiology workup and treatment. He had no personal history of known heart disease, no family history of sudden cardiac death. His cardiovascular risk factors were represented by smoking (40 packs-year) and age >55 years old. He was on no chronic medication.

At physical exam, his blood pressure was 130/76 mmHg, heart rate of 68 bpm, $SpO_2 = 97\%$ breathing room air, heart sounds were regular, there was no audible heart murmur, there were no signs of heart failure, pulmonary auscultation was normal.

His ECG is presented in Fig. 12.1.

A transthoracic echocardiography was performed, showing a non-dilated LV, absence of LV hypertrophy, with a preserved EF% of 55% (Fig. 12.2). It also showed normal diastolic function, a non-dilated left atrium (surface of 15 cm^2, antero-posterior diameter in parasternal long axis of 30 mm), absence of significant valve disease, a non-dilated right ventricle, trivial tricuspid regurgitation, absence of pulmonary hypertension, a non-dilated IVC, no pericardial effusion, a non-dilated aorta.

His biological workup showed a Hb level of 14.0 g/dl, leucocytes $7.8 \times 10^9/L$, platelets $205 \times 10^9/L$, CRP <3 mg/L, BUN 6.0 mmol/L, creatinine 86 μmol/L, glycemia 6.0 mmol/L, Na+ 138 mmol/L, K+ 4.9 mmol/L, total proteins 71 g/L.

Question 1: Are there any clues on the 12-lead ECG suggesting a specific diagnosis?

A. No. This is a normal ECG.

B. Yes. Epsilon wave in V1 in favor of arrhythmogenic cardiomyopathy.

C. Yes. The incomplete right bundle branch block in V1 suggests type 2 Brugada Syndrome.

D. Yes. Short QT interval, in favor of Short QT Syndrome.

E. Yes. Ventricular pre-excitation.

Figure 12.1 shows sinus rhythm with a heart rate of 72 bpm, QRS axis at +60°, possible LV hypertrophy (R wave of 26 mV in V4), incomplete RBBB, short PR of 120 ms, positive delta wave in V3-V6 and in leads II, III, aVF, absence of q waves in V5, V6 (explanation below), in favor of ventricular pre-excitation

R. Le Bouar (✉) · C. Muresan
Cardiology Department, "Emile Muller" Hospital,
Mulhouse, France
e-mail: LEBOUARR@ghrmsa.fr

M. George · E. Gain
Biosense Webster, Mulhouse, France

© The Author(s), under exclusive license to Springer Nature Switzerland AG 2022
L. Muresan (ed.), *Clinical Cases in Cardiac Electrophysiology: Supraventricular Arrhythmias*,
https://doi.org/10.1007/978-3-031-07357-1_12

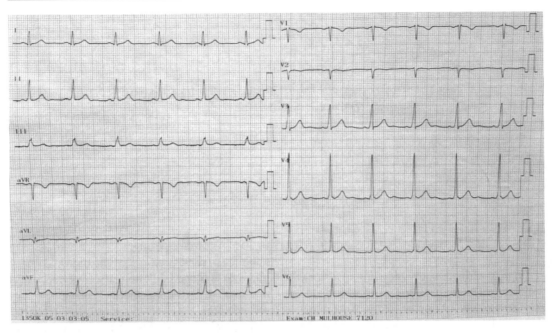

Fig. 12.1 A 12-lead ECG showing sinus rhythm with a heart rate of 72 bpm, QRS axis at +60°, possible LV hypertrophy (R wave of 26 mV in V4), absence of ischemia, PR of 120 ms, QRS duration of 110 ms, incomplete RBBB

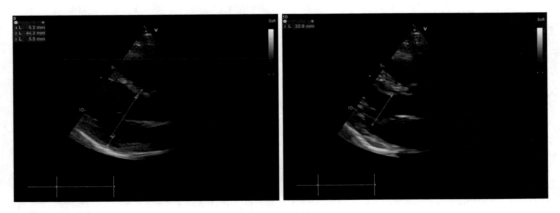

Fig. 12.2 *Left panel*: Echocardiography image in parasternal long axis view showing a non-dilated LV with an end diastolic diameter of 44 mm. *Right panel*: Parasternal long axis view showing an end diastolic diameter of 32 mm. These measures correspond to a LV EF% of 55% (Teicholz method)

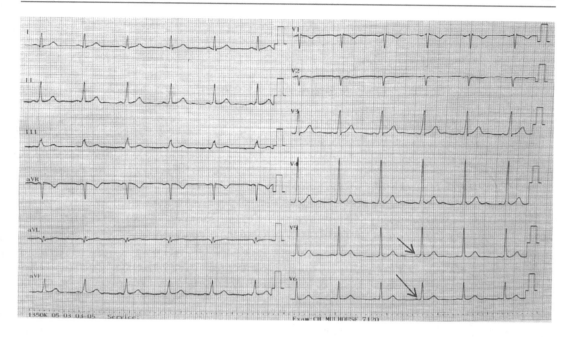

Figure 12.1 **(explained)**. A 12-lead ECG showing sinus rhythm with a heart rate of 72 bpm, QRS axis at +60°, possible LV hypertrophy (R wave of 26 mV in V4), incomplete RBBB, short PR of 120 ms, positive delta wave in V3-V6 and in leads II, III, aVF, absence of q waves in V5, V6 (red arrow).

> **Question 2: Where is the accessory pathway situated?**
> A. Left lateral.
> B. Left postero-septal.
> C. Right postero-septal.
> D. Right lateral.
> E. Right antero-septal.

Given the presence of palpitations and the ECG aspect in favor of ventricular pre-excitation, the diagnosis of WPW Syndrome was established. An electrophysiological study was subsequently offered and performed.

12.2 Electrophysiological Study and RF Catheter Ablation Procedure

The electrophysiological study was performed under local anesthesia and conscious sedation. Vascular access was obtained using the modified Seldinger technique, under Doppler ultrasound guidance.

A 6F quadripolar steerable catheter (Dynamic Extrem, Microport®) was introduced in a 9F 20 cm vascular sheath and was subsequently advanced via the right common femoral vein up to the bundle of His. Another 6F quadripolar steerable catheter (Dynamic Extrem, Microport®) was introduced in a 6F 20 cm vascular sheath and placed via the right common femoral vein in the coronary sinus, with the distal poles at the level of the lateral mitral annulus. A bipolar non-steerable catheter (Viking, Boston Scientific®) was introduced in a 6F 20 cm vascular sheath and was subsequently advanced via the right common femoral vein up to the right ventricular apex.

Atrial and ventricular pacing were carried out at twice the diastolic threshold using the EP-4™ Cardiac Stimulator (Abbott®) system.

Surface ECG and intracavitary ECGs were recorded by the WorkMate Claris™ System (Abbott®).

Radiofrequency ablation was delivered using a Biosense Webster® SmartTouch SF open-irrigated 3.5 mm tip with D curve. The CARTO® 3 electro-anatomic mapping system (Biosense Webster, Johnson & Johnson) was used to guide mapping and ablation of the accessory pathway.

Baseline AH was 70 ms, the HV interval was 26 ms, confirming the presence of ventricular pre-excitation.

The anterior effective refractory period of the accessory pathway was 290 ms.

Programmed atrial stimulation initiated an orthodromic tachycardia (Fig. 12.3), with the earliest retrograde atrial depolarization situated at the level of the lateral mitral annulus (Fig. 12.4).

Access to the mitral valve was obtained using an antegrade approach. A single transseptal punc-ture was performed under fluoroscopic guidance using an 8.5F 67cm Swartz SL0™ transseptal sheath (Abbott®) and a BRK™ XS 71 cm needle (Abbott®).

After the transseptal puncture, anticoagulation was obtained with unfractionated Heparin 70 IU/kg given as bolus, followed by continuous infu-sion of 12 IU/kg/h, with a target ACT of 300 s.

Once the access to the left atrium was granted, the SmartTouch SF roving/ablation catheter was introduced in the SL0 transseptal sheath. An ana-tomical map of the left atrium was first created. Activation mapping of the atrial myocardium around the mitral valve was then performed dur-ing orthodromic tachycardia, with emphasis on the retrograde atrial activation. The earliest local atrial activation was recorded in the lateral region of the annulus, corresponding to the 3'clock position, where the local atrial electro-gram preceded the atrial electrogram recorded by the distal poles of the coronary sinus by 25 ms. At this level, the local V and A electro-grams were fused (Fig. 12.4).

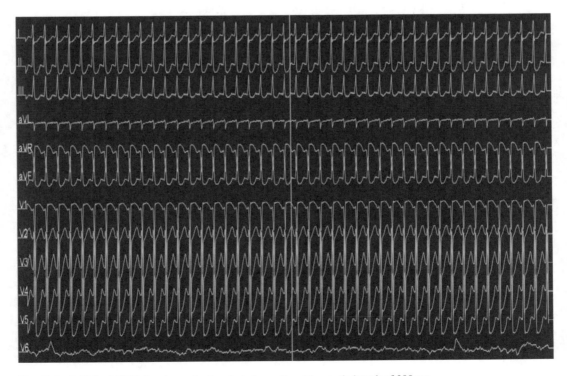

Fig. 12.3 A 12-lead ECG showing orthodromic tachycardia with a cycle length of 290 ms

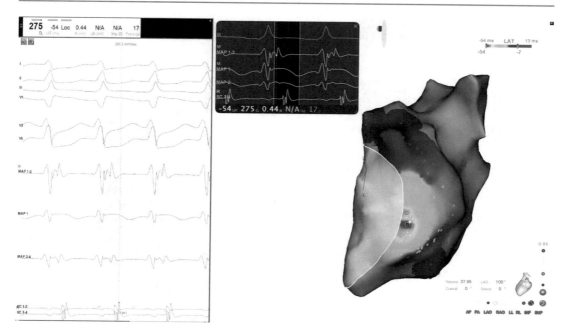

Fig. 12.4 *Right side of the image*: CARTO image in LAO 122° caudal 2° showing the activation map of the left atrium during orthodromic AVRT, with the earliest local atrial activation recorded in a narrow area at the level of the mitral annulus (red area), where fusion between the local V and A is recorded (MAP 1–2). *Left side of the image*: Surface ECG leads I, II, III, V1, V3, V5, and intra-

cavitary recordings from the distal bipolar electrode of the roving/ablation catheter (MAP 1–2), (MAP 3–4), unipolar recording from the distal electrode of the roving/ablation catheter (M1), and bipolar recordings from the quadripolar catheter placed inside the coronary sinus (SC 1–2 and SC 3–4) during orthodromic tachycardia

A second activation map was then created during sinus rhythm, with careful recording of the local activation of the ventricular myocardium around the mitral annulus. The earliest local ventricular activation was found in the lateral region of the mitral annulus, at the 3 o'clock position, corresponding to a very small area situated slightly higher than the area of the earliest local atrial depolarization during ORT (Fig. 12.5). This is explained most likely by an oblique course of the accessory pathway. At this site, the A and the V electrograms were fused, with a possible accessory pathway potential recorded in between (Fig. 12.4). The unipolar electrogram recorded by the distal pole of the roving/ablation catheter recorded a "QS" signal at this site. The local bipolar ventricular electrogram preceded the onset of the QRS complex by 15 ms.

Target ablation parameters were a power of 30 W, with a target duration of RF application of 60 s.

Application of RF energy at the site of the earliest local ventricular activation where the sharp local potential was recorded (Fig. 12.6) promptly eliminated the conduction over the accessory pathway.

Ventricular pacing after the RF application demonstrated absence of retrograde conduction over the accessory pathway.

There was no complication related to the procedure.

The 12-lead ECG recorded after the catheter ablation procedure is presented in Fig. 12.7.

The patient was discharged from the hospital 24 h later, on no antiarrhythmic medication

ANSWERS TO:
Question 1: E. Yes. Ventricular pre-excitation.
Question 2: A. Left Lateral.

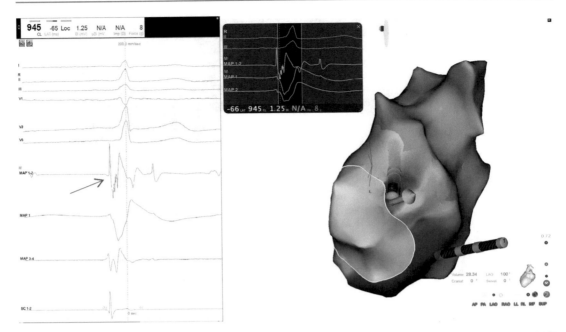

Fig. 12.5 *Right side of the image*: CARTO image in LAO 87° cranial 3° showing the activation map of the left atrium during sinus rhythm, with the earliest local ventricular activation recorded in a narrow area at the level of the mitral annulus (red area), where fusion between the local A and V is recorded (MAP 1–2). *Left side of the image*: Surface ECG leads I, II, III, V1, V3, V5, and intracavitary recordings from the distal bipolar electrode of the roving/ablation catheter (MAP 1–2), (MAP 3–4), unipolar recording from the distal electrode of the roving/ablation catheter (M1) and bipolar recordings from the quadripolar catheter placed inside the coronary sinus (SC 1–2 and SC 3–4). It is worth noting that the unipolar ventricular electrogram recorded from the distal electrode of the roving/ablation catheter has an initial negative component with a steep negative deflection (its beginning is marked by the dotted yellow line). The red arrow indicated a local pathway potential. One should also note that the earliest retrograde atrial activation during ORT recorded in Fig. 12.3 is slightly inferior compared to the earliest ventricular activation during sinus rhythm, a finding in favor of an oblique course of the accessory pathway

12.3   Commentary

The present case illustrates an RF ablation procedure of a manifest left lateral accessory pathway in a 58-year-old male patient with WPW syndrome using an antegrade (transseptal) approach of the mitral valve. Several observations can be made about the present case.

The interpretation of the 12-lead ECG in a young patient complaining of palpitations suggesting a paroxysmal tachycardia should be done patiently and systematically. One should look for signs of ventricular pre-excitation: short PR interval, the presence of delta waves, which, like in the present case, can be very subtle, and an enlarged QRS duration; ST segment elevation with a negative T wave in lead V1 in favor of a

Brugada type 1 or type 2 pattern should be sought; epsilon waves should be looked for, especially in lead V1, suggesting arrhythmogenic cardiomyopathy; the QT interval should be systematically measured, looking for long or short QT syndrome; and last but not least, signs of ischemia such as pathologic q waves, T wave inversion, ST segment elevation, or ST segment depression.

The incidence of ventricular pre-excitation or WPW pattern on the 12-lead ECG is between 0.1% and 0.3% in the general population [1].

For left lateral manifest accessory pathways, such as in the present case, besides a short PR interval and the presence of delta waves, the absence of q waves in V5 and V6 should raise suspicion of ventricular pre-excitation.

Fig. 12.6 CARTO image in LAO 45° view showing the activation map of the left atrium during ORT with superposed RF lesions (pink and red dots) at the level of the successful ablation site

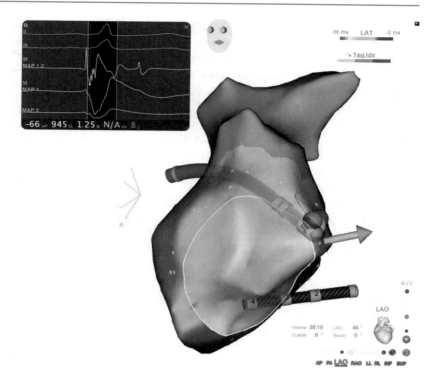

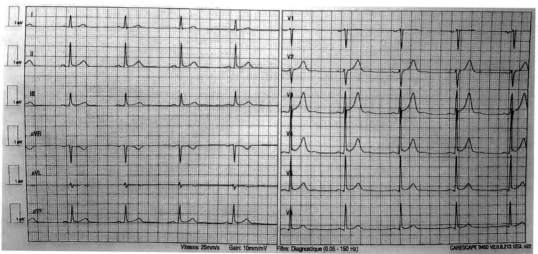

Fig. 12.7 A 12-lead ECG recorded after the RF ablation procedure showing sinus rhythm with a heart rate of 58 bpm, QRS axis at +60°, incomplete RBBB, PR of 150 ms, absence of delta wave (different compared to the ECG at admission) q waves in V5, V6 (which were not present on the admission ECG)

Orthodromic tachycardia is the most common form of arrhythmia in patients with WPW syndrome accounting for more than 90% of arrhythmias, followed by pre-excited atrial fibrillation and antidromic tachycardia, the latter occurring in 3–8% of WPW patients [2]. The treatment of choice is catheter ablation of the accessory pathway. For a left lateral accessory pathway, this can be accomplished either by an antegrade (transeptal) approach of the mitral valve or by a retrograde transaortic approach. Both techniques have a similar success rate when magnetically guided ablation is used [3]. Otherwise, the antegrade approach has a slightly higher (but significantly) success rate compared to the transaortic approach: 98% vs. 94%. The retrograde approach is associated with a slightly higher incidence of vascular complications. There is no significant difference in the procedure time and the fluoroscopy time between the 2 approaches. Recurrences after a successful procedure are rare and do not significantly differ between the 2 approaches [4].

Ablation of a manifest accessory pathway can be performed during sinus rhythm, ventricular pacing, or AV reentry tachycardia. In this patient, we chose to perform catheter ablation during sinus rhythm, given the manifest pre-excitation and the identification of an accessory pathway potential during sinus rhythm at the level of the mitral annulus (see Fig. 12.4). The alternatives are represented by ablation during ventricular pacing, for patients who present retrograde conduction over the accessory pathway, or during orthodromic/antidromic tachycardia. As explained in the commentary section of case 10, the most common problem associated with ablation of the accessory pathway during tachycardia is catheter movement immediately after the termination of the tachycardia. This is due to a first prolonged diastole after interruption of the tachycardia circuit and a subsequent "vigorous" systole, which determines a slight catheter movement. However, with the use of an electro-anatomically mapping system, this problem can be overcome since recording of the ablation catheter position at the successful site is done automatically and its repositioning to the successful ablation site is usually not a problem.

Learning Point
- A careful analysis of the 12-lead ECG is necessary in patients with paroxysmal episodes of palpitations since pre-excitation may be easily missed in patients with WPW syndrome and a rapid conduction through the AV node associating the presence of an accessory pathway situated far from the AV node, such as the case of left lateral accessory pathways.
- The absence of q waves in leads V5 and V6 in such patients suggests the presence of ventricular pre-excitation, with a left-sided situated accessory pathway.

References

1. Page RL, Joglar JA, Caldwell MA, et al. 2015 ACC/AHA/HRS Guideline for the Management of Adult Patients With Supraventricular Tachycardia: A Report of the American College of Cardiology/American Heart Association Task Force on Clinical Practice Guidelines and the Heart Rhythm Society. J Am Coll Cardiol. 2016;67:e27–e115.
2. Brugada J, Katritsis DG, Arbelo E, et al. 2019 ESC Guidelines for the management of patients with supraventricular tachycardiaThe Task Force for the management of patients with supraventricular tachycardia of the European Society of Cardiology (ESC). Eur Heart J. 2020;41:655–720.
3. Schwagten B, Jordaens L, Rivero-Ayerza M, et al. A randomized comparison of transseptal and transaortic approaches for magnetically guided ablation of left-sided accessory pathways. Pacing Clin Electrophysiol. 2010;33:1298–303.
4. Anselmino M, Matta M, Saglietto A, et al. Transseptal or retrograde approach for transcatheter ablation of left sided accessory pathways: a systematic review and meta-analysis. Int J Cardiol. 2018;272:202–7.

Case 13

Justine Havard, Frédéric Halbwachs, Ronan Le Bouar, and Tarek El Nazer

13

13.1 Case Presentation

A 56-year-old male patient with a long history of paroxysmal episodes of palpitations, with duration of several minutes up to 20 min, several times per year, accompanied by anxiety, is addressed by his treating cardiologist to the Cardiology Department for evaluation and treatment. He had no relevant past medical history, no structural heart disease, no family history of sudden cardiac death. His cardiovascular risk factors were represented by smoking (10 packs-year), grade 2 obesity, and age >55 years old. He was on no chronic medication. At physical exam, his blood pressure was 126/ 82 mmHg, heart rate of 67 bpm, SpO_2 98%, $H = 180$ cm, $W = 114$ kg, $BMI = 35.18$ kg/m^2 breathing room air, heart sounds were regular, there was no audible heart murmur, there were no signs of heart failure, pulmonary auscultation was normal. His ECG at admittance is presented in Fig. 13.1.

A transthoracic echocardiography was performed, showing a non-dilated LV, absence of LV hypertrophy, with a cardiac output of 6.4 l/min (Fig. 13.2). It also showed a normal diastolic function, a non-dilated left atrium, absence of significant valve disease, a non-dilated right ventricle, trivial tricuspid regurgitation, absence of pulmonary hypertension, a non-dilated IVC, a non-dilated aorta, absence of pericardial effusion.

His biological workup showed a Hb level of 15.2 g/dl, leucocytes 11.8×10^9/L, platelets 316×10^9/L, CRP <3 mg/L, BUN 5.8 mmol/L, creatinine 94 µmol/L, glycemia 6.2 mmol/L, Na+ 142 mmol/L, K+ 4.8 mmol/L, total proteins 77 g/L.

Question 1: Are there any clues on the 12-lead ECG suggesting a specific diagnosis?

A. No. This is a normal ECG.

B. Yes. Q waves in lead III, VF suggesting remote inferior wall myocardial infarction.

C. Yes. Delta waves suggesting ventricular pre-excitation.

D. Yes. Negative T waves in I, aVL, suggesting LV lateral wall ischemia.

E. Yes. Short QT interval suggesting short QT syndrome.

J. Havard (✉) · F. Halbwachs
Biosense Webster, Mulhouse, France

R. Le Bouar · T. El Nazer
Cardiology Department, "Emile Muller" Hospital, Mulhouse, France
e-mail: LEBOUARR@ghrmsa.fr; tarek.elnazer@ghrmsa.fr

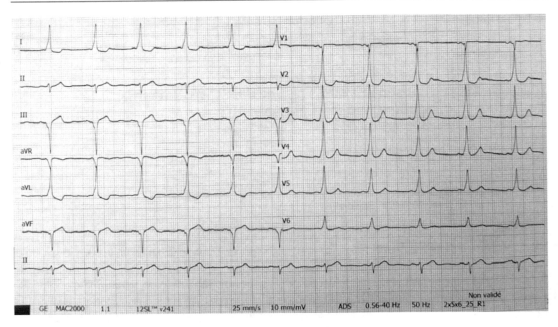

Fig. 13.1 A 12-lead ECG at admittance to the Cardiology Department

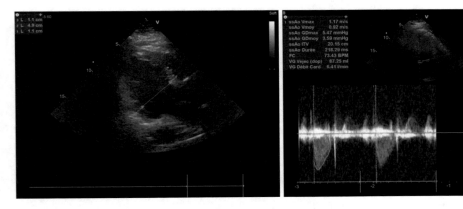

Fig. 13.2 *Left panel:* Echocardiography image in para-sternal long axis view showing a non-dilated LV with an end diastolic diameter of 49 mm, normal IVS and poste-rior wall thickness. *Right panel:* preserved stroke volume and normal cardiac output of 6.4 l/min

Figure 13.1 shows sinus rhythm with a heart rate of 70 bpm, QRS axis at −40°, short PR interval of 100 ms, with overt pre-excitation: presence of negative delta waves in lead II, III, aVF, and V1, positive in lead I, aVL, V2-V6

Question 2: Where is the accessory pathway situated?
A. Left lateral.
B. Left postero-septal.
C. Right postero-septal.
D. Right lateral.
E. Right antero-septal.

An electrophysiological study was scheduled and subsequently performed.

13.2   Electrophysiological Study and RF Catheter Ablation Procedure

The electrophysiological study was performed under local anesthesia and conscious sedation. Vascular access was obtained using the modified Seldinger technique, under Doppler ultrasound guidance. A 6F quadripolar steerable catheter (Dynamic Extrem, Microport®) was introduced in a 9F 20 cm vascular sheath and was subsequently advanced via the right common femoral vein up to the bundle of His. Another 6F quadripolar steerable catheter (Dynamic Extrem, Microport®) was introduced in a 6F 20 cm vascular sheath and placed via the right common femoral vein in the coronary sinus, with the distal poles at the level of the lateral mitral annulus. A bipolar non-steerable catheter (Viking, Boston Scientific®) was introduced in a 6F 20 cm vascular sheath and was subsequently advanced via the right common femoral vein up to the right ventricular apex. Atrial and ventricular pacing were

carried out at twice the diastolic threshold using the EP-4™ Cardiac Stimulator (Abbott®) system. Surface ECG and intracavitary ECGs were recorded by the WorkMate Claris™ System (Abbott®).

Radiofrequency ablation was delivered using a Biosense Webster® SmartTouch SF open-irrigated 3.5 mm tip with D curve. The CARTO ® 3 electro-anatomic mapping System (Biosense Webster, Johnson & Johnson) was used to guide mapping and ablation of the accessory pathway. The 12-lead ECG at the beginning of the procedure is shown in Fig. 13.3.

Baseline AH was 80 ms, the HV interval was 15 ms, confirming the presence of ventricular pre-excitation. The anterior effective refractory period of the accessory pathway was 200 ms, in favor of a malignant accessory pathway (Fig. 13.4).

Programmed atrial stimulation initiated an orthodromic tachycardia, with a cycle length of 320 ms, with the earliest retrograde atrial depolarization situated at the level of the proximal coronary sinus. The VA interval during tachycardia was 98 ms (Fig. 13.5). The spontaneous termination of the tachycardia is shown in Fig. 13.6.

Manipulation of the SmartTouch SF roving/ablation catheter in the right atrium initiated

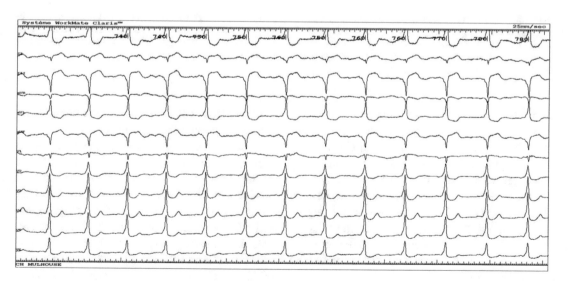

Fig. 13.3 Surface ECG recorded at the beginning of the electrophysiological study, showing sinus rhythm with a heart rate of 78 bpm, QRS axis at −40°, short PR interval of 100 ms, with over pre-excitation, an aspect similar to

the ECG from Fig. 13.1. The rS aspect in lead V1 is in favor of a right postero-septal location, but this always needs to be confirmed during the electrophysiological study

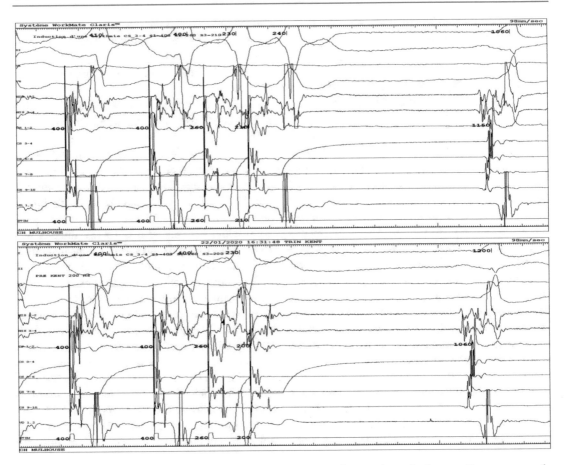

Fig. 13.4 *Upper panel*: Surface ECG leads I, II, V1, and V6 and intracavitary leads recorded from the distal (1, 2) and proximal (3, 4) electrodes of the His catheter, coronary sinus catheter (CS 1–2 to 9–10), and distal electrodes of the right ventricular catheter (VD 1–2) showing the presence of antegrade conduction over the accessory pathway at a coupling interval of 210 ms. *Lower panel*: Same leads as above, showing an ERP of the accessory pathway of 200 ms

atrial fibrillation. With the help of the CARTO system, an anatomical map of the right atrium was first created. Activation mapping of the atrial myocardium around the tricuspid valve was then performed during AF, with emphasis on the earliest antegrade ventricular activation. This was recorded in the postero-septal region of the annulus, corresponding to the 4'clock position, where the local ventricular electrogram preceded the surface QRS complex by 10 ms (Fig. 13.7).

In order to perform a more accurate mapping of the right postero-septal region, electrical

cardioversion was performed, after administration of propofol 1 mg/kg (Fig. 13.8).

A new activation map of the right postero-septal region was performed during sinus rhythm. The earliest local ventricular activation was recorded outside and lateral to the ostium of the coronary sinus (Fig. 13.9), where the local electrogram preceded the onset of the QRS onset by 9 ms. The unipolar local electrogram had a "QS" morphology.

Application of RF energy with a target power of 30 W and a target ablation index of 450 at this level interrupted the conduction over the accessory pathway (Figs. 13.10 and 13.11).

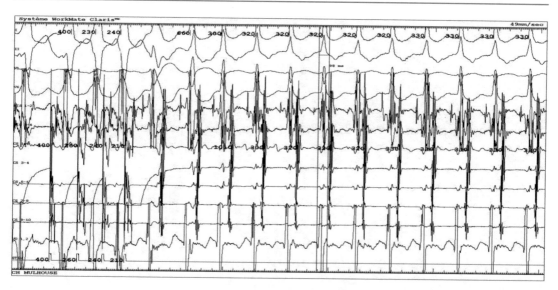

Fig. 13.5 Surface ECG leads I, II, V1, and V6 and intracavitary leads same as in Fig. 13.3 showing initiation of orthodromic AVRT with a cycle length of 320 ms. The earliest retrograde atrial activation is recorded at the level of the poles 7–8 of the coronary sinus catheter, corresponding to the postero-septal region

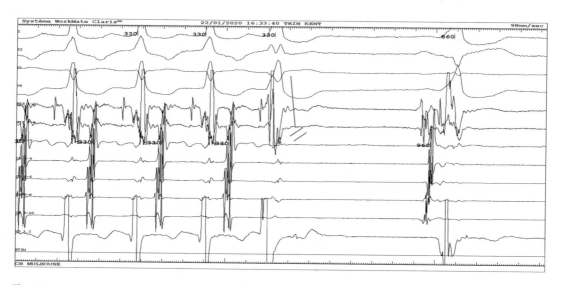

Fig. 13.6 Surface ECG leads I, II, V1, and V6 and intracavitary leads same as in Fig. 13.3 showing spontaneous termination of the tachycardia in the retrograde limb, with block in the accessory pathway (indicated by the red lines)

Ventricular pacing after the RF application demonstrated absence of retrograde conduction over the accessory pathway.

There were no complications related to the ablation procedure.

Adenosine administration after a waiting period of 30 min after the ablation of the accessory pathway demonstrated absence of conduction over the Kent pathway (Fig. 13.12).

The 12-lead ECG recorded after the ablation procedure is presented in Fig. 13.13. It shows sinus rhythm, absence of ventricular pre-excitation, negative T waves in lead II, III, and aVF, or so-called T wave memory.

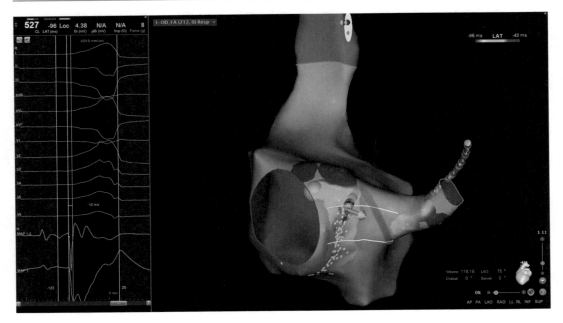

Fig. 13.7 *Right side of the image:* CARTO image in LAO 120° showing the activation map of the right atrium during pre-excited AF, with the earliest local ventricular activation recorded in a narrow area at the level of the tricuspid annulus (red area), in the postero-septal region, between the coronary sinus ostium and the tricuspid valve, where the earliest local ventricular activation precedes the QRS onset by 10 ms. *Left side of the image:* Surface ECG leads and intracavitary recordings from the distal bipolar electrode of the roving /ablation catheter (MAP 1–2), and the unipolar recording from the distal electrode of the roving / ablation catheter (M1)

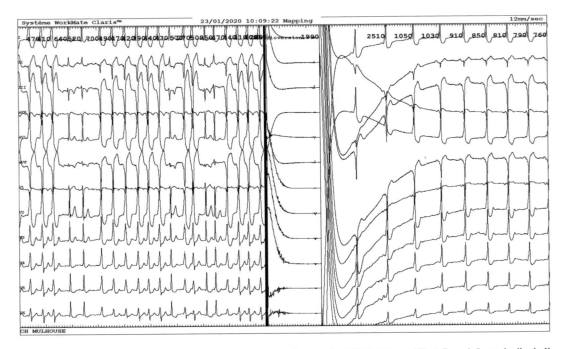

Fig. 13.8 A 12-lead ECG showing in the first part of the tracing an irregular tachycardia with narrow QRS complexes alternating with wide QRS complexes, the latter having the "FBI" pattern: "Fast, Broad, Irregular," a hallmark of pre-excited atrial fibrillation. Electrical cardioversion is performed, with conversion to sinus rhythm

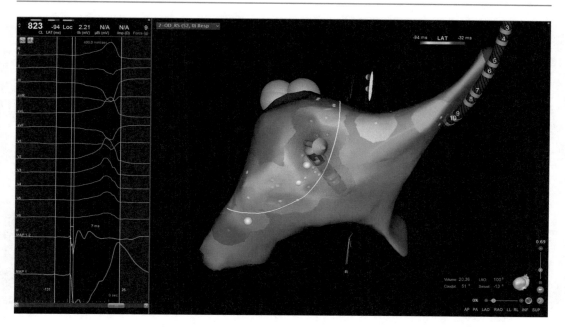

Fig. 13.9 *Right side of the image:* CARTO image inferior view showing the activation map of the right atrium during sinus rhythm, with the earliest local ventricular activation recorded in a narrow area in the postero-septal region, lower than the earliest local activation during atrial fibrillation, where the earliest local ventricular activation precedes the QRS onset by 9 ms. *Left side of the image:* Surface ECG leads and intracavitary recordings from the distal bipolar electrode of the roving/ablation catheter (MAP 1–2), and the unipolar recording from the distal electrode of the roving/ablation catheter (MAP 1)

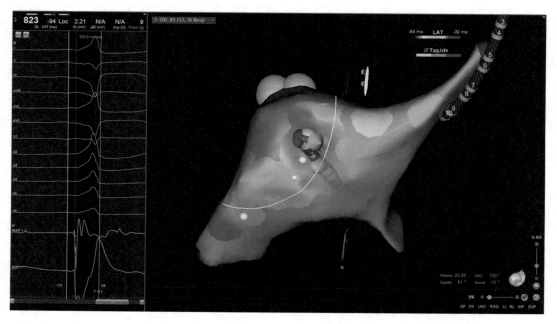

Fig. 13.10 Same image as in Fig. 13.6, with RF ablation lesions (red and pink dots) applied at the level of the earliest endocardial ventricular activation during sinus rhythm

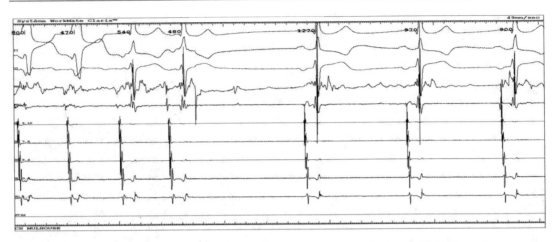

Fig. 13.11 Surface ECG leads I, II, V1, V6, and intra-cavitary leads recorded from the distal (ABL d) and proximal (Abl p) electrodes of the ablation catheter and the coronary sinus catheter (SC 9–10 to 1–2). The tracing is recorded during RF ablation in the area presented in Figs. 13.6 and 13.7. The first 2 QRS complexes are pre-excited, starting with the third QRS complex the pre-excitation is absent as a consequence of successful RF ablation of the accessory pathway

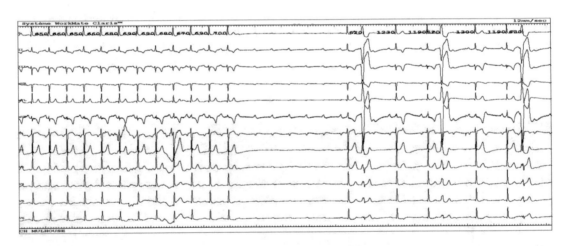

Fig. 13.12 A 12-lead ECG recorded during 20 mg of iv adenosine administration showing transient AV block with no conduction over the accessory pathway (see text for further explanation)

The patient was discharged from the hospital 24 h later.

> **ANSWER TO:**
> **Question 1: C. Yes. Delta waves suggesting ventricular pre-excitation.**
> **Question 2: C. Right postero-septal.**

13.3 Commentary

The present case illustrates a RF ablation procedure of a manifest right postero-septal accessory pathway in a 56-year-old male patient with WPW syndrome. Several observations merit further discussion.

Postero-septal accessory pathways represent around 23% of all accessory pathways, with the rest being represented by left lateral in around 58% of cases, right free wall in 9%, right antero-septal in 7%, and other areas in 3% of cases [1]. Among postero-septal accessory pathways, about two-thirds are ablated from the left postero-septal region and one-third from the right postero-septal region (64% vs. 36%) [2]. There is no gender difference in the prevalence of postero-septal accessory pathways. Differentiating between right postero-septal and left-postero-septal accessory pathways using the 12-lead ECG is not always possible with a high accuracy, but several criteria have currently been published [3–5], which can help the operator suspect a right or a left postero-septal accessory pathway before starting the EP study. The presence of a "QS" aspect in lead V1 is in favor of a right postero-septal accessory pathway; the presence of a unique "R" wave in lead V1 is in favor of a left postero-septal accessory pathway.

When ablating a postero-septal accessory pathway, mapping should always be commenced in the right postero-septal region. If suboptimal ablation criteria are found in this region, the next areas to map are the coronary venous system and the left postero-septal region. For bidirectional conducting accessory pathways, mapping can be performed either during sinus rhythm, targeting the earliest ventricular activation site, during antidromic tachycardia if present; during ventric-ular pacing, targeting the earliest retrograde atrial depolarization; or during orthodromic tachycardia, also targeting the earliest retrograde atrial activation. In the present case, mapping was first carried out during atrial fibrillation, which is challenging since, in this case, antegrade activation of the ventricular myocardium is a fusion between different degrees of depolarization using the His-Purkinje system and the accessory pathway. This is the main reason for which the activation map can be less accurate compared to an activation map performed in antidromic tachycardia or in sinus rhythm.

Adenosine may unmask dormant conduction after pulmonary vein isolation [6]. Its administration may also be useful in identifying dormant conduction after an apparent successful ablation of an accessory pathway [7]. By transiently blocking the AV node, in the case of an incomplete ablation of an accessory pathway, conduction over it may transiently recover, with the ECG recording pre-excited QRS complexes. A positive adenosine test strongly predicts recurrence of conduction over the accessory pathway, requiring a redo procedure [8]. Nevertheless, a negative test does not necessarily imply the absence of future recurrence [9].

The repolarization changes observed on the ECG from Fig. 13.13, recorded after the ablation procedure, showing negative T waves in

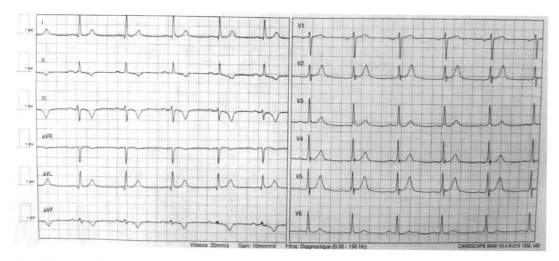

Fig. 13.13 A 12-lead ECG recorded after the RF ablation procedure showing sinus rhythm with a heart rate of 70 bpm, QRS axis at −40°, PR interval of 140 ms, absence of pre-excitation, with negative T waves in leads II, III, aVF ("T wave-memory," see text)

leads II, III, and aVF are compatible with "cardiac memory." They mimic ischemia and are not associated with myocardial injury [10]. As previously described, this refers to transient repolarization changes occurring during sinus rhythm after a period of modified ventricular depolarization and is a form of electrical remodeling of the ventricle. These changes usually disappear completely 3 months after the ablation of the accessory pathway. Accessory pathways from the right posteroseptal region have the highest percentage of showing cardiac memory after their ablation [11]. Interestingly, their presence is associated with long-term success of the ablation procedure [11].

Learning Point

- Postero-septal accessory pathways are characterized by the presence of negative delta waves in the inferior leads.
- An electroanatomical mapping system is very useful in guiding the ablation procedure in patients with WPW syndrome, especially in those who develop atrial fibrillation during the electrophysiological study.

References

1. Birati EY, Eldar M, Belhassen B. Gender differences in accessory connections location: an Israeli study. J Interv Cardiac Electrophysiol. 2012;34:227–9.
2. Wen MS, Yeh SJ, Wang CC, et al. Radiofrequency ablation therapy of the posteroseptal accessory pathway. Am Heart J. 1996;132:612–20.
3. Payami B, Shafiee A, Shahrzad M, et al. Posteroseptal accessory pathway in association with coronary sinus diverticulum: electrocardiographic description and result of catheter ablation. J Interv Cardiac Electrophysiol. 2013;38:43–9.
4. Arruda MS, McClelland JH, Wang X, et al. Development and validation of an ECG algorithm for identifying accessory pathway ablation site in Wolff-Parkinson-White syndrome. J Cardiovasc Electrophysiol. 1998;9:2–12.
5. Li HY, Chang SL, Chuang CH, et al. A novel and simple algorithm using surface electrocardiogram that localizes accessory conduction pathway in Wolff-Parkinson-White syndrome in pediatric patients. Acta Cardiol Sinica. 2019;35:493–500.
6. Chen YH, Lin H, Xie CL, et al. Role of adenosine-guided pulmonary vein isolation in patients undergoing catheter ablation for atrial fibrillation: a meta-analysis. Europace. 2017;19:552–9.
7. Walker KW, Silka MJ, Haupt D, et al. Use of adenosine to identify patients at risk for recurrence of accessory pathway conduction after initially successful radiofrequency catheter ablation. Pacing Clin Electrophysiol. 1995;18:441–6.
8. Spotnitz MD, Markowitz SM, Liu CF, et al. Mechanisms and clinical significance of adenosine-induced dormant accessory pathway conduction after catheter ablation. Circ Arrhythm Electrophysiol. 2014;7:1136–43.
9. Pegoraro V, Paiva B, AlTurki A, et al. The use of adenosine to identify dormant conduction after accessory pathway ablation: a single center experience and literature review. Am J Cardiovasc Dis. 2019;9:84–90.
10. Kalbfleisch SJ, Sousa J, el-Atassi R, et al. Repolarization abnormalities after catheter ablation of accessory atrioventricular connections with radiofrequency current. J Am Coll Cardiol. 1991;18:1761–6.
11. Trajkov I, Poposka L, Kovacevic D, et al. Cardiac memory (t-wave memory) after ablation of posteroseptal accessory pathway. Prilozi. 2008;29:167–82.

Case 14

14

Frédéric Halbwachs, Ronan Le Bouar,
Didier Bresson, Mihaela Calcaianu,
and Aubrietia Lawson

14.1 Case Presentation

A 51-year-old male patient with no significant past medical history presents to the Cardiology Department for an episode of pre-syncope in a context of palpitations with sudden onset and irregular rhythm, which had started 20 min prior to his presentation to the hospital. His only cardiovascular risk factor was represented by overweight. He had no personal history of syncope or known arrhythmia, there was no family history of sudden cardiac death. He denied smoking, consumption of alcohol or illicit drugs. He was on no chronic medication.

At physical exam, his blood pressure was 100/70 mmHg, heart rate of 170 bpm, SpO$_2$ 98% breathing room air, H = 185 cm, W = 100 kg, BMI = 29.21 kg/m^2, heart sounds were rapid and irregular, there was no audible heart murmur, there were no signs of congestive heart failure, pulmonary auscultation was normal.

His ECG is presented in Fig. 14.1.

Transthoracic echocardiography showed a non-dilated LV with a preserved LV EF%, mild septal LV hypertrophy, no significant valve dis-

ease, non-dilated right ventricle, absence of pericardial fluid (Fig. 14.2).

Figure 14.3 shows the 12-lead ECG after administration of iv Flecainide 2 mg/kg.

A few minutes later, the ECG in Fig. 14.4 was recorded.

His biological workup showed a Hb level of 14.3 g/dl, leucocytes 7.6 × 10^9/L, platelets 302 × 10^9/L, CRP <3 mg/L, BUN 3.9 mmol/L, creatinine 90 μmol/L, glycemia 6.7 mmol/L, Na+ 140 mmol/L, K+ 3.7 mmol/L, total proteins 81 g/L, TSH 2.1 IU/L, NT pro-BNP < 30 pg/ml.

> **Question 1. What is the nature of the tachycardia presented in Fig. 14.1?**
> A. Ventricular tachycardia
> B. Supraventricular tachycardia with bundle branch block
> C. Pre-excited atrial fibrillation
> D. Bundle branch reentry tachycardia
> E. Torsade des pointes

Figure 14.4 shows sinus rhythm with ventricular pre-excitation, with positive delta waves in leads V1-V6, negative in lead II, positive in lead III and aVF.

"FBI tachycardia" stands for "Fast, Broad, Irregular." It corresponds to atrial fibrillation in patients with WPW syndrome. The variation in the QRS width is explained by different degrees

F. Halbwachs (✉)
Biosense Webster, Mulhouse, France

R. Le Bouar · D. Bresson · M. Calcaianu · A. Lawson
Cardiology Department, "Emile Muller" Hospital,
Mulhouse, France

© The Author(s), under exclusive license to Springer Nature Switzerland AG 2022
L. Muresan (ed.), *Clinical Cases in Cardiac Electrophysiology: Supraventricular Arrhythmias*,
https://doi.org/10.1007/978-3-031-07357-1_14

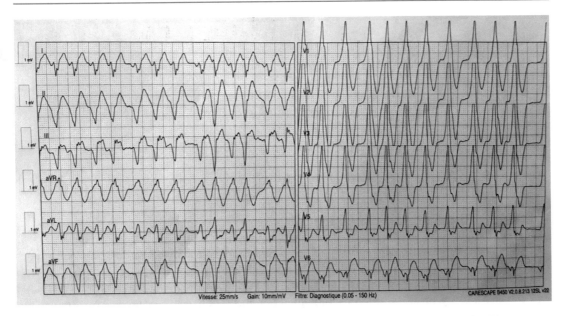

Fig. 14.1 A 12-lead ECG showing "FBI" tachycardia: Fast, Broad, Irregular, with a heart rate of 170–180 bpm

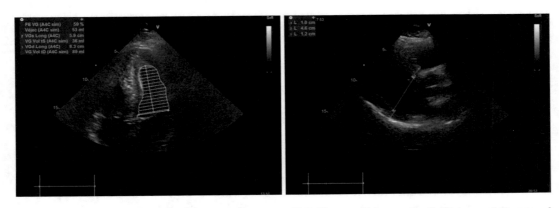

Fig. 14.2 *Left panel:* Transthoracic echocardiography image in apical 4 chamber view axis showing a non-dilated LV with preserved systolic function, a LVEF% of 59% (Simpson biplane method). *Right panel:* Parasternal long axis view showing a non-dilated left ventricle, with an end-systolic diameter of 46 mm

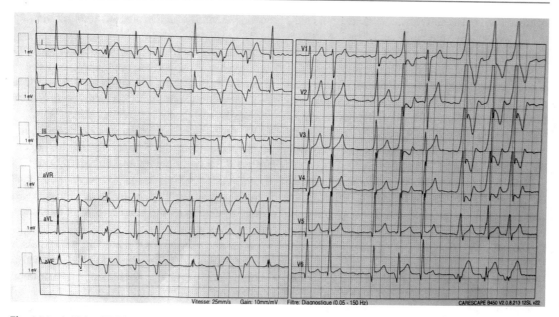

Fig. 14.3 A 12-lead ECG showing a rapid an irregular rhythm with alternating narrow and wide QRS complexes, with a heart rate of 90–100 bpm

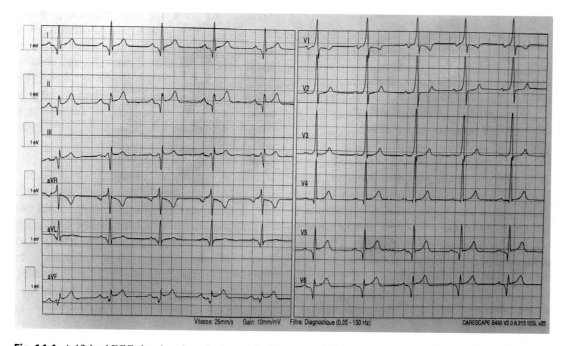

Fig. 14.4 A 12-lead ECG showing sinus rhythm with a heart rate of 64 bpm, QRS axis at −25°

of fusion between the ventricular activation using the His-Purkinje network and the accessory pathway.

Figure 14.3 shows atrial fibrillation with alternating narrow and wide QRS complexes. The refractory period of the accessory pathway was prolonged by flecainide administration; therefore, some of the ventricular depolarizations take place entirely via the His-Purkinje network, resulting in narrow QRS complexes.

The diagnosis of WPW syndrome was established, having pre-exited atrial fibrillation as the first clinical manifestation. An electrophysiological study was offered and subsequently accepted by the patient.

Question 2: Where is the accessory pathway located?
A. Left lateral
B. Left postero-septal
C. Right postero-septal
D. Right lateral
E. Right antero-septal

14.2 Electrophysiological Study and RF Catheter Ablation Procedure

The electrophysiological study was performed 48 h after the flecainide administration, under local anesthesia and conscious sedation. Vascular access was obtained using the modified Seldinger technique, under Doppler ultrasound guidance. A 6F quadripolar steerable catheter (Dynamic Extrem, Microport®) was introduced in a 9F 20 cm vascular sheath and was subsequently advanced via the right common femoral vein up to the bundle of His. A 6F decapolar steerable catheter (Inquiry, Abbott®) was introduced in a 6F 20 cm vascular sheath and placed via the right common femoral vein in the coronary sinus, with the proximal poles at the level of the coronary sinus ostium. A bipolar non-steerable catheter (Viking, Boston Scientific®) was introduced in a 6F 20 cm vascular sheath and was subsequently

advanced via the right common femoral vein up to the right ventricular apex.

Atrial and ventricular pacing were carried out at twice the diastolic threshold using the EP-4™ Cardiac Stimulator (Abbott®) system. Surface ECG and intracavitary ECGs were recorded by the WorkMate Claris™ System (Abbott®).

Radiofrequency ablation was delivered using a Biosense Webster® SmartTouch SF open-irrigated 3.5 mm tip with double curve (D and F). The CARTO ® 3 electroanatomic mapping system (Biosense Webster, Johnson & Johnson) was used to guide mapping and ablation of the accessory pathway.

Measurement of basal conduction intervals is shown in Fig. 14.5. The recorded HV interval is short (<35 ms), confirming ventricular pre-excitation.

The antegrade effective refractory period of the accessory pathway was <270 ms, value which corresponded to the atrial refractory period (Fig. 14.6).

Given the presence of symptomatic atrial fibrillation in this patient, the possibility of a malignant accessory pathway (ERP undetermined exactly but shorter than 270 ms), a decision to perform RF ablation was taken. The aspect of the QRS complex during maximal pre-excitation showed a unique "R wave" from V1-V4, suggesting a left-sided accessory pathway (Fig. 14.7).

Mapping of the right postero-septal region was briefly performed during sinus rhythm, but with suboptimal ablation criteria in this region (the earliest local ventricular activation did not precede the beginning of the QRS complex on surface ECG, there was an "rS" aspect recorded by the unipolar electrogram of the distal electrode of the roving/ablation catheter). Therefore, a decision to map the mitral annulus was taken.

Access to the mitral valve was obtained using an antegrade approach. A single transseptal puncture was performed under fluoroscopic guidance using an 8.5F 67cm Swartz SL0™ transseptal sheath (Abbott®) and a BRK ™ XS 71 cm needle (Abbott®).

After the transseptal puncture, anticoagulation was obtained with unfractionated heparin 70 IU/

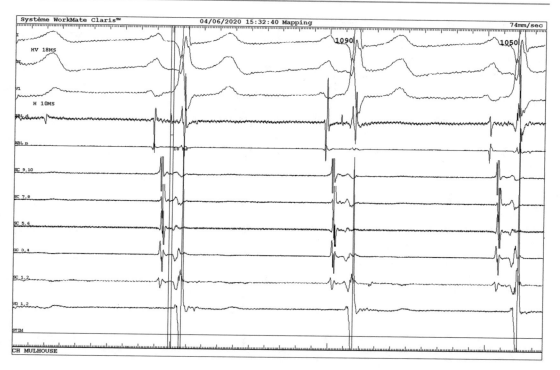

Fig. 14.5 Surface ECG leads I, II, and V1, together with intracavitary leads recorded from the distal and the proximal electrodes of the roving/ablation catheter (Abl d, Abl p), coronary sinus catheter (SC 9–10, 7–8, 5–6, 3–4, and 1–2), and the right ventricular apex catheter (VD 1–2), showing a short HV interval, of 18 ms, confirming ventricular pre-excitation

kg given as bolus, followed by continuous infusion of 12 IU/kg/h, with a target ACT of 300 s.

Once the access to the left atrium was granted, the SmartTouch SF roving/ablation catheter was introduced in the SL0 transseptal sheath and mapping of the mitral valve was performed. An anatomical map of the left atrium was first created.

An activation map targeting the earliest local ventricular activation was subsequently created during atrial pacing, in order to obtain maximal pre-excitation, with careful analysis of the local ventricular electrograms recorded around the mitral annulus. The earliest local ventricular activation was recorded in the lateral region of the annulus, corresponding to the 2'clock position, where the local ventricular electrogram preceded the onset of the surface QRS complex by 10 ms. A sharp potential in-between the local atrial and ventricular potential was recorded at this level,

possibly corresponding to an accessory pathway potential (Fig. 14.8).

The anatomical map of the right and left atrium with the activation map recorded during atrial pacing is presented in Figs. 14.9 and 14.10.

The 12-lead ECG during RF ablation of the accessory pathway is presented in Fig. 14.11. This was carried out during atrial stimulation, in order to obtain maximum pre-excitation. Target ablation parameters were a power of 30 W and an ablation index of 450. Application of RF energy at the site of the earliest local ventricular activation, where the sharp local potential was recorded, interrupted the conduction over the accessory pathway 3.2 s after the application onset (Fig. 14.11).

There were no complications related to the procedure.

The 12-lead ECG recorded after the catheter ablation procedure is presented in Fig. 14.12.

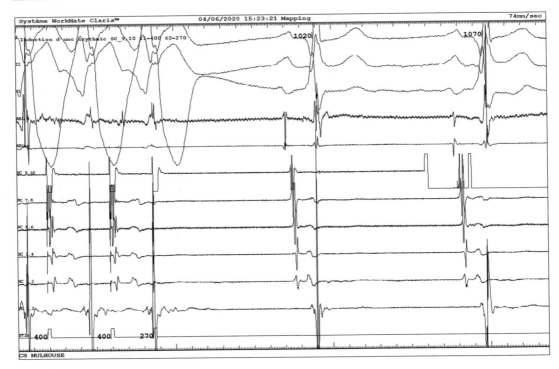

Fig. 14.6 Surface ECG leads I, II, and V1, together with intracavitary leads recorded from the distal and the proximal electrodes of the roving/ablation catheter (Abl d, Abl p), coronary sinus catheter (SC 9–10, 7–8, 5–6, 3–4, and 1–2), and the right ventricular apex catheter (VD 1–2), showing a refractory period of the accessory pathway

<270 ms. Note that the extrastimulus delivered at a coupling interval of 270 ms is blocked at the level of the atrium (no atrial electrogram visible after the spike), so the refractory period of the accessory pathway is actually shorter than this value

The patient was discharged from the hospital 24 h later, on no antiarrhythmic medication.

His 24-hour Holter ECG performed 5 weeks after the ablation procedure showed the absence of recurrence of WPW pattern and no significant atrial of ventricular arrhythmia (Fig. 14.13).

> **ANSWERS TO:**
> **Question 1: C. Pre-excited atrial fibrillation.**
> **Question 2: A. Left lateral.**

14.3 Commentary

The present case illustrates a RF ablation procedure of a manifest left lateral accessory pathway using an antegrade (transseptal) approach in a 51-year-old male patient with WPW syndrome. Several observations can be made about the present case.

Determining the localization of the accessory pathway using the 12-lead is an important step before the ablation procedure, which allows the operator to properly prepare before starting the EP study. Several algorithm have been described which help localize the accessory pathway location using the 12-lead ECG [1–6]. However, all

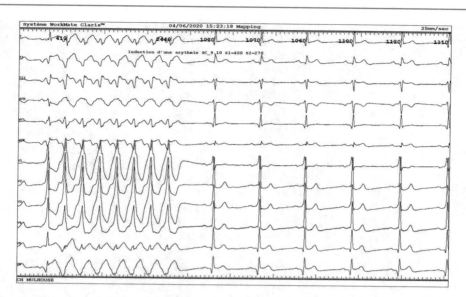

Fig. 14.7 A 12-lead surface ECG showing the aspect of the QRS complex during atrial pacing at a fixed cycle length of 600 ms (first 8 QRS complexes) corresponding to the maximal pre-excitation and the aspect of the QRS complex during sinus rhythm (last 6 QRS complexes), which is a fusion of conduction using the His-Purkinje network and conduction using the accessory pathway. The aspect of the QRS complex during maximal pre-excitation shows a unique "R wave" from V1-V4, suggesting a left-sided accessory pathway

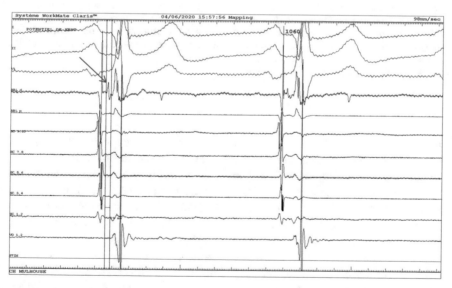

Fig. 14.8 Surface ECG leads I, II, and V1, together with intracavitary leads recorded from the distal and the proximal electrodes of the roving/ablation catheter (Abl d, Abl p), coronary sinus catheter (SC 9–10, 7–8, 5–6, 3–4 and 1–2), and the right ventricular apex catheter (VD 1–2). The roving/ablation catheter is positioned at the lateral part of the mitral annulus (Fig. 14.8), where the local ventricular electrogram precedes the beginning of the QRS complex on surface ECG by 10 ms. Note the presence of a sharp potential in-between the local atrial and ventricular potential was recorded at this level, possibly corresponding to an accessory pathway potential (red arrow)

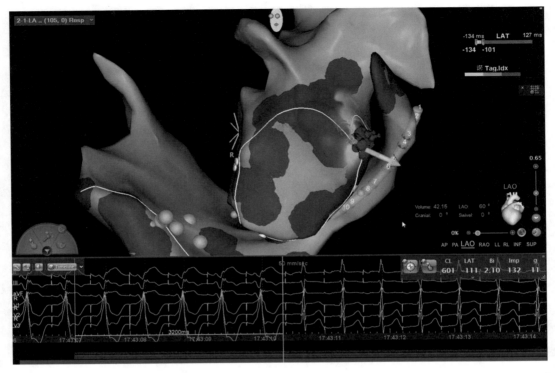

Fig. 14.9 CARTO image in LAO 75° showing the activation map of the right and left atrium and of the coronary sinus during coronary sinus pacing. The orange dots in the right atrium represent the region where a His potential was recorded by the roving/ablation catheter. The area of the earliest antegrade ventricular activation is recorded in the antero-lateral region of the mitral valve (red area), where the shortest AV was recorded. The bottom part of the image: surface ECG leads II, III, aVF, V1, V2, and V3 during the first RF application at the site of the earliest antegrade ventricular activation with rapid interruption of the antegrade conduction at the level of the accessory pathway

these algorithms have potential shortcomings in accurately predicting the localization of the accessory pathway, this being related to the existing subtle variations in the anatomy of the heart, variations in the position of the heart within the thorax and the presence of multiple accessory pathways. The present case illustrates the limitations of such algorithms, since the negative delta waves observed on the 12-lead ECG during maximal pre-excitation would suggest a postero-septal accessory pathway, which was not the case in this patient. This shows once again the fact that a careful and patient mapping phase during the EP study should precede the RF ablation, with activation recorded in several regions of the mitral valve, in order to limit the number of unnecessary RF applications and avoid potential complications.

Atrial fibrillation occurs in up to 50% of patients with WPW syndrome [7]. In cases of malignant accessory pathways (ERP < 250 ms), it can precipitate ventricular fibrillation and cause sudden cardiac death. Ablation of the accessory pathway is the treatment of choice for atrial fibrillation in this particular setting. Interestingly, pulmonary vein isolation in addition to accessory pathway ablation is not recommended since it is not associated with a reduced AF recurrence after catheter ablation [8].

Another point worth making is that the aspect of "FBI" tachycardia should strongly raise the suspicion of pre-excited atrial fibrillation. The

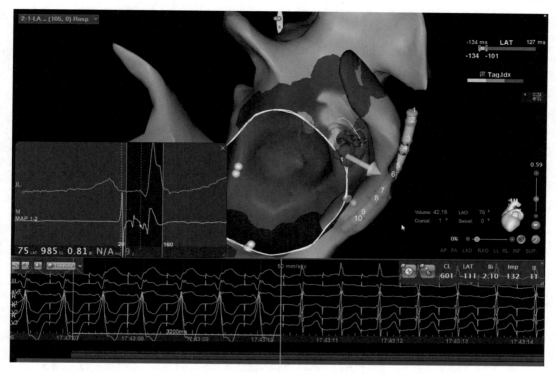

Fig. 14.10 CARTO image in LAO 75°, same as in Fig. 14.6, showing the local potential recorded by the roving/ablation catheter (MAP 1–2) together with surface ECG lead II at the level of the accessory pathway (red area). The ablation catheter records an atrial potential, a ventricular potential, and in between a potential that could correspond to an accessory pathway potential. Application of RF energy at this site rapidly interrupted the conduction at the level of the accessory pathway

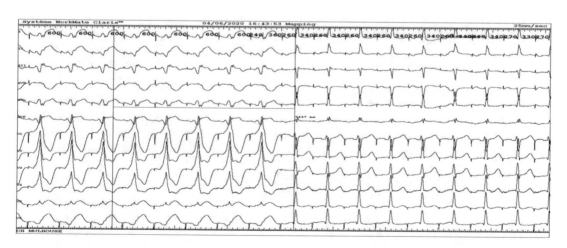

Fig. 14.11 A 12-lead ECG showing disappearance of ventricular pre-excitation during RF ablation of the accessory pathway (middle part of the tracing). This was carried out during atrial pacing, in order to obtain maximum pre-excitation

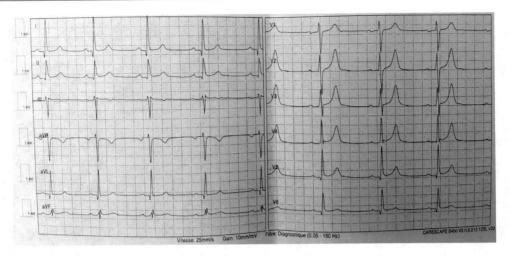

Fig. 14.12 A 12-lead ECG recorded after the RF ablation procedure showing sinus rhythm with a heart rate of 54 bpm, QRS axis at 0°, absence on LV hypertrophy, absence of ischemia, no sign of ventricular pre-excitation

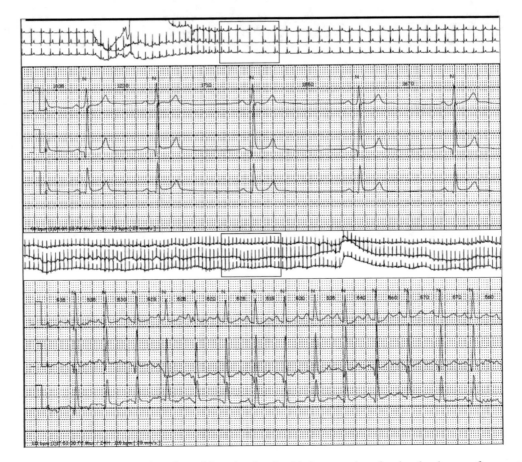

Fig. 14.13 A 24-hour Holter ECG performed 5 weeks after the ablation procedure showing the absence of recurrence of WPW pattern and no significant atrial of ventricular arrhythmia

differential diagnosis includes polymorphic ventricular tachycardia. An ECG during sinus rhythm can be helpful in orienting the correct diagnosis: in the case of WPW syndrome, ventricular pre-excitation can be observed in sinus rhythm, while in patients with polymorphic VT signs of ischemia might be present, such as ST segment elevation or depression, or negative T waves. Whatever the case, in the emergency department, if the positive diagnosis cannot be established, the treatment is the same for both arrhythmias, especially if the patient is hemodynamically unstable: electrical cardioversion.

Learning Point

- "FBI" tachycardia stands for "Fast, Broad and Irregular" and characterizes atrial fibrillation in patients with pre-excitation syndromes.
- Catheter ablation of the accessory pathway is the treatment of choice.
- A three-dimensional electroanatomical mapping system is very helpful in reducing the fluoroscopy time and dose throughout the procedure and accurately identifies its location.

References

1. Arruda MS, McClelland JH, Wang X, et al. Development and validation of an ECG algorithm for identifying accessory pathway ablation site in Wolff-Parkinson-White syndrome. J Cardiovasc Electrophysiol. 1998;9:2–12.
2. Frank R, Chandon E, Deschamps JP, et al. [Revision of criteria for locating the accessory pathway by electrocardiogram in Wolff-Parkinson-White syndrome. A new algorithm]. Ann Cardiol Angeiol. 1990;39:225–231.
3. Giorgi C, Nadeau R, Primeau R, et al. Comparative accuracy of the vectorcardiogram and electrocardiogram in the localization of the accessory pathway in patients with Wolff-Parkinson-White syndrome: validation of a new vector cardiographic algorithm by intraoperative epicardial mapping and electrophysiologic studies. Am Heart J. 1990;119:592–8.
4. Li HY, Chang SL, Chuang CH, et al. A novel and simple algorithm using surface electrocardiogram that localizes accessory conduction pathway in Wolff-Parkinson-White Syndrome in pediatric patients. Acta Cardiol Sin. 2019;35:493–500.
5. Rantner LJ, Stuhlinger MC, Nowak CN, et al. Localizing the accessory pathway in ventricular pre-excitation patients using a score based algorithm. Methods Inf Med. 2012;51:3–12.
6. Saidullah S, Shah B, Ullah H, et al. Localization of accessory pathway in patients with Wolff-Parkinson-White syndrome from surface ECG using arruda algorithm. J Ayub Med Coll Abbottabad. 2016;28:441–4.
7. Brugada J, Katritsis DG, Arbelo E, et al. 2019 ESC Guidelines for the management of patients with supraventricular tachycardia The Task Force for the management of patients with supraventricular tachycardia of the European Society of Cardiology (ESC). Eur Heart J. 2020;41:655–720.
8. Kawabata M, Goya M, Takagi T, et al. The impact of B-type natriuretic peptide levels on the suppression of accompanying atrial fibrillation in Wolff-Parkinson-White syndrome patients after accessory pathway ablation. J Cardiol. 2016;68:485–91.

Case 15

Ronan Le Bouar, Frédéric Halbwachs,
Arthur Kohler, and Maxime Tissier

15.1 Case Presentation

A 29-year-old African-American male patient with a past medical history of palpitations with sudden onset and offset, non-related to physical effort, with a duration of maximum 20 min presents to the Cardiology Department for an episode of malaise and lightheadedness in a context of palpitations with sudden onset and regular rhythm, which had a few minutes prior to his presentation to the hospital. He had no cardiovascular risk factors. He had no personal history of syncope, and there was no family history of sudden cardiac death. He denied smoking, consumption of alcohol of illicit drugs. He was on no chronic medication.

At physical exam, his blood pressure was 124/73 mmHg, heart rate of 75 bpm, SpO$_2$ 99% breathing room air, $H = 172$ cm, $W = 63$ kg, BMI $= 21.29$ kg/m^2, heart sounds were regular, there was no audible heart murmur, there were no signs of congestive heart failure, pulmonary auscultation was normal.

His ECG is presented in Fig. 15.1.

Transthoracic echocardiography showed a non-dilated LV with a preserved LV EF%, absence of LV hypertrophy, no significant valve disease, non-dilated right ventricle, absence of pericardial fluid (Fig. 15.2).

His biological workup showed a Hb level of 15.0 g/dl, leucocytes 8.5 × 10^9/L, platelets 351 × 10^9/L, CRP <3 mg/L, BUN 4.0 mmol/L, creatinine 83 μmol/L, glycemia 6.2 mmol/L Na+ 139 mmol/L, K+ 3.9 mmol/L, total proteins 85 g/L, TSH = 2.2 IU/L, NT pro-BNP < 30 pg/ml.

> **Question 1: What does the ECG in Fig. 15.1 show?**
> A. Normal ECG.
> B. Pre-excitation syndrome: Wolff-Parkinson-White.
> C. Sinus rhythm with incomplete left bundle branch block.
> D. Sinus rhythm with old anterior myocardial infarction.
> E. Accelerated idioventricular rhythm.

Figure 15.1 shows sinus rhythm with a heart rate of 74 bpm, QRS axis at +60°, with short PR interval of 80 ms, positive delta waves in leads II, III, aVF, I, aVL, a QRS transition in V4, an enlarged QRS complex, in favor of ventricular pre-excitation.

R. Le Bouar (✉)
Cardiology Department, "Emile Muller" Hospital,
Mulhouse, France
e-mail: LEBOUARR@ghrmsa.fr

F. Halbwachs · A. Kohler · M. Tissier
Biosense Webster, Mulhouse, France

© The Author(s), under exclusive license to Springer Nature Switzerland AG 2022
L. Muresan (ed.), *Clinical Cases in Cardiac Electrophysiology: Supraventricular Arrhythmias*,
https://doi.org/10.1007/978-3-031-07357-1_15

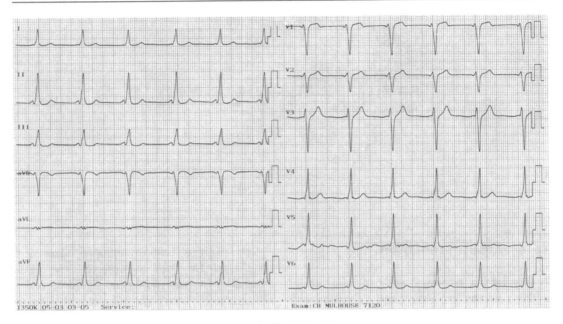

Fig. 15.1 A 12-lead ECG recorded at admittance to the Cardiology Department

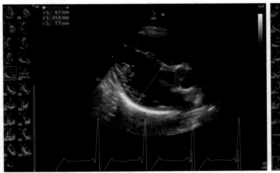

Fig. 15.2 *Left panel:* Transthoracic echocardiography in parasternal long axis view showing a non-dilated LV, with an end-diastolic diameter of 42 mm. *Right panel:* Transthoracic echocardiography in apical 4 chamber view showing a non-dilated left atrium and a non-dilated right atrium, with a surface of 18.2 cm² and 14.0 cm², respectively

An exercise stress test was performed in order to assess in a non-invasive manner the effective refractory period of the accessory pathway and to assess the initiation of arrhythmias during physical effort. The stress test demonstrated an effective refractory period of the accessory pathway of 430 ms, in favor of a benign accessory pathway (Fig. 15.3). There were no arrhythmias initiated during the test.

Question 2: Where is the accessory pathway located?
A. Left lateral
B. Left postero-septal
C. Right postero-septal
D. Right lateral
E. Right antero-septal

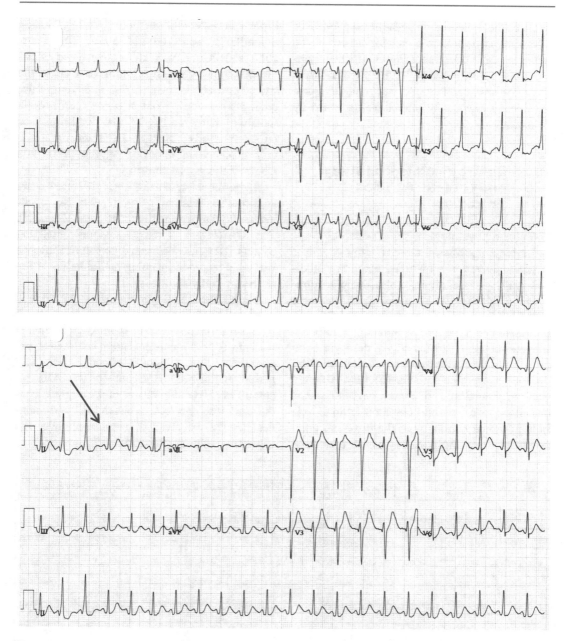

Fig. 15.3 Exercise stress test showing the abrupt disappearance of ventricular pre-excitation at a heart rate of 140 bpm (red arrow), corresponding to an effective refractory period of the accessory pathway of 430 ms, in favor of a benign accessory pathway

Given the presence of palpitations suggestive of a paroxysmal tachycardia and the aspect of the ECG in Fig. 15.1 showing ventricular pre-excitation, the diagnosis of Wolff-Parkinson-White syndrome was established. An electrophysiological study was subsequently offered and accepted by the patient.

15.2 Electrophysiological Study and Catheter Ablation Procedure

The electrophysiological study was performed under local anesthesia and conscious sedation. Vascular access was obtained using the modified Seldinger technique, under Doppler ultrasound guidance. A 6F quadripolar steerable catheter (Dynamic Extrem, Microport®) was introduced in a 9F 20 cm vascular sheath and was subsequently advanced via the right common femoral vein up to the bundle of His. A 6F decapolar steerable catheter (Inquiry, Abbott®) was introduced in a 6F 20 cm vascular sheath and placed via the right common femoral vein in the coronary sinus, with the proximal poles at the level of the coronary sinus ostium. A bipolar non-steerable catheter (Viking, Boston Scientific®) was introduced in a 6F 20 cm vascular sheath and was subsequently advanced via the right common femoral vein up to the right ventricular apex. Atrial and ventricular pacing were carried out at twice the diastolic threshold using the EP-4™ Cardiac Stimulator (Abbott®) system. Surface ECG and intracavitary ECGs were recorded by the WorkMate Claris™ System (Abbott®).

Radiofrequency ablation was delivered using a Biosense Webster® SmartTouch SF open-irrigated 3.5 mm tip with double curve (D and F). The CARTO ® 3 electroanatomic mapping System (Biosense Webster, Johnson & Johnson) was used to guide mapping and ablation of the accessory pathway.

The ECG at the beginning of the EP study is presented in Fig. 15.4.

Baseline measurements were AH = 53 ms, H = 15 ms, HV = 27 ms, confirming ventricular pre-excitation. The antegrade effective refractory period of the accessory pathway was 450 ms, confirming its benign character. Retrograde conduction was present, concentric, and non-decremental, in favor of conduction over the accessory pathway (Figs. 15.5, 15.6, and 15.7).

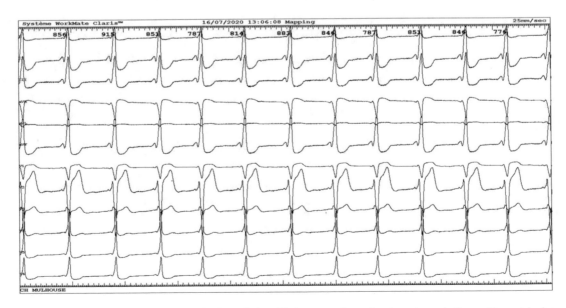

Fig. 15.4 A 12-lead ECG at the beginning of the ablation procedure showing sinus rhythm with ventricular pre-excitation

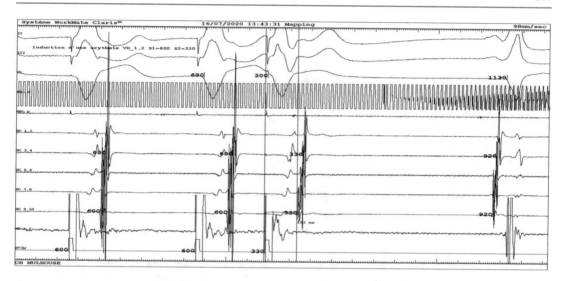

Fig. 15.5 Surface ECG leads II, III, and V6, together with intracavitary leads recorded from the 10 electrodes of the coronary sinus catheter (SC 1–2 to SC 9–10) and the bipolar electrodes of the RV catheter (VD 1–2) show-ing the presence of concentric retrograde conduction, with a VA interval of 152 ms for a coupling interval of 330 ms

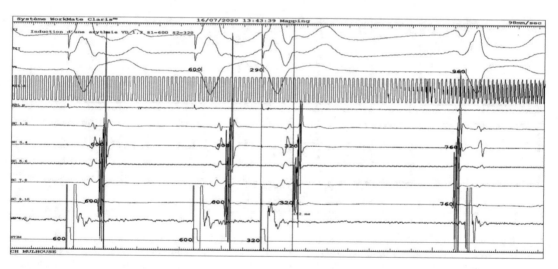

Fig. 15.6 Surface ECG leads II, III, and V6, together with intracavitary leads recorded from the 10 electrodes of the coronary sinus catheter (SC 1–2 to SC 9–10) and the bipolar electrodes of the RV catheter (VD 1–2) show-ing the presence of concentric retrograde conduction, with the same VA interval of 152 ms, this time for a coupling interval of 320 ms, in favor of a non-decremental character

Mechanically induced PACs initiated the tachycardia in Fig. 15.8.

The spontaneous termination of the tachycardia is shown in Fig. 15.9.

PPI – TCL at the RV apex was 80 ms, in favor of an ORT. Given the symptomatic nature of the tachy-cardia and the patient's history of repeated episodes of palpitations, ablation of the accessory pathway was discussed with the patient, explaining the risks and the benefits of such an ablation procedure. The patient opted for the accessory ablation since long-term antiarrhythmic treatment was not desired.

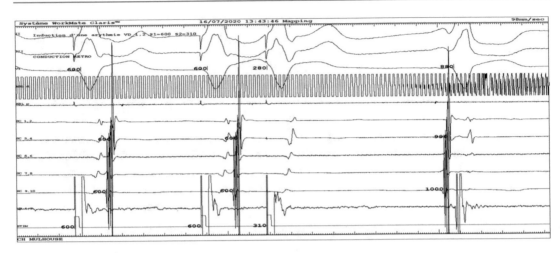

Fig. 15.7 Surface ECG leads II, III, and V6, together with intracavitary leads recorded from the 10 electrodes of the coronary sinus catheter (SC 1–2 to SC 9–10) and the bipolar electrodes of the RV catheter (VD 1–2) showing the absence of retrograde conduction for a coupling interval of 310 ms

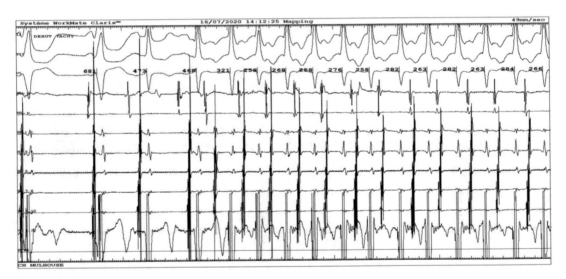

Fig. 15.8 Surface ECG leads II, III, and V6, together with intracavitary leads recorded from the distal and the proximal electrodes of the ablation catheter (Abl d, Abl p), from the 10 electrodes of the coronary sinus catheter (SC 1–2 to SC 9–10) and the bipolar electrodes of the RV catheter (VD 1–2) showing initiation of a narrow-QRS complex tachycardia with a cycle length of 260 ms, with the earliest atrial depolarization recorded by the roving / ablation catheter, situated at the level of the high inter-atrial septum, followed by the proximal coronary sinus, middle and distal coronary sinus

An anatomical map of the right atrium was initially created with the roving/ablation catheter. This showed a non-dilated right atrium of 70 ml.

Next, an activation map of the myocardium adjacent to the tricuspid annulus was created, with emphasis on the antero-septal area, targeting the earliest ventricular activation during sinus rhythm. This is presented in Fig. 15.10. The earliest ventricular activation was recorded at 10 mm lateral and superior to the His region, corresponding to the 12 o'clock area of the tricuspid annulus when view in LAO 45° (T12).

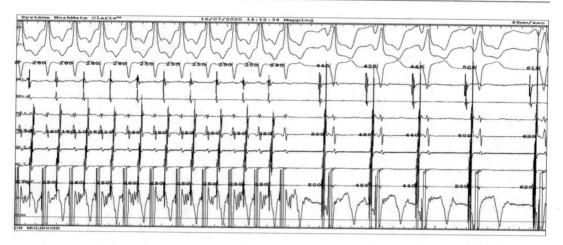

Fig. 15.9 Surface ECG leads II, III, and V6, together with intracavitary leads recorded from the distal and the proximal electrodes of the ablation catheter (Abl d, Abl p), from the 10 electrodes of the coronary sinus catheter (SC 1–2 to SC 9–10) and the bipolar electrodes of the RV catheter (VD 1–2) showing termination of the narrow-QRS complex tachycardia with the sequence "A-V"

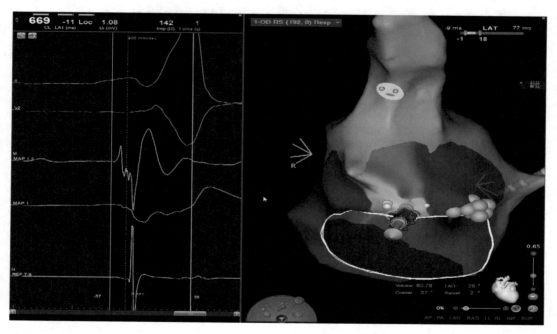

Fig. 15.10 *Right side of the image:* CARTO image in LAO 26° cranial 37° view showing the activation map of the right atrium during sinus rhythm, with the earliest local ventricular activation recorded in a narrow area in the antero-septal region, where the earliest local ventricular activation precedes the QRS onset by 27 ms. *Left side of the image:* Surface ECG leads II and V2 and intracavitary recordings from the distal bipolar electrode of the roving/ablation catheter (MAP 1–2), and the unipolar recording from the distal electrode of the roving/ablation catheter (MAP 1) and the coronary sinus catheter electrodes 7–8 showing a sharp potential recorded by the ablation catheter at this site, between the atrial and the ventricular potential, likely corresponding to an accessory pathway potential

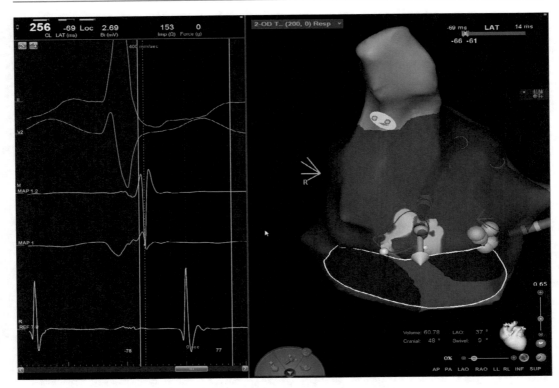

Fig. 15.11 CARTO image in LAO 26° cranial 48° view showing the activation map of the right atrium during ORT, with the earliest local atrial activation recorded in a narrow area in the antero-septal region, corresponding to the 12 o'clock area of the tricuspid annulus. Left side of the image: surface ECG leads II and V2 and intracavitary recordings from the distal bipolar electrode of the roving/ablation catheter (MAP 1–2), and the unipolar recording from the distal electrode of the roving/ablation catheter (MAP 1) and the coronary sinus catheter electrodes 7–8 showing the short VA interval at this level

Next, programmed atrial stimulation was repeated, and the narrow-QRS tachycardia presented in Figs. 15.8 and 15.9 was reinitiated. An activation map of the right atrium was created during tachycardia which confirmed its orthodromic nature, with the earliest retrograde atrial depolarization at the level of the superior part of the tricuspid annulus, 13 mm lateral and superior to the His region, corresponding to the 12 o'clock area of the tricuspid annulus when view in LAO 45° (T12), just above the earliest ventricular activation site during sinus rhythm (Fig. 15.11).

The anatomical relationship between the earliest retrograde atrial depolarization site during ORT and the earliest ventricular depolarization site during sinus rhythm is presented in Figs. 15.12 and 15.13

Placing the roving/ablation catheter at the level of the earliest ventricular activation site during sinus rhythm bumped the accessory pathway, with transient interruption of the conduction over the accessory pathway (Fig. 15.13).

RF ablation was applied with energy titration from 10 W to 30 W and a target ablation index of 450, with a force between 5 and 30 g. The conduction over the accessory pathway disappeared rapidly after the beginning of the ablation, but due to poor catheter stability, conduction reappeared at the end of the RF application. An Agilis (Abbott®) deflectable 8.5F medium curve sheath was used to improve catheter stability. RF re-application at the site of the earliest ventricular activation during sinus rhythm, 27 ms before the beginning of the QRS complex on the surface ECG, where the local unipolar electrogram had a

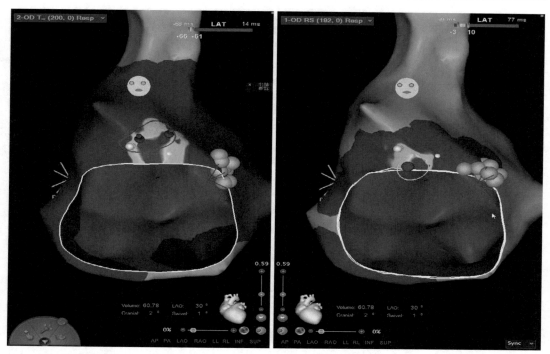

Fig. 15.12 CARTO image in LAO 26° cranial 48° view showing the activation map of the right atrium during ORT, with the earliest local atrial activation recorded in a narrow area in the antero-septal region, corresponding to the 12 o'clock area of the tricuspid annulus (left panel) and the activation map of the right atrium during sinus rhythm, with the earliest local ventricular activation recorded just below the area of the earliest retrograde atrial activation during ORT

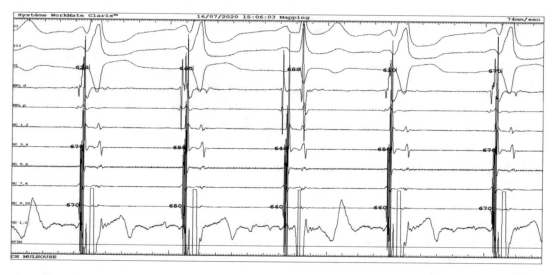

Fig. 15.13 Surface ECG leads II, III, and V6, together with intracavitary leads recorded from the distal and the proximal electrodes of the ablation catheter (Abl d, Abl p), from the 10 electrodes of the coronary sinus catheter (SC 1–2 to SC 9–10) and the bipolar electrodes of the RV catheter (VD 1–2) showing catheter bump of the accessory pathway (third complex), with transient interruption of the conduction over the accessory pathway, confirming the location of the accessory pathway at this level

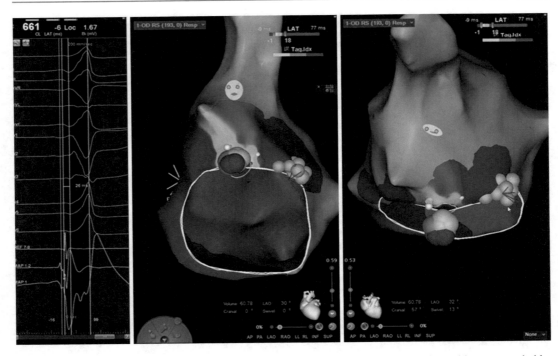

Fig. 15.14 *Left panel*: A 12-lead ECG together with intracavitary recordings from the electrodes 7–8 of the coronary sinus catheter and the bipolar and unipolar electrodes of the mapping/ablation catheter (Map 1–2, Map 1) showing the local electrograms recorded by the ablation catheter at the successful ablation site. The local bipolar electrogram precedes the beginning of the QRS complex on the surface ECG by 27 ms, and the unipolar ventricular electrogram has a "QS" aspect. *Middle panel*: CARTO image in LAO 30° view showing the activation map of the right atrium during sinus rhythm, with superposed ablation lesions at the site of the earliest local ventricular activation. *Right panel*: CARTO image in LAO 32° cranial 57° view showing the activation map of the right atrium during sinus rhythm, with superposed ablation lesions at the site of the earliest local ventricular activation. Note that these lesions were applied on the ventricular side of the tricuspid annulus, in order to minimize the risk of AV node injury

"QS" aspect resulted in elimination of the conduction over the accessory pathway (Figs. 15.14 and 15.15). There was no prolongation of the AH interval at any point during ablation.

The HV interval after the ablation measured 43 ms (Fig. 15.16).

There was no retrograde conduction after the ablation of the accessory pathway (Fig. 15.17).

Administration of 20 mg of adenosine resulted in transient complete AV block, demonstrating no antegrade "dormant" conduction over the ablated accessory pathway (Fig. 15.18).

The ECG at the end of the ablation procedure is presented in Fig. 15.19.

There were no complications related to the procedure. The ECG recorded 24 h after the ablation procedure, before the patient's discharge is shown in Fig. 15.20.

ANSWERS TO:
Question 1: B. Pre-excitation syndrome: Wolff-Parkinson-White.
Question 2: E. Right antero-septal.

15.3   Commentary

The present case presents a RF catheter ablation procedure of an antero-septal accessory pathway (T12) with bidirectional conduction properties in a 29-year-old male patient with no structural heart disease. Several observations can be made about the present case.

Antero-septal accessory pathways represent around 7% to 9% of all accessory pathways [1–3].

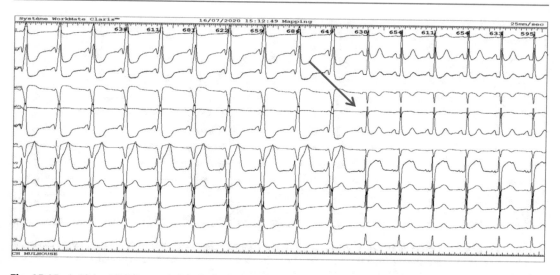

Fig. 15.15 A 12-lead ECG recorded during RF ablation of the accessory pathway showing abrupt disappearance of conduction over the accessory pathway and abrupt narrowing of the QRS complex (red arrow)

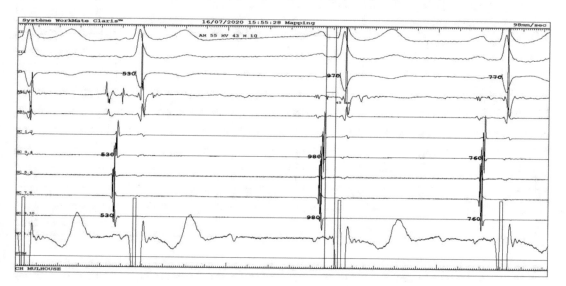

Fig. 15.16 Surface ECG leads II, III, and V6, together with intracavitary leads recorded from the 10 electrodes of the coronary sinus catheter (SC 1–2 to SC 9–10) and the bipolar electrodes of the RV catheter (VD 1–2) showing an HV interval of 43 ms (Abl 1–2) recorded by the distal electrode of the ablation catheter

ECG characteristics suggesting an antero-septal location of the accessory pathway include positive delta waves in leads II, III, aVF, and iso-electric/negative delta waves in V1.

RF ablation of antero-septal accessory pathways can be attempted using RF energy or, in order to minimize the risk of inadvertent AV block, with cryo energy [3, 4]. Ablation of the accessory pathway should be attempted targeting its ventricular insertion (as shown in Fig. 15.14, right panel), since the fibrous tissue isolating the bundle of His protects the conduction tissue at this level from thermal injury; ablation should not target the atrial insertion of the accessory

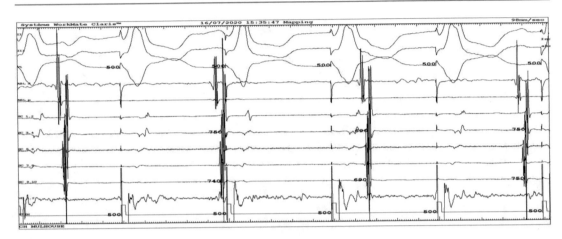

Fig. 15.17 Surface ECG leads II, III, and V6, together with intracavitary leads recorded from the 10 electrodes of the coronary sinus catheter (SC 1–2 to SC 9–10) and the bipolar electrodes of the RV catheter (VD 1–2) showing the absence of retrograde conduction at a coupling interval of 400 ms

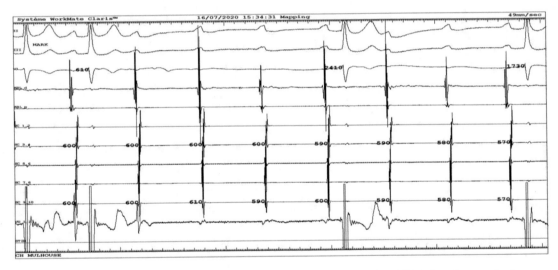

Fig. 15.18 Surface ECG leads II, III, and V6, together with intracavitary leads recorded from the 10 electrodes of the coronary sinus catheter (SC 1–2 to SC 9–10) and the bipolar electrodes of the RV catheter (VD 1–2) showing transient complete AV block and no conduction over an accessory pathway after the iv administration of 20 mg of adenosine

pathway, since this can be in close proximity to the compact AV node, and ablation attempts in this area can produce complete AV block.

Another ablation issue of antero-septal accessory pathway is catheter instability. A good contact between the ablation catheter and the accessory pathway is crucial in order to perform successful ablation and to avoid recurrences.

Frequently, a stabilizing sheath is required in order to improve catheter stability in this region.

Using an electroanatomical mapping system to guide mapping and ablation of antero-septal pathways has the advantage of reducing the fluoroscopy time and dose throughout the procedure, and to allow assessment of proper catheter positioning at the optimal ablation site. Contact force

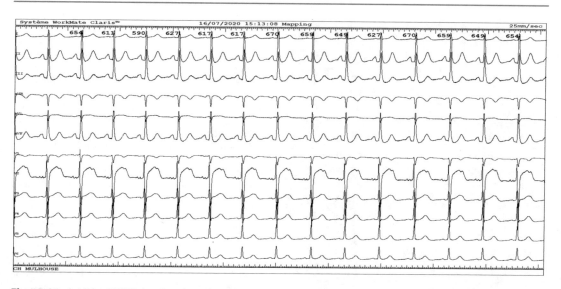

Fig. 15.19 A 12-lead ECG showing sinus rhythm with a heart rate of 91 bpm, QRS axis at +75°, absence of ventricular pre-excitation

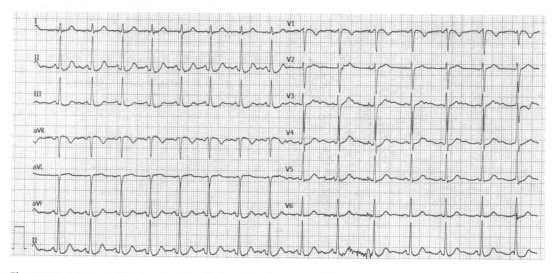

Fig. 15.20 A 12-lead ECG showing sinus rhythm with a heart rate of 80 bpm, QRS axis at +75°, absence of ventricular pre-excitation, presence of U wave

evaluation before ablating the accessory pathway is also an advantage. It is our experience to titrate RF energy from 10 to 15 W and increase the target power up to 25 to 30 W in this region if conduction block at the level of the accessory pathway but not at the level of the normal conduction system is observed during the first 10 s of RF application. Up to date, there is no ablation index suggested value as a definite end-point for the ablation. The value that we use is 450. Additional "consolidating" RF lesions can be applied at the successful ablation site, in order to minimize the risk of recurrence, but always weighing the risk/benefit ratio for any extra lesion in this area.

Some authors have suggested and successfully performed RF ablation of antero-septal pathways from the non-coronary aortic cusp [5, 6].

Learning Point

- Catheter ablation of right antero-septal accessory pathways can be accomplished with a high success rate and a low complication rate.
- When bidirectional conduction is present via the accessory pathway, performing 2 activation maps (that of the earliest atrial activation during V pacing/ORT and that of the earliest ventricular activation site during sinus rhythm/atrial pacing/ART) is very useful, since they provide information about both the atrial and the ventricular insertion site of the accessory pathway. Ablation should be done in between the atrial and the ventricular insertion site, to maximize the success rate.
- If the AP is dangerously close to the His bundle, RF energy should be applied on the ventricular part of the annulus, in order to minimize the risk of inadvertent AV node injury (at a site where the amplitude of the local V electrogram >amplitude of the local A electrogram).
- When ablating antero-septal accessory pathways, catheter stability is an issue. This can be improved by using a long deflectable sheath that confers a better contact between the catheter tip and the myocardium.

References

1. Birati EY, Eldar M, Belhassen B. Gender differences in accessory connections location: an Israeli study. J Interv Cardiac Electrophysiol. 2012;34(3):227–9.
2. Schaffer MS, Silka MJ, Ross BA, Kugler JD. Inadvertent atrioventricular block during radiofrequency catheter ablation. Results of the Pediatric Radiofrequency Ablation Registry. Pediatric Electrophysiology Society. Circulation. 1996;94(12):3214–20.
3. Mandapati R, Berul CI, Triedman JK, Alexander ME, Walsh EP. Radiofrequency catheter ablation of septal accessory pathways in the pediatric age group. Am J Cardiol. 2003;92(8):947–50.
4. Collins KK, Rhee EK, Kirsh JA, Cannon BC, Fish FA, Dubin AM, et al. Cryoablation of accessory pathways in the coronary sinus in young patients: a multicenter study from the Pediatric and Congenital Electrophysiology Society's Working Group on Cryoablation. J Cardiovasc Electrophysiol. 2007;18(6):592–7.
5. Letsas KP, Efremidis M, Vlachos K, Georgopoulos S, Karamichalakis N, Saplaouras A, et al. Catheter ablation of anteroseptal accessory pathways from the aortic cusps: a case series and a review of the literature. J Arrhythm. 2016;32(6):443–8.
6. Huang H, Wang X, Ouyang F, Antz M. Catheter ablation of anteroseptal accessory pathway in the non-coronary aortic sinus. Europace. 2006;8(12):1041–4.

Frédéric Halbwachs, Charline Daval,
Justine Havard, and Crina Muresan

16.1 Case Presentation

A 59-year-old male patient with a past medical history of COPD, recurrent undocumented episodes of palpitations with sudden onset and a regular rhythm, presents to the Emergency Department for another episode of palpitations with regular rhythm, which had started 20 min prior to his presentation to the hospital. His cardiovascular risk factors were represented by age >55 years, grade 1 obesity, smoking, and dyslipidemia. He had no personal history of syncope, no family history of sudden cardiac death. He consumed alcohol up to 750 ml of whiskey per day but denied consumption of illicit drugs. He was on no chronic medication. At physical exam, his blood pressure was 137/90 mmHg, heart rate of 200 bpm, SpO_2 93% breathing room air, $H = 175$ cm, $W = 85$ kg, BMI = 27.75 kg/m^2, heart sounds were rapid and regular, there was no audible heart murmur, there were no signs of heart failure, pulmonary auscultation revealed bilateral sibilant rales. His ECG recorded in the Emergency Department is presented in Fig. 16.1.

Twenty mg of intravenous adenosine was administered, after which the ECG in Fig. 16.2 was recorded. The patient was subsequently hospitalized in the Cardiology Department.

His biological workup showed a Hb level of 16.9 g/dl, leucocytes 9.74×10^9/L, platelets 143×10^9/L, CRP 11 mg/L, BUN 3.1 mmol/L, creatinine 88 μmol/L, glycemia 6.0 mmol/L, Na+ 135 mmol/L, K+ 3.6 mmol/L, total proteins 69 g/L, D-dimers 581 ng/ml, TSH 3.5 IU/L, NT pro-BNP 284 pg/ml.

Transthoracic echocardiography showed a non-dilated LV with a preserved LV EF% of 52%, absence of LV hypertrophy, no significant valve disease, non-dilated right ventricle, absence of pericardial fluid (Fig. 16.3).

> **Question 1: Are there any clues on the 12-lead ECG in Fig. 16.2 suggesting a specific diagnosis?**
> A. No. This is a normal ECG.
> B. Yes. Q waves in lead III, aVF suggesting remote inferior wall myocardial infarction.
> C. Yes. Delta waves suggesting ventricular pre-excitation.
> D. Yes. Negative T waves in I, aVL, suggesting LV lateral wall ischemia.
> E. Yes. Incomplete RBBB suggesting arrhythmogenic cardiomyopathy.

F. Halbwachs (✉) · J. Havard
Biosense Webster, Mulhouse, France

C. Daval · C. Muresan
Cardiology Department, "Emile Muller" Hospital, Mulhouse, France

© The Author(s), under exclusive license to Springer Nature Switzerland AG 2022
L. Muresan (ed.), *Clinical Cases in Cardiac Electrophysiology: Supraventricular Arrhythmias*,
https://doi.org/10.1007/978-3-031-07357-1_16

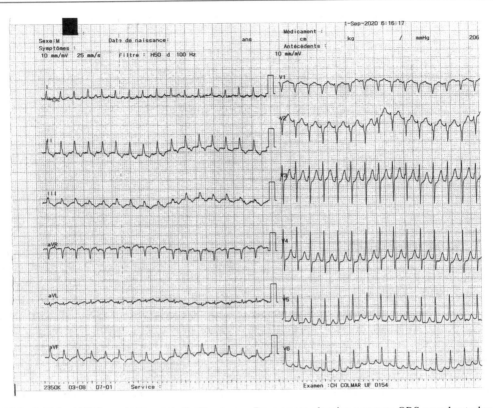

Fig. 16.1 A 12-lead ECG at admittance to the Emergency Department, showing a narrow QRS complex tachycardia with a heart rate of 206 bpm

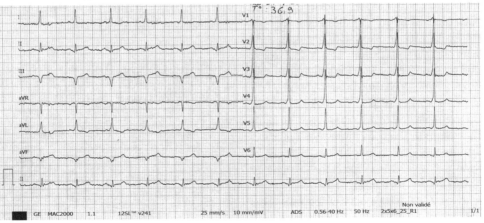

Fig. 16.2 A 12-lead ECG showing sinus rhythm with a heart rate of 75 bpm, QRS axis a −15°

Figure 16.2 shows sinus rhythm with a heart rate of 75 bpm, QRS axis a −15°, with overt ventricular pre-excitation, with positive delta waves in lead V1 to V6, lead I, aVL, negative in lead II, III and aVF. The diagnosis was therefore WPW syndrome.

Question 2: Where is the accessory pathway located?
A. Left lateral.
B. Left postero-septal.
C. Right postero-septal.
D. Right lateral.
E. Right antero-septal.

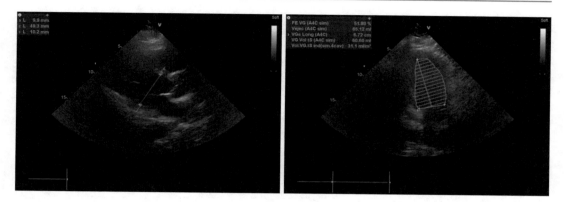

Fig. 16.3 *Left panel:* Transthoracic echocardiography image in parasternal long axis view showing a non-dilated LV with an ESD of 48 mm. *Right panel:* Apical 4 chamber view showing a LV EF% of 52%

An electrophysiological study was subsequently offered and accepted by the patient.

16.2 Electrophysiological study and RF Catheter Ablation Procedure

The electrophysiological study was performed under local anesthesia and conscious sedation. Vascular access was obtained using the modified Seldinger technique, under Doppler ultrasound guidance. A 6F quadripolar steerable catheter (Dynamic Extrem, Microport®) was introduced in a 9F 20 cm vascular sheath and was subsequently advanced via the right common femoral vein up to the bundle of His. A decapolar steerable catheter (Inquiry, Abbott®) was introduced in a 6F 20 cm vascular sheath and placed via the right common femoral vein in the coronary sinus, with the distal poles at the level of the lateral mitral annulus and the proximal poles at the level of the CS ostium. A bipolar non-steerable catheter (Viking, Boston Scientific®) was introduced in a 6F 20 cm vascular sheath and was subsequently advanced via the right common femoral vein up to the right ventricular apex.

Atrial and ventricular pacing were carried out at twice the diastolic threshold using the EP-4™ Cardiac Stimulator (Abbott®) system. Surface ECG and intracavitary ECGs were recorded by the WorkMate Claris™ System (Abbott®).

Radiofrequency ablation was delivered using a Biosense Webster® SmartTouch SF open-irrigated 3.5 mm tip with dual curve (D/F). The CARTO ® 3 electro-anatomic mapping System (Biosense Webster, Johnson & Johnson) was used to guide mapping and ablation of the accessory pathway.

The ECG at the beginning of the electrophysiological study is presented in Fig. 16.4.

Baseline AH was 99 ms, the HV interval was −10 ms, confirming the diagnosis of ventricular pre-excitation.

Retrograde conduction was present, concentric, non-decremental, with the earliest local atrial electrogram recorded at the level of the CS electrodes 7–8.

The effective anterograde refractory period of the accessory pathway at a coupling interval of 600 ms was <260 ms (value of the effective atrial refractory period), and at 400 ms it was < 260 ms (value of the effective atrial refractory period) (Fig. 16.5).

Catheter manipulation initiated the narrow QRS complex tachycardia in Fig. 16.6, with a cycle length of 320 ms, with a concentric atrial activation sequence, with the earliest atrial depolarization situated at the level of the coronary sinus catheter electrodes 7–8, corresponding to the postero-septal region. The tachycardia was terminated by 3 atrial ectopic beats (Fig. 16.7).

At the end of ventricular pacing at a fixed coupling interval of 300 ms, the return sequence was

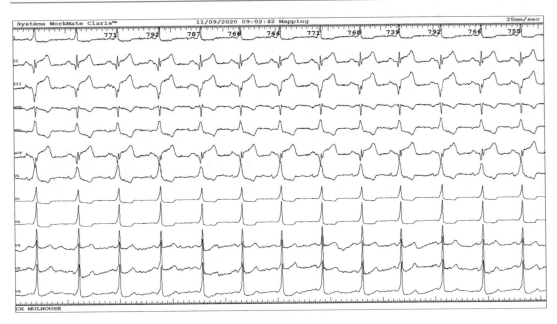

Fig. 16.4 A 12-lead ECG recorded at the beginning at the ablation procedure, showing sinus rhythm with ventricular pre-excitation, with a heart rate of 76 bpm

V-A-V, excluding an atrial tachycardia. A single ventricular extrastimulus during His refractoriness advanced the tachycardia with 15 ms. PPI at the apex of the right ventricle—TCL = 60 ms, confirming the diagnosis of AVRT using a manifest postero-septal accessory pathway.

Given the antegrade refractory period of <260 ms and the presence of repeated symptomatic episodes of ORT, a decision to ablate the accessory pathway was taken.

Mapping of the right postero-septal region was performed first, during sinus rhythm.

An anatomical map of the right atrium was first created, carefully identifying key structures such as the superior and inferior vena cava, the right atrial appendage and the bundle of His. Subsequently, an activation map of the ventricular myocardium around the tricuspid annulus was then performed, targeting the earliest local ventricular activation site during sinus rhythm. This was found to be at about 1 cm inside the coronary sinus (Fig. 16.8), where the local ventricular electrogram preceded the onset of the QRS complex by 15 ms. The local AV interval was short, and the local unipolar ventricular electrogram had a "QS" aspect.

Question 3: Is this a good ablation site?
A. Yes. The bipolar EGM precedes the surface ECG by 15 ms.
B. Yes. The unipolar EGM shows a "QS" aspect.
C. Yes. The local AV is short.
D. No. The surface ECG suggests a left postero-septal origin.
E. No. The local bipolar EGM is not the earliest local EGM that can be recorded in this patient.

Application of RF energy at this level interrupted the conduction over the accessory pathway 5 s after the initiation of RF delivery (Fig. 16.9). However, 30 s after the end of the RF delivery, pre-excitation spontaneously appeared on the ECG (Fig. 16.10). Three more RF applications were performed at the successful ablation site (Fig. 16.11), but after each RF application, the conduction over the accessory pathway reappeared.

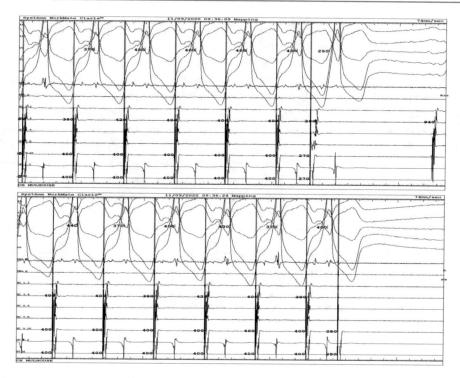

Fig. 16.5 Surface ECG leads I, II, III, V1, V2, and V3 together with intracavitary leads recorded from the distal and the proximal bipolar electrodes of the ablation catheter (Abl d, Abl p) and from the bipolar electrodes of the coronary sinus catheter (SC 1–2 to S-C 9–10) showing the effective antegrade refractory period of the accessory pathway at a coupling interval of 400 ms, of <260 ms. The effective antegrade refractory period of the atrium is 260 ms

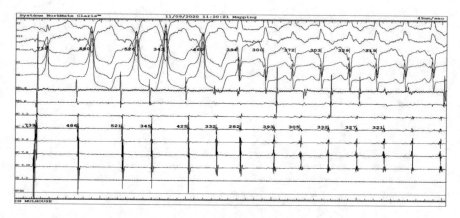

Fig. 16.6 Surface ECG leads I, II, III, V1, V2, and V3 together with intracavitary leads recorded from the distal and the proximal bipolar electrodes of the ablation catheter (Abl d, Abl p) and from the bipolar electrodes of the coronary sinus catheter (SC 1–2 to S-C 9–10) showing the initiation of a narrow QRS complex tachycardia with the earliest atrial depolarization situated at the postero-septal region

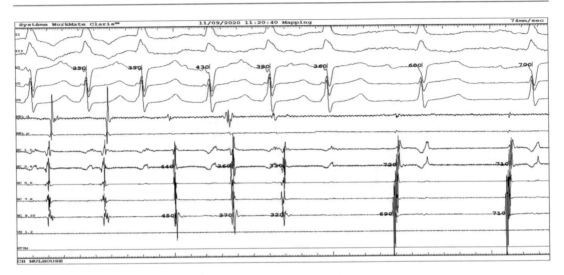

Fig. 16.7 Surface ECG leads I, II, III, V1, V2, and V3 together with intracavitary leads recorded from the distal and the proximal bipolar electrodes of the ablation catheter (Abl d, Abl p) and from the bipolar electrodes of the coronary sinus catheter (SC 1–2 to S-C 9–10) showing termination of the narrow QRS complex tachycardia by 3 atrial ectopic beats

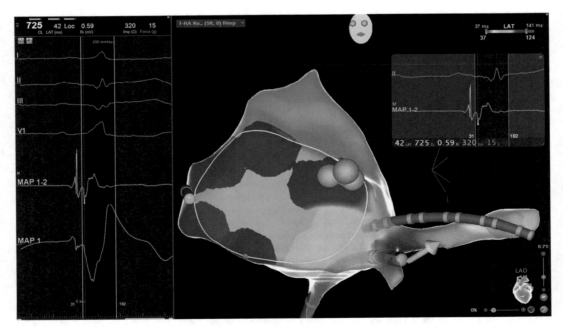

Fig. 16.8 CARTO image in LAO 45° showing the activation map of the right atrium during sinus rhythm, with the earliest local ventricular activation recorded in a narrow area in the right postero-septal region, inside the coronary sinus, where the earliest local ventricular activation precedes the QRS onset by 15 ms. Left side of the image: surface ECG leads I, II, III, V1, and intracavitary recordings from the distal bipolar electrode of the roving/ablation catheter (MAP 1–2), and the unipolar recording from the distal electrode of the roving/ablation catheter (M1), showing a "QS" aspect

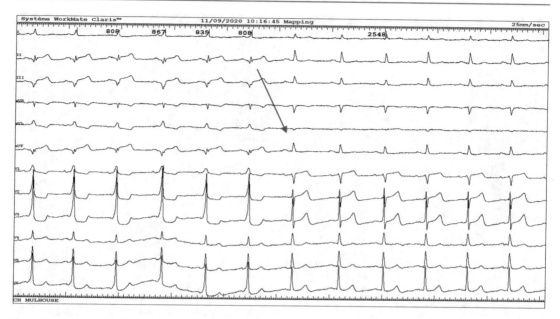

Fig. 16.9 A 12-lead ECG showing disappearance of conduction over the accessory pathway during RF application (red arrow)

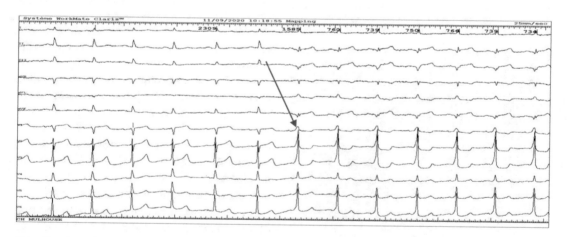

Fig. 16.10 A 12-lead ECG showing recurrence of conduction over the accessory pathway at the end of the RF application (red arrow)

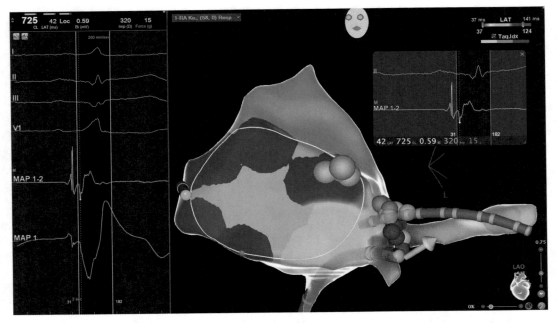

Fig. 16.11 CARTO image in LAO 45° (same as in Fig. 16.8) showing the activation map of the right atrium during sinus rhythm, with the earliest local ventricular activation recorded in a narrow area in the right postero-septal region, inside the coronary sinus, where the earliest local ventricular activation precedes the QRS onset by 15 ms, with superposed RF ablation lesions. Left side of the image: surface ECG leads I, II, III, V1, and intracavitary recordings from the distal bipolar electrode of the roving/ablation catheter (MAP 1–2), and the unipolar recording from the distal electrode of the roving/ablation catheter (M1), showing a "QS" aspect

---

Question 4: What is the next best step at this point of the procedure?

A. Increase power to 40 W.

B. Increase RF application time to an ablation index of at least 550.

C. Map the CS venous system for a better ablation site.

D. Ameliorate the local contact by taking a deflectable sheath.

E. Map the left postero-septal region.

Given the unsatisfactory result of the RF ablation in the right postero-septal region, and the aspect of the surface ECG (the presence of an R wave in lead V1 in Figs. 16.2 and 16.4), a decision to map the left postero-septal region was taken.

Access to the mitral valve was obtained using an antegrade approach. A single transseptal puncture was performed under fluoroscopic guidance using an 8.5F 67cm Swartz SL0™ transseptal sheath (Abbott®) and a BRK™ XS 71 cm needle (Abbott®).

After the transseptal puncture, anticoagulation was obtained with unfractionated heparin 70 IU/kg given as bolus, followed by continuous infusion of 12 IU/kg/h, with a target ACT of 300 s.

Once the access to the left atrium was granted, the SmartTouch SF roving/ablation catheter was introduced in the SL0 transseptal sheath and mapping of the mitral valve was performed.

An anatomical map of the left atrium was first created, showing a non-dilated LA of 94 ml. An activation map targeting the earliest local ventricular activation was subsequently created during sinus rhythm, careful analysis of the local ventricular electrograms recorded around the mitral annulus. The earliest local ventricular activation was recorded in the postero-septal region of the annulus, corresponding to the 7'clock position, where the local ventricular electrogram preceded the onset of the surface QRS complex by 25 ms. A sharp potential in-between the local

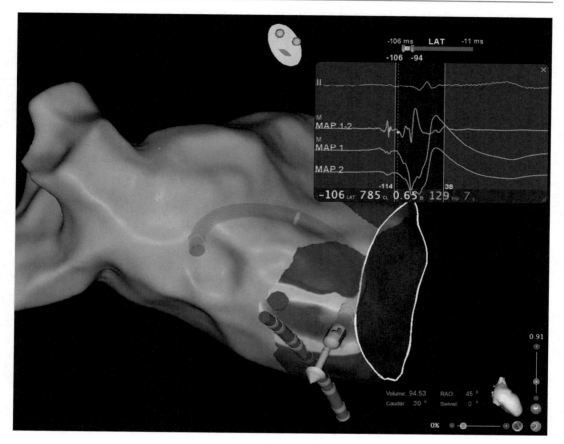

Fig. 16.12 CARTO image in RAO 47° showing the activation map of the left atrium during sinus rhythm. The area of the earliest antegrade ventricular activation is recorded in the postero-septal region of the mitral valve (red area), where the shortest AV was recorded. Of note, the electrodes 7–8 of the coronary sinus catheter are situated adjacent to this site

atrial and ventricular potential was recorded at this level, possibly corresponding to an accessory pathway potential (Fig. 16.12).

> **Question 5: Is this a better ablation site than the one in Fig. 16.8?**
> A. Yes. The bipolar EGM precedes the surface ECG by 25 ms.
> B. Yes. The unipolar EGM shows a "QS" aspect.
> C. Yes. The local AV is short.
> D. Yes. An accessory pathway potential can be seen at this site.
> E. All of the above.

The anatomical relationship between the earliest ventricular activation site during sinus rhythm recorded in the right atrium and the earliest ventricular activation site in the left atrium is presented in Fig. 16.13.

RF application at the site or earliest ventricular activation in the LA eliminated anterior conduction over the accessory pathway in less than 2 s (Figs. 16.14 and 16.15). Target power was set at 30 W, with a target ablation index of 450. Four additional RF applications were delivered at the successful ablation site, with no recurrence of the anterograde or retrograde conduction over the accessory pathway over a waiting period of 30 min.

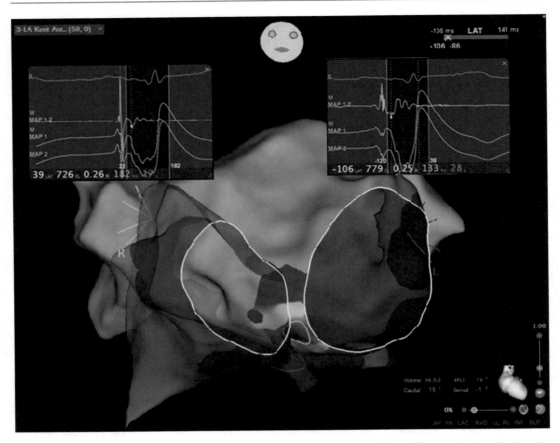

Fig. 16.13 CARTO image in antero-posterior view showing the anatomical relationship between the earliest ventricular activation site during sinus rhythm recorded in the right atrium and the earliest ventricular activation site in the left atrium. The recorded local electrograms are shown in the upper part of the image

The anatomical relationship between the RF application sites in the right and in the left postero-septal region is shown in Fig. 16.16.

The ECG at the end of the ablation procedure is shown in Fig. 16.17.

The ECG recorded 24 h after the ablation procedure is shown in Fig. 16.18.

The patient was discharged from the hospital 24 h later.

ANSWERS TO:
Question 1: C. Yes. Delta waves suggesting ventricular pre-excitation
Question 2: B. Left postero-septal
Question 3:
   D. No. The surface ECG suggests a left postero-septal origin

No. The local bipolar EGM is not the earliest local EGM that can be recorded in this patient.
Question 4: E. Map the left postero-septal region
Question 5: E. All of the above

16.3 Commentary

This case presents a catheter ablation procedure of a malignant left postero-septal accessory pathway with bidirectional conduction properties in a 59-year-old male patient with WPW syndrome. Several aspects related to the electrophysiological study and the ablation procedure deserve comments.

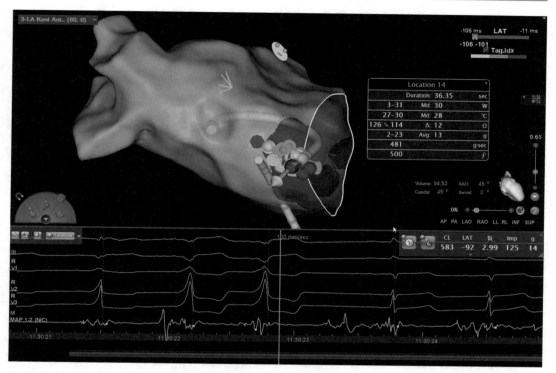

Fig. 16.14 CARTO image in RAO 45°, caudal 45° showing the position of the roving/ablation catheter at the successful ablation site in the left postero-septal region. The bottom part of the tracing shows disappearance of antegrade conduction over the accessory pathway during RF delivery

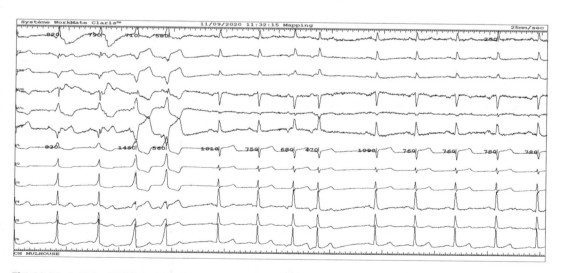

Fig. 16.15 A 12-lead ECG showing disappearance of conduction over the accessory pathway during the first RF application in the left postero-septal region

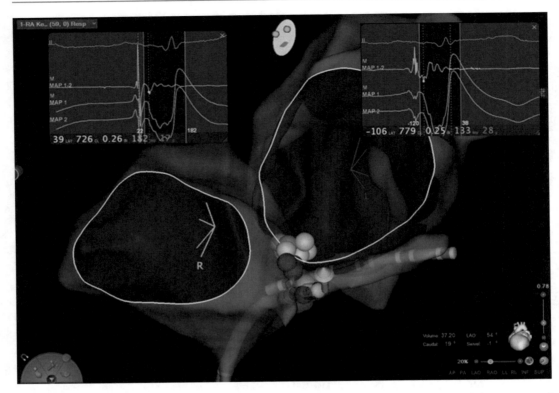

Fig. 16.16 CARTO image in LAO showing the anatomical relationship between the right and the left postero-septal regions, with superposed RF application lesions

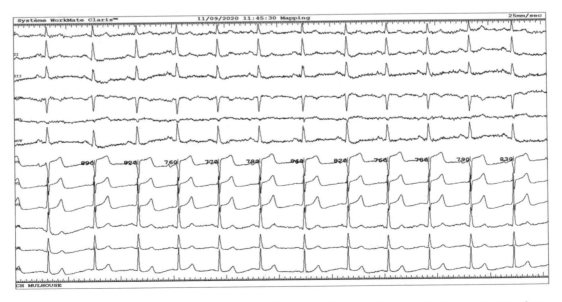

Fig. 16.17 A 12-lead ECG recorded at the end of the ablation procedure, showing sinus rhythm and absence of ventricular pre-excitation

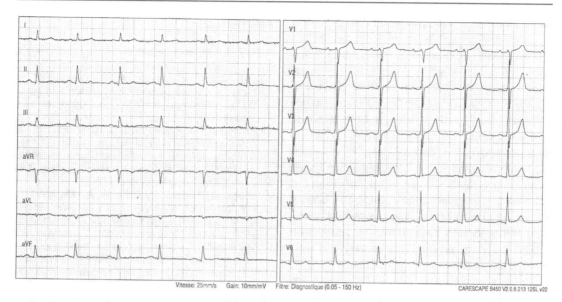

Fig. 16.18 A 12-lead ECG recorded 24 h after the ablation procedure, showing sinus rhythm with a heart rate of 75 bpm, QRS axis at +60° and absence of ventricular pre-excitation

As mentioned before, the localization of the accessory pathway using the 12-lead ECG should be the first step in the management of the patient when preparing for a catheter ablation procedure, and several algorithms have been developed to help the physician identify its location [1–6]. Postero-septal accessory pathways are characterized by the presence of negative delta waves in the inferior leads. Distinguishing left postero-septal pathways from right postero-septal pathways usually requires a careful analysis of the delta waves in lead V1. A positive delta wave in lead V1 is usually associated with the presence of a left postero-septal pathway, while a negative delta wave in lead V1 indicates the presence of a right postero-septal accessory pathway. Exception do exist and these must be kept in mind, such as the presence of multiple accessory pathways, the absence of maximal pre-excitation and an accelerated conduction through the AV node, where the ECG aspect can be misleading. An understanding of the anatomy of the postero-septal region of the annuli is extremely important before performing a catheter ablation procedure [7]. Distinguishing left-sided postero-septal pathways from right-sided postero-septal pathways is sometimes challenging [8]. An electro-anatomical mapping system can be very helpful in localizing the accessory pathway, in helping avoiding unnecessary, repeated RF ablation in suboptimal ablation sites, reproduce catheter positioning in desired ablation sites [9–11] and, when using contact sensor-equipped catheters, such as the SmartTouch SF catheter, provide valuable information on the contact between the ablation catheter and the atrial/ventricular tissue at the desired ablation site [12]. It should be kept in mind that when ablation of a postero-septal accessory pathway fails in the right postero-septal region, repeated RF lesions should not be attempted, since there is an increased risk of damaging surrounding anatomical structures (such as the circumflex coronary artery or the compact AV node) and mapping of the left postero-septal region should be attempted. As shown in Fig. 16.16, the optimal ablation site may be situated just a few mm away from a previously failed ablation site, but in the other atrium.

Another aspect worth mentioning is the fact that distinguishing between the benign or malignant character of an accessory pathway is usually based on the shortest pre-excited RR interval (SPERRI) during atrial fibrillation. A SPERRI <250 ms characterizes malignant accessory pathways, since these pathways are capable of rapidly conducting electrical impulses from the atria to the ventricles and precipitate ventricular fibrillation and sudden cardiac death [13, 14]. Some authors propose a value of less than 220 ms in children [15] or less than 200 ms after isoprenaline infusion [16, 17]. Other authors have proposed that an effective refractory period of the accessory pathway of less than 250 ms [18] be associated with a higher risk of developing malignant ventricular arrhythmias. However, this is not as relevant as the shortest pre-excited RR interval during atrial fibrillation, since malignant accessory pathways with an ERP >250 ms have been reported, and because the ERP of the AP is not a fixed value and can vary in time [19].

In the above-presented case, RF application in the right postero-septal region temporarily interrupted conduction over the accessory pathway. However, conduction over the accessory pathway recurred rapidly after the termination of RF application, since the location of the accessory pathway was situated in the left postero-septal region. Application of RF energy in the left postero-septal region definitively interrupted conduction over the accessory pathway.

Learning Point

- When ablating postero-septal accessory pathways, mapping should be commenced at the level of the tricuspid annulus. However, if ablation fails at this site, mapping of the postero-septal region of the mitral annulus should be performed.
- The use of an electro-anatomical mapping system is very useful in finding the optimal ablation site and in reducing the fluoroscopy time and dose throughout the ablation procedure.

References

1. Arruda MS, McClelland JH, Wang X, Beckman KJ, Widman LE, Gonzalez MD, et al. Development and validation of an ECG algorithm for identifying accessory pathway ablation site in Wolff-Parkinson-White syndrome. J Cardiovasc Electrophysiol. 1998;9(1):2–12.

2. Frank R, Chandon E, Deschamps JP, Leclerc JF, Fontaine G. [Revision of criteria for locating the accessory pathway by electrocardiogram in Wolff-Parkinson-White syndrome. A new algorithm]. Ann Cardiol Angeiol 1990;39(4):225–231.

3. Giorgi C, Nadeau R, Primeau R, Campa MA, Cardinal R, Shenasa M, et al. Comparative accuracy of the vectorcardiogram and electrocardiogram in the localization of the accessory pathway in patients with Wolff-Parkinson-White syndrome: validation of a new vectorcardiographic algorithm by intraoperative epicardial mapping and electrophysiologic studies. Am Heart J. 1990;119(3 Pt 1):592–8.

4. Li HY, Chang SL, Chuang CH, Lin MC, Lin YJ, Lo LW, et al. A novel and simple algorithm using surface electrocardiogram that localizes accessory conduction pathway in Wolff-Parkinson-White syndrome in pediatric patients. Acta Cardiol Sin. 2019;35(5):493–500.

5. Rantner LJ, Stuhlinger MC, Nowak CN, Spuller K, Etsadashvili K, Stuhlinger X, et al. Localizing the accessory pathway in ventricular preexcitation patients using a score based algorithm. Methods Inf Med. 2012;51(1):3–12.

6. Saidullah S, Shah B, Ullah H, Aslam Z, Khan MA. Localization of accessory pathway in patients with Wolff-Parkinson-White syndrome from surface ECG using Arruda Algorithm. J Ayub Med Coll Abbottabad. 2016;28(3):441–4.

7. Jazayeri MR, Dhala A, Deshpande S, Blanck Z, Sra J, Akhtar M. Posteroseptal accessory pathways: an overview of anatomical characteristics, electrocardiographic patterns, electrophysiological features, and ablative therapy. J Interv Cardiol. 1995;8(1):89–101.

8. Liu E, Shehata M, Swerdlow C, Amorn A, Cingolani E, Kannarkat V, et al. Approach to the difficult septal atrioventricular accessory pathway: the importance of regional anatomy. Circ Arrhythm Electrophysiol. 2012;5(3):e63–6.

9. Drago F, Grifoni G, Remoli R, Russo MS, Righi D, Pazzano V, et al. Radiofrequency catheter ablation of left-sided accessory pathways in children using a new fluoroscopy integrated 3D-mapping system. Europace. 2017;19(7):1198–203.

10. Raatikainen MJ, Pedersen AK. Catheter ablation of a difficult accessory pathway guided by coronary

sinus venography and 3D electroanatomical mapping. Europace. 2010;12(8):1200–1.

11. Ishizu T, Seo Y, Igarashi M, Sekiguchi Y, Machino-Ohtsuka T, Ogawa K, et al. Noninvasive localization of accessory pathways in wolff-parkinson-white syndrome by three-dimensional speckle tracking echocardiography. Circ Cardiovasc Imaging. 2016;9(6):e004532.

12. Page SP, Dhinoja M. SmartTouch - the emerging role of contact force technology in complex catheter ablation. Arrhythmia Electrophysiol Rev. 2012;1(1):59–62.

13. Klein GJ, Bashore TM, Sellers TD, Pritchett EL, Smith WM, Gallagher JJ. Ventricular fibrillation in the Wolff-Parkinson-White syndrome. N Engl J Med. 1979;301(20):1080–5.

14. Al-Khatib SM, Arshad A, Balk EM, Das SR, Hsu JC, Joglar JA, et al. Risk Stratification for Arrhythmic Events in Patients With Asymptomatic Pre-Excitation: A Systematic Review for the 2015 ACC/AHA/HRS Guideline for the Management of Adult Patients With Supraventricular Tachycardia: A Report of the American College of Cardiology/American Heart Association Task Force on Clinical Practice Guidelines and the Heart Rhythm Society. J Am Coll Cardiol. 2016;67(13):1624–38.

15. Bromberg BI, Lindsay BD, Cain ME, Cox JL. Impact of clinical history and electrophysiologic characterization of accessory pathways on management strategies to reduce sudden death among children with Wolff-Parkinson-White syndrome. J Am Coll Cardiol. 1996;27(3):690–5.

16. Brembilla-Perrot B, Terrier de la Chaise A, Marcon F, Cherrier F, Pernot C. [Should the Isuprel test be performed systematically in Wolff-Parkinson-White syndrome?]. Arch Mal Coeur Vaiss. 1988;81(10):1227–1233.

17. Wellens HJ, Durrer D. Wolff-Parkinson-White syndrome and atrial fibrillation. Relation between refractory period of accessory pathway and ventricular rate during atrial fibrillation. Am J Cardiol. 1974;34(7):777–82.

18. Santinelli V, Radinovic A, Manguso F, Vicedomini G, Ciconte G, Gulletta S, et al. Asymptomatic ventricular preexcitation: a long-term prospective follow-up study of 293 adult patients. Circ Arrhythm Electrophysiol. 2009;2(2):102–7.

19. Oliver C, Brembilla-Perrot B. Is the measurement of accessory pathway refractory period reproducible? Indian Pacing Electrophysiol J. 2012;12(3):93–101.

Frédéric Halbwachs, Justine Havard, Ronan Le Bouar, and Jacques Levy

17.1 Case Presentation

A 42-year-old male patient with a history of repeated episodes of palpitations with sudden onset, with alternating regular and irregular rhythm, of variable duration from several minutes to 1 h, presented to the Cardiology Department for another episode of palpitations with sudden onset and irregular rhythm, which had started 30 min prior to his presentation to the hospital. His only cardiovascular risk factor was represented by active smoking. He had no personal history of syncope, and there was no family history of sudden cardiac death. He denied consumption of alcohol or illicit drugs. He was on no chronic medication. His CHA_2DS_2-VASc score was 0, his HAS-BLED score was 0.

At physical exam, his blood pressure was 111/77 mmHg, heart rate of 111 bpm, SpO_2 96% breathing room air, $H = 173$ cm, $W = 66$ kg, BMI $= 22$ kg/m^2, heart sounds were rapid and irregular, there was no audible heart murmur, there were no signs of congestive heart failure, pulmonary auscultation was normal.

His ECG is presented in Fig. 17.1.

Transthoracic echocardiography performed in the Emergency Department showed a non-dilated LV with a preserved LV EF%, absence of LV hypertrophy, no significant valve disease, non-dilated right ventricle, absence of pericardial fluid (Fig. 17.2).

His ECG obtained after the administration of 2 mg/kg iv of flecainide is presented in Fig. 17.3.

His biological workup showed a Hb level of 13.1 g/dl, leucocytes 4.4×10^9/L, platelets 237×10^9/L, CRP <3 mg/L, BUN 3.6 mmol/L, creatinine 88 µmol/L, glycemia 6.0 mmol/L, Na+ 141 mmol/L, K+ 4.5 mmol/L, total proteins 71 g/L, TSH 1.9 IU/L, NT pro-BNP < 30 pg/ml.

> **Question 1. What is the nature of the tachycardia presented in Fig. 17.1?**
> A. Ventricular tachycardia.
> B. Supraventricular tachycardia with bundle branch block.
> C. Pre-excited atrial fibrillation.
> D. Bundle branch reentry ventricular tachycardia.
> E. Torsade des pointes.

Figure 17.1 shows "FBI tachycardia" that stands for "Fast, Broad, Irregular." It corresponds to atrial fibrillation in patients with ventricular pre-excitation. The variation in the QRS width is explained by different degrees of fusion between

F. Halbwachs (✉) · J. Havard
Biosense Webster, Mulhouse, France

R. Le Bouar · J. Levy
Cardiology Department, "Emile Muller" Hospital, Mulhouse, France

L. Muresan (ed.), *Clinical Cases in Cardiac Electrophysiology: Supraventricular Arrhythmias*, https://doi.org/10.1007/978-3-031-07357-1_17

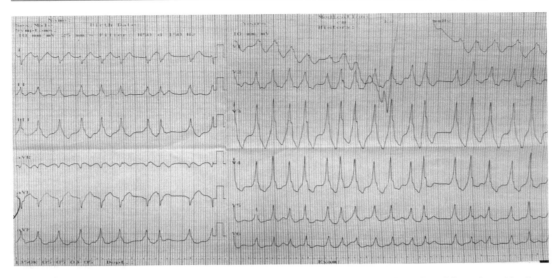

Fig. 17.1 ECG recorded in the Emergency Department showing "FBI" tachycardia: Fast, Broad, Irregular, with a heart rate of 170–180 bpm

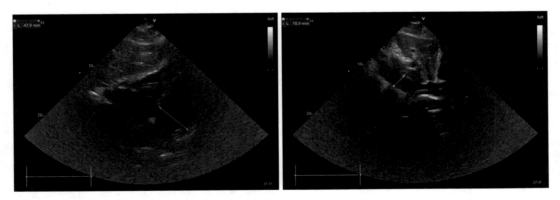

Fig. 17.2 *Left panel:* Transthoracic echocardiography image in subcostal view showing a non-dilated LV, with an ESD of 48 mm. *Right panel:* Subcostal view showing a non-dilated IVC, with a diameter of 19 mm

the ventricular activation using the His-Purkinje network and the accessory pathway.

Figure 17.2 shows sinus rhythm with ventricular pre-excitation, with positive delta waves in leads V1-V6, lead II, III and aVF, negative in lead I and aVL.

The diagnosis of WPW syndrome was established, the arrhythmia being pre-exited atrial fibrillation. An electrophysiological study was offered and subsequently accepted by the patient.

Question 2: Where is the accessory pathway located?
A. Left lateral.
B. Left postero-septal.
C. Right postero-septal.
D. Right lateral.
E. Right antero-septal.

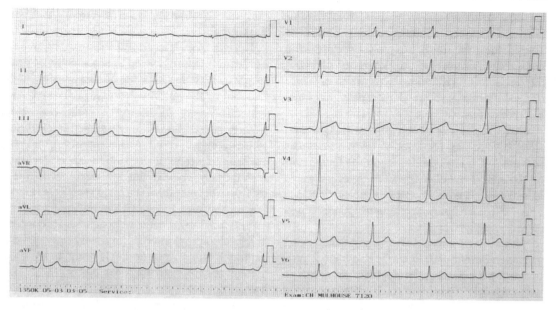

Fig. 17.3 A 12-lead ECG at admittance to the Cardiology department, showing sinus rhythm with a heart rate of 59 bpm

17.2   Electrophysiological Study and RF Catheter Ablation Procedure

The electrophysiological study was performed 48 h after the flecainide administration, under local anesthesia and conscious sedation. Vascular access was obtained using the modified Seldinger technique, under Doppler ultrasound guidance. A 6F quadripolar steerable catheter (Dynamic Extrem, Microport®) was introduced in a 9F 20 cm vascular sheath and was subsequently advanced via the right common femoral vein up to the bundle of His. A second 6F quadripolar steerable catheter (Dynamic Extrem, Microport®) was introduced in a 6F 20 cm vascular sheath and placed via the right common femoral vein in the coronary sinus, with the proximal poles at the level of the coronary sinus ostium. A bipolar non-steerable catheter (Viking, Boston Scientific®) was introduced in a 6F 20 cm vascular sheath and was subsequently advanced via the right common femoral vein up to the right ventricular apex.

Atrial and ventricular pacing were carried out at twice the diastolic threshold using the EP-4™

Cardiac Stimulator (Abbott®) system. Surface ECG and intracavitary ECGs were recorded by the WorkMate Claris™ System (Abbott®).

Radiofrequency ablation was delivered using a Biosense Webster® SmartTouch SF open-irrigated 3.5 mm tip with double curve (D and F). The CARTO ® 3 electro-anatomic mapping System (Biosense Webster, Johnson & Johnson) was used to guide mapping and ablation of the accessory pathway.

Measurement of basal conduction intervals found a HV interval of 10 ms, confirming ventricular pre-excitation.

Retrograde conduction was present, concentric, decremental, confirming the absence of conduction over an accessory pathway, being compatible with conduction over the AV node.

The antegrade effective refractory period of the accessory pathway while pacing the distal coronary sinus electrodes at a coupling interval of 600 ms was 260 ms. The antegrade effective refractory period of the accessory pathway while pacing the distal coronary sinus electrodes at a coupling interval of 400 ms was 230 ms, confirming the malignant character of the accessory pathway. At this coupling interval, atrial fibrillation was induced. After a waiting period of 30 min, the atrial fibrillation persisted. Given the malignant character of the accessory pathway, the presence of symptomatic recurrent episodes of atrial fibrillation, a decision to ablate the accessory pathway was taken.

Given the aspect of the 12-lead ECG during sinus rhythm, the localization of the accessory pathway was considered to be in the lateral part of the mitral annulus (positive delta waves in leads V1-V6, lead II, III and aVF, negative in lead I and aVL). Mapping of the mitral annulus was subsequently performed.

Access to the mitral valve was obtained using an antegrade approach. A single transseptal puncture was performed under fluoroscopic guidance using an 8.5F 67cm Swartz SL0™ transseptal sheath (Abbott®) and a BRK ™ XS 71 cm needle (Abbott®).

After the transseptal puncture, anticoagulation was obtained with unfractionated Heparin 70 IU/kg given as bolus, followed by continuous infusion of 12 IU/kg/h, with a target ACT of 300 seconds.

Once the access to the left atrium was granted, the SmartTouch SF roving/ablation catheter was introduced in the SL0 transseptal sheath, and mapping of the mitral valve was performed. An anatomical map of the left atrium was first created, which showed a non-dilated felt atrium with a volume of 65 ml. An activation map targeting the earliest local ventricular activation was subsequently created during atrial fibrillation, with careful analysis of the local ventricular electrograms recorded around the mitral annulus. The earliest local ventricular activation was recorded in the lateral region of the annulus, corresponding to the 2'clock position, where the local ventricular electrogram preceded the onset of the surface QRS complex by 15 ms (Fig. 17.4).

Ablation was carried out during atrial fibrillation. Target ablation parameters were a power of 30 W and an ablation index of 450. Application of RF energy at the site of the earliest local ventricular activation interrupted the conduction

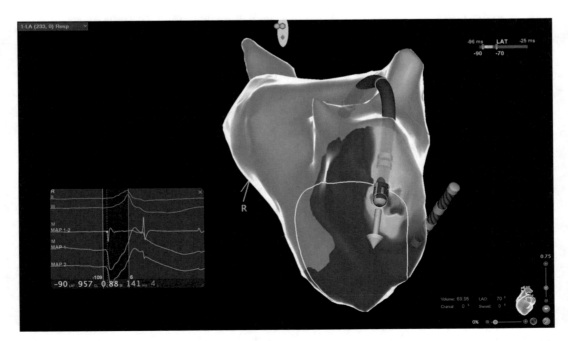

Fig. 17.4 CARTO image in LAO 70° showing the activation map of the left atrium during atrial fibrillation. The area of the earliest antegrade ventricular activation is recorded in the antero-lateral region of the mitral valve (red area), where the shortest AV was recorded. At this site, the local bipolar ventricular electrogram preceded the surface ECG QRS complex by 15 ms. The local unipolar electrogram had a QS aspect

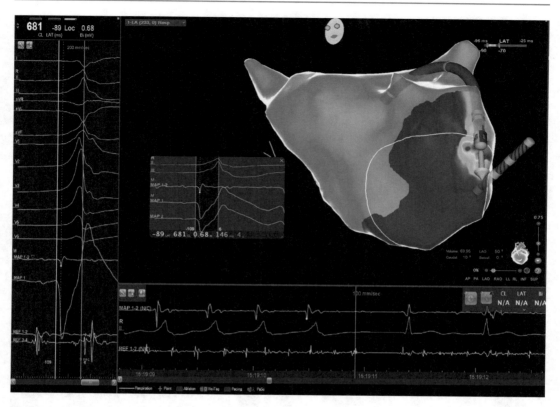

Fig. 17.5 CARTO image in LAO showing the position of the roving/ablation catheter at the successful ablation site at the level of the lateral part of the mitral annulus. The local bipolar electrogram recorded by the roving/ablation catheter (MAP 1–2) together with surface ECG lead II and the distal coronary sinus electrograms are shown below (REF 1, 2). The ablation catheter records a high amplitude ventricular potential and a very low amplitude atrial potential. Application of RF energy at this site rapidly interrupted the conduction at the level of the accessory pathway, with disappearance of conduction after the fourth QRS complex. The distal coronary sinus catheter shows persistence of atrial fibrillation despite disappearance of antegrade conduction over the accessory pathway

over the accessory pathway in less than 2 s after the second RF application onset (Fig. 17.5). However, despite the successful ablation of the accessory pathway, atrial fibrillation persisted.

The activation map of the LA with superposed RF lesions at the successful ablation site is shown in Fig. 17.6.

Question 3: Where is the next best step in the management of this patient at this point of the procedure, given the persistence of atrial fibrillation after the successful ablation of the accessory pathway?
A. Administer Flecainide 2 mg/kgc.
B. Administer Amiodarone 300 mg iv.

C. Terminate the ablation procedure.
D. Perform PVI.
E. I don't know.

Given the persistence of atrial fibrillation after the successful ablation of the accessory pathway, the possibility of atrial fibrillation being non-related to the accessory pathway was taken into consideration. A bipolar map of the left atrium was subsequently performed, which showed a voltage > 0.5 mV in all areas of the left atrium (Fig. 17.7), suggesting the absence of an arrhythmic substrate at this level.

Considering the possibility of atrial fibrillation arising from the pulmonary veins, the persis-

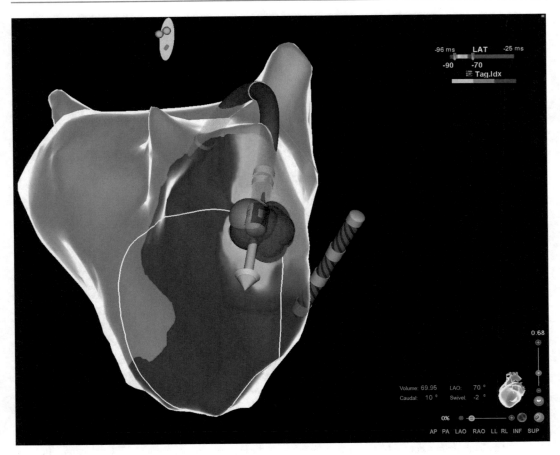

Fig. 17.6 CARTO image in LAO 70° (same as in Fig. 17.4) showing the activation map of the left atrium during atrial fibrillation with superposed RF ablation lesions at the successful ablation site (red dots)

tence of atrial fibrillation at this point of the procedure, a decision to perform PVI was taken. This was performed with a target power of 30 W and an ablation index of 450 for the anterior LA wall and 350 for the posterior LA wall (Figs. 17.8 and 17.9).

The ECG recorded after PVI is presented in Fig. 17.10.

There were no complications related to the procedure.

The patient was discharged from the hospital 24 h later, on no antiarrhythmic medication, but on anticoagulant treatment. Given his CHADS-VASc score of 0, the recommended duration of the anticoagulant treatment was 3 months.

ANSWERS TO:
Question 1: C. Pre-excited atrial fibrillation
Question 2: A. Left lateral
Question 3: Open for discussion.

17.3 Commentary

The present case illustrates a catheter ablation procedure of a left lateral accessory pathway and PVI in a 42-year-old male patient with WPW syndrome and atrial fibrillation, in whom atrial

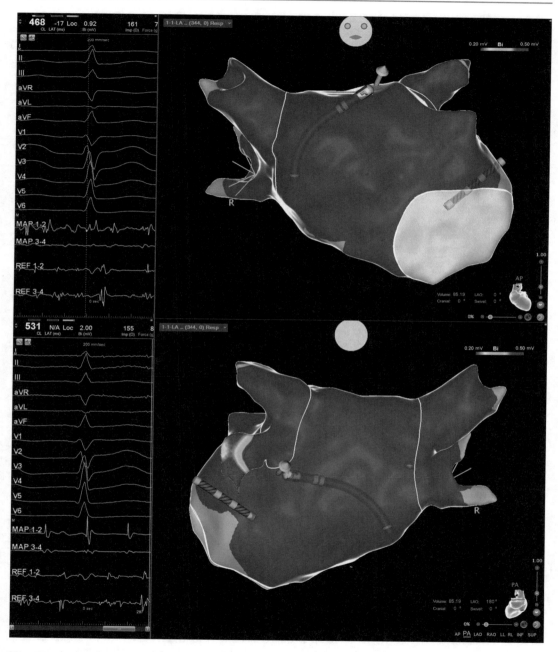

Fig. 17.7 CARTO image in antero-posterior view (upper panel) and postero-anterior view (lower panel) showing the bipolar voltage map of the left atrium during atrial fibrillation. The red areas represent atrial tissue with low voltage (<0.2 mV), the purple area represents atrial tissue with normal voltage (>0.5 mV), and green/blue areas represent atrial tissue with borderline voltage (0.2–0.5 mV). The left atrial tissue has a high voltage in all areas, argument in favor of absence of an arrhythmic substrate

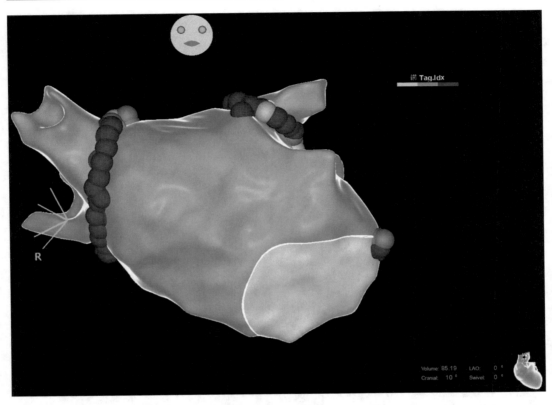

Fig. 17.8 CARTO image in AP view showing the anatomical map of the LA with superposed RF lesions after the ablation of the accessory pathway (lateral part of the mitral annulus) and after successful PVI

fibrillation persisted after successful RF ablation of the accessory pathway. This observation and its possible management strategies merit further discussion.

Atrial fibrillation occurs in up to 50% of patients with WPW syndrome [1]. The mechanism of atrial fibrillation in patients with WPW syndrome is different from that of AF in structural heart disease [2, 3]. Several hypotheses have been proposed, such as multiple intra-atrial wavefront collision [4], AP-mediated premature atrial contractions initiating AF in patients with multiple accessory pathways [5], abnormal electrical impulse circulation due to the presence of atrial double potentials [6], PVC with retrograde conduction induced AF [7], micro-reentry within the branching networks of the accessory pathway [2], maintenance of atrial reentry by increased structural heterogeneity due to the presence of the AP [8], accessory pathway related atrial refractoriness dispersion [2]. Even though elucidation of the exact mechanism has not yet been

accomplished, there is much less ambiguity about its treatment.

The treatment of atrial fibrillation in patients with WPW is ablation of the accessory pathway. This is sufficient in most cases to prevent atrial fibrillation recurrence [9], and no further RF lesion is generally necessary during the ablation procedure. However, in some patients, such as in the above presented case, atrial fibrillation may persist despite successful accessory pathway ablation. The persistence of atrial fibrillation in these cases might be explained by an underlying heart disease causing atrial fibrillation, coexisting with the presence of the AP [10]. Treatment of atrial fibrillation in these cases is not well established, and no consensus currently exists. However, a couple of studies exist in the literature treating this subject. In the experience of Kawabata et al., pulmonary vein isolation in addition to accessory pathway ablation was not associated with a reduced AF recurrence after catheter ablation [11]. In their population of 96

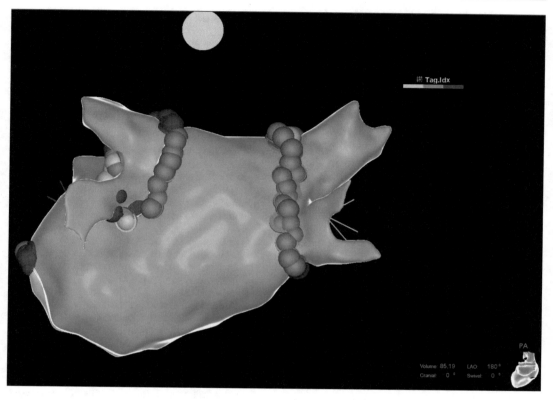

Fig. 17.9 CARTO image in PA view showing the anatomical map of the LA with superposed RF lesions after the ablation of the accessory pathway (lateral part of the mitral annulus) and after successful PVI

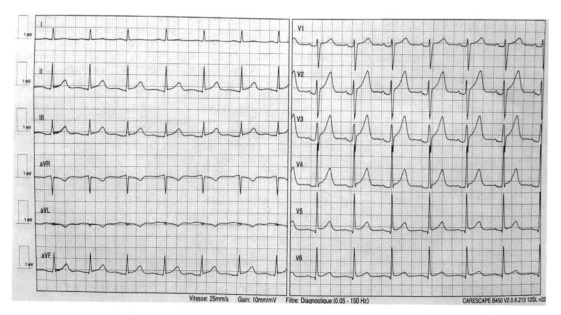

Fig. 17.10 A 12-lead ECG recorded after the ablation procedure showing sinus rhythm with a heart rate of 76 bpm, QRS axis at +60°, absence of LV hypertrophy, absence of ischemia, and absence of ventricular pre-excitation

patients, 64 underwent ablation of the accessory pathway alone and 32 underwent ablation of the accessory pathway + PVI. At follow-up, the recurrence rate of atrial fibrillation did not significantly differ between the two groups (18.8% in the AP ablation + PVI vs. 25% in the AP ablation only, $p = 0.53$). Freedom from AF at 3 months post-catheter ablation was 87.5%, after 1 year 85.5%, and after 5 years 64.6% in the accessory pathway ablation-only group, while in the AP ablation + PVI group it was 90.6% after 3 months, 87.1% after 1 year, and 77.8% after 5 years ($p = $ ns).

In the second study, Wu et al. recently reported their experience with additional PVI in patients who underwent accessory pathway ablation [12]. Compared to patients with WPW syndrome and atrial fibrillation who underwent ablation of the accessory pathway alone, the recurrence rate of atrial fibrillation after additional PVI was not significantly different (15.5% vs 10.5%, respectively; $P = 0.373$). Furthermore, PVI was not associated with the risk of atrial fibrillation recurrence ($H = 0.66$; 95% CI, 0.26–1.68; $P = 0.380$). Atrial fibrillation recurrence was lower only in those patients who presented advanced interatrial block on the surface ECG.

Further studies on larger populations are needed in order to establish the optimal treatment strategy in patients with WPW and atrial fibrillation in whom atrial fibrillation persists after successful catheter ablation of the accessory pathway.

Learning Point

- Atrial fibrillation of patients with WPW is usually related to the presence of the accessory pathway.
- In the majority of cases, ablation of the accessory pathway alone is sufficient for the treatment of atrial fibrillation.
- In the case of AF persistence after successful catheter ablation of the accessory pathway, AF may be non-AP mediated and its treatment should be discussed on a case-by-case basis.

References

1. Brugada J, Katritsis DG, Arbelo E, Arribas F, Bax JJ, Blomstrom-Lundqvist C, et al. 2019 ESC Guidelines for the management of patients with supraventricular tachycardiaThe Task Force for the management of patients with supraventricular tachycardia of the European Society of Cardiology (ESC). Eur Heart J. 2020;41(5):655–720.
2. Centurion OA. Atrial Fibrillation in the Wolff-Parkinson-White Syndrome. J Atr Fibrillation. 2011;4(1):287.
3. Centurion OA, Shimizu A, Isomoto S, Konoe A. Mechanisms for the genesis of paroxysmal atrial fibrillation in the Wolff Parkinson-White syndrome: intrinsic atrial muscle vulnerability vs. electrophysiological properties of the accessory pathway. Europace. 2008;10(3):294–302.
4. Ong JJ, Cha YM, Kriett JM, Boyce K, Feld GK, Chen PS. The relation between atrial fibrillation wavefront characteristics and accessory pathway conduction. J Clin Invest. 1995;96(5):2284–96.
5. Sharma AD, Klein GJ, Guiraudon GM, Milstein S. Atrial fibrillation in patients with Wolff-Parkinson-White syndrome: incidence after surgical ablation of the accessory pathway. Circulation. 1985;72(1):161–9.
6. Hsieh MH, Tai CT, Chiang CE, Tsai CF, Chen YJ, Chan P, et al. Double atrial potentials recorded in the coronary sinus in patients with Wolff-Parkinson-White syndrome: a possible mechanism of induced atrial fibrillation. J Interv Cardiac Electrophysiol. 2004;11(2):97–103.
7. Iesaka Y, Yamane T, Takahashi A, Goya M, Kojima S, Soejima Y, et al. Retrograde multiple and multifiber accessory pathway conduction in the Wolff-Parkinson-White syndrome: potential precipitating factor of atrial fibrillation. J Cardiovasc Electrophysiol. 1998;9(2):141–51.
8. Frame LH, Page RL, Hoffman BF. Atrial reentry around an anatomic barrier with a partially refractory excitable gap. A canine model of atrial flutter. Circ Res. 1986;58(4):495–511.
9. Haissaguerre M, Fischer B, Labbe T, Lemetayer P, Montserrat P, d'Ivernois C, et al. Frequency of recurrent atrial fibrillation after catheter ablation of overt accessory pathways. Am J Cardiol. 1992;69(5):493–7.
10. Fujimura O, Klein GJ, Yee R, Sharma AD. Mode of onset of atrial fibrillation in the Wolff-Parkinson-White syndrome: how important is the accessory pathway? J Am Coll Cardiol. 1990;15(5):1082–6.
11. Kawabata M, Goya M, Takagi T, Yamashita S, Iwai S, Suzuki M, et al. The impact of B-type natriuretic peptide levels on the suppression of accompanying atrial fibrillation in Wolff-Parkinson-White syndrome patients after accessory pathway ablation. J Cardiol. 2016;68(6):485–91.
12. Wu JT, Zhao DQ, Li FF, Zhang LM, Hu J, Fan XW, et al. Effect of pulmonary vein isolation on atrial fibrillation recurrence after accessory pathway ablation in patients with Wolff-Parkinson-White syndrome. Clin Cardiol. 2020;43(12):1511–6.

Case 18

Ronan Le Bouar, Frédéric Halbwachs,
Matthieu George, Serban Schiau,
and Thomas Robein

18

18.1 Case Presentation

An 18-year-old male patient with a past medical history of recurrent undocumented episodes of palpitations with sudden onset and offset, with a regular rhythm, variable duration up to 1 h, presents to the Emergency Department for another episode of palpitations with regular rhythm, which had started 20 min prior to his presentation to the hospital, and that had suddenly terminated short before his arrival in the Emergency Department. He had a diagnosis of WPW syndrome established a few months prior and of prolactinoma. He had no cardiovascular risk factors. He had no personal history of syncope, no family history of sudden cardiac death. He denied consumption of alcohol or illicit drugs. His medication at home consisted of flecainide 100 mg. At physical exam, his blood pressure was 115/79 mmHg, heart rate of 75 bpm, SpO$_2$ 99% breathing room air, H = 187 cm, W = 84 kg, BMI = 24.02 kg/m^2, heart sounds were regular, there was no audible heart murmur, there were no signs of heart failure, pulmonary auscultation was nor-mal. His ECG recorded in the Emergency Department is presented in Fig. 18.1.

The patient was transferred to the Cardiology Department for further investigations and management.

Transthoracic echocardiography showed a non-dilated LV with normal systolic and diastolic function, absence of LV hypertrophy, no significant valve disease, non-dilated RV, absence of pulmonary hypertension, absence of pericardial effusion (Figs. 18.2 and 18.3).

His biological workup showed a Hb level of 14.4 g/dl, leucocytes 5.26 × 10^9/L, platelets 231 × 10^9/L, CRP <3 mg/l, BUN 3.1 mmol/l, creatinine 61 μmol/l, glycemia 5.1 mmol/l, Na+ 141 mmol/l, K+ 4.0 mmol/l, total proteins 75 g/l, TSH 1.63 IU/L, troponin <0.015 ng/ml, NT pro-BNP < 30 pg/ml.

> **Question 1: Where is the accessory pathway situated?**
> A. Right antero-septal.
> B. Right lateral.
> C. Right postero-septal.
> D. Left postero-septal.
> E. Parahisian.

R. Le Bouar (✉) · S. Schiau
Cardiology Department, "Emile Muller" Hospital,
Mulhouse, France
e-mail: LEBOUARR@ghrmsa.fr

F. Halbwachs · M. George · T. Robein
Biosense Webster, Mulhouse, France

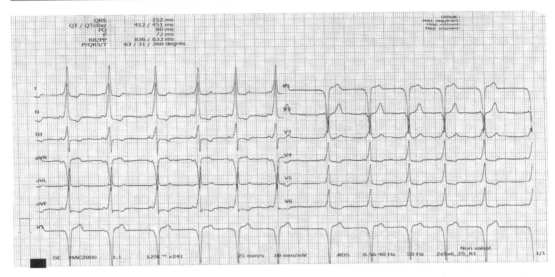

Fig. 18.1 A 12-lead ECG at admittance to the cardiology department showing sinus rhythm with a heart rate of 75 bpm, QRS axis at +30°, a short pR interval of 86 ms, the presence of delta waves, negative T waves in leads V3-V6, I, aVL, II, III, and aVF, compatible with ventricular pre-excitation

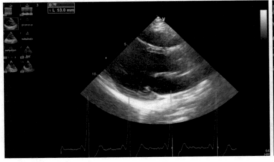
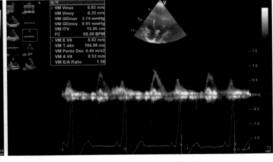

Fig. 18.2 *Left panel:* Transthoracic echocardiography image in parasternal long axis view showing a non-dilated LV with an end diastolic diameter of 52 mm, absence of LV hypertrophy. *Right panel:* Pulsed Doppler interrogation of the transmitral flow showing a normal diastolic function (E/A>1)

Question 2. What is the next best step in the stratification of the arrhythmic risk of this patient?

A. Perform a physical stress test to non-invasively assess the effective refractory period of the AP.

B. Perform a 7-day Holter ECG to document possible episodes of atrial fibrillation.

C. Perform epinephrine stress test.

D. Perform a transesophageal non-invasive electrophysiological study.

E. Perform an invasive electrophysiological study.

An exercise stress test was considered the next best step in the stratification of the arrhythmic risk of this patient. This was carried out 72 h after the interruption of flecainide, up to 120 W, 6.2 METS, when it was stopped do to fatigue, reaching a maximum heart rate of 179 bpm, BP = 147/78 mmHg, with no sudden disappearance of ventricular pre-excitation on the 12-lead ECG (Fig. 18.4). No conclusion regarding the benign or malignant character of the accessory pathway could be drawn from this test.

Given the aspect of pre-excitation on the 12-lead ECG, showing negative delta waves in lead V1, aVL, positive delta waves in leads II, III

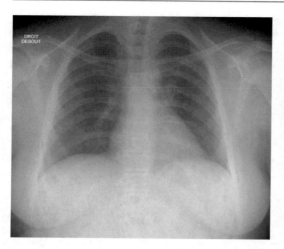

Fig. 18.3 Chest X-ray in postero-anterior view showing a normal cardiac silhouette, no signs of pulmonary hypertension, no pleural effusion, no signs of parenchymal infection, gynecomastia

and aVF and a QRS transition in lead V4, an antero-septal or parahisian location was suspected.

An invasive electrophysiological study was offered and accepted by the patient.

18.2   Electrophysiological Study and RF Catheter Ablation Procedure

The electrophysiological study was performed under local anesthesia and conscious sedation, 5 days after the interruption of flecainide. Vascular access was obtained using the modified Seldinger technique, under Doppler ultrasound guidance. A 6F quadripolar steerable catheter (Dynamic Extrem, Microport®) was introduced in a 9F 20 cm vascular sheath and was subsequently advanced via the right common femoral vein up to the bundle of His. A decapolar steerable catheter (Inquiry, Abbott®) was introduced in a 6F 20 cm vascular sheath and placed via the right common femoral vein in the coronary sinus, with the distal poles at the level of the lateral mitral annulus and the proximal poles at the level of the CS ostium. A bipolar non-steerable catheter (Viking, Boston Scientific®) was introduced in a 6F 20 cm vascular sheath and was subsequently

advanced via the right common femoral vein up to the right ventricular apex.

Atrial and ventricular pacing were carried out at twice the diastolic threshold using the EP-4™ Cardiac Stimulator (Abbott®) system. Surface ECG and intracavitary ECGs were recorded by the WorkMate Claris™ System (Abbott®).

Radiofrequency ablation was delivered using a Biosense Webster® SmartTouch SF open-irrigated 3.5 mm tip with D curve. The CARTO ® 3 electro-anatomic mapping System (Biosense Webster, Johnson & Johnson) was used to guide mapping and ablation of the accessory pathway.

The ECG at the beginning of the electrophysiological study is presented in Fig. 18.5. The presence of a "QS" aspect in lead V1 was an argument in favor of a parahisian rather than an antero-septal location.

Baseline AH was 100 ms, the HV interval was −20 ms, confirming the diagnosis of ventricular pre-excitation.

Retrograde conduction was present, concentric, non-decremental, with the earliest local atrial electrogram recorded at the level of the His catheter.

The effective anterograde refractory period of the accessory pathway at a coupling interval of 600 ms was 290 ms (Fig. 18.6).

The effective anterograde refractory period of the accessory pathway at a coupling interval of 400 ms was 260 ms.

Programmed atrial stimulation repeatedly initiated the tachycardia in Fig. 18.7.

At the end of ventricular pacing at a fixed coupling interval of 290 ms, the return sequence was V-A-V, excluding an atrial tachycardia. A single ventricular extrastimulus during His refractoriness advanced the tachycardia by 10 ms. PPI at the apex of the right ventricle – TCL = 60 ms. SA – VA during tachycardia was <85 ms, confirming the diagnosis of ORT using a manifest accessory pathway. The spontaneous termination of the tachycardia is shown in Figs. 18.8 and 18.9.

Given the symptomatic nature of the tachycardia and the presence of several episodes during the past months, ablation was offered to the patient, after having discussed all the potential complications related to the procedure.

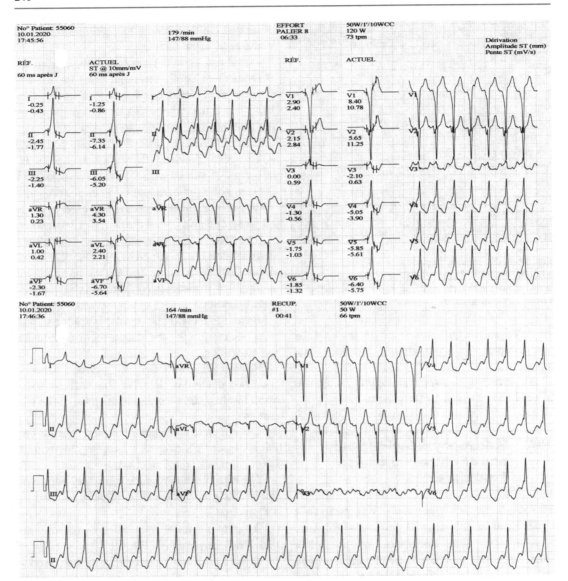

Fig. 18.4 Exercise stress test carried out up to 120 W, 6.2 METS, stopped do to fatigue, reaching a maximum heart rate of 179 bpm, BP = 147/78 mmHg (upper panel), with no sudden disappearance of ventricular pre-excitation on the 12-lead ECG. The lower panel shows the first recovery stage of the stress test showing marked ventricular pre-excitation

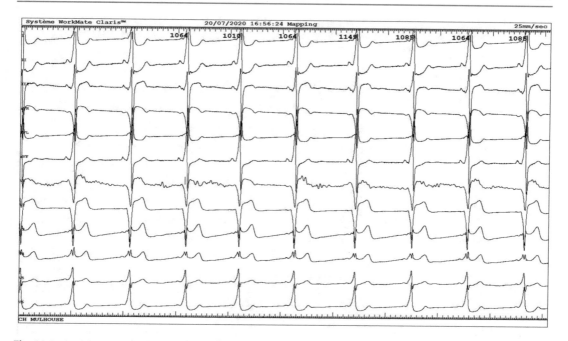

Fig. 18.5 A 12-lead ECG at the beginning of the ablation procedure showing sinus rhythm with ventricular pre-excitation with negative delta waves in lead V1, aVL, positive delta waves in leads II, III, and aVF and a QRS transition in lead V4. These, together with a "QS" aspect in lead V1 are in favor of a parahisian location

Mapping of the right antero-septal region was performed first, during sinus rhythm, using the CARTO system.

An anatomical map of the right atrium was first created, carefully identifying key structures such as the superior and inferior vena cava, the right atrial appendage, and the bundle of His. Subsequently, an activation map of the ventricular myocardium around the tricuspid annulus was then performed, targeting the earliest local ventricular activation site during sinus rhythm. This was found to be at 3 mm distance from the bundle of His (Fig. 18.10), where the local ventricular electrogram preceded the onset of the QRS complex by 25 ms. The local AV interval was short (Fig. 18.11), and the local unipolar ventricular electrogram had a "QS" aspect. A sharp local electrogram was recorded between the atrial and the ventricular electrogram, possibly corresponding to an accessory pathway potential.

Catheter positioning at the level of the earliest local ventricular activation site bumped the accessory pathway, with temporarily inhibiting conduction over it (Figs. 18.12, 18.13, 18.14, and 18.15).

Given the presence of symptomatic episodes of ORT, catheter ablation was subsequently performed. This was carried out at the level of the earliest ventricular activation site during sinus rhythm, starting with a power of 10 W with a target power of 20 W (Fig. 18.16).

Seven seconds after the beginning of the RF application, disappearance of conduction over the accessory pathway was noticed, but with appearance of a complete RBBB pattern (Fig. 18.17).

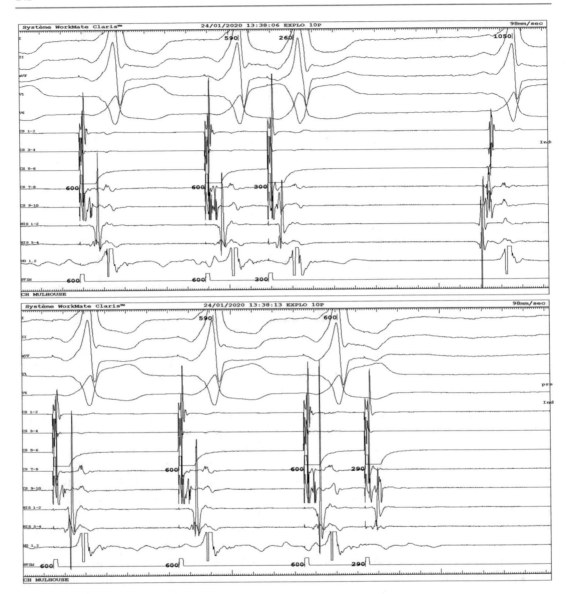

Fig. 18.6 Surface ECG leads I, II, aVF V1, and V6, together with intracavitary leads recorded from the bipolar electrodes of the coronary sinus catheter (SC 1–2 to SC 9–10), from the His catheter (His 1–2, His 3–4) and from the right ventricular catheter (VD 1,2) showing the antegrade effective refractory period of the accessory pathway of 290 ms, argument in favor of a benign accessory pathway

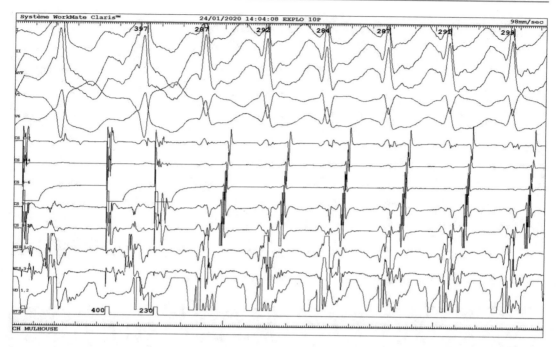

Fig. 18.7 Surface ECG leads I, II, aVF, V1, and V6, together with intracavitary leads recorded from the bipolar electrodes of the coronary sinus catheter (SC 1–2 to SC 9–10), from the His catheter (His 1–2, His 3–4) and from the right ventricular catheter (VD 1,2) showing the initiation of a narrow QRS complex tachycardia with a cycle length of 300 ms

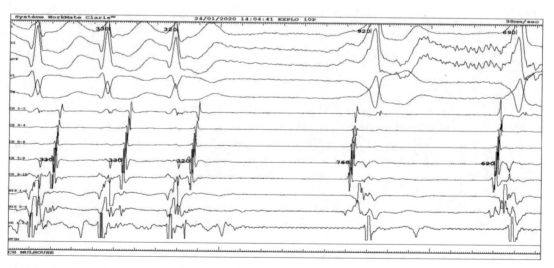

Fig. 18.8 Surface ECG leads I, II, aVF, V1, and V6, together with intracavitary leads recorded from the bipolar electrodes of the coronary sinus catheter (SC 1–2 to SC 9–10), from the His catheter (His 1–2, His 3–4) and from the right ventricular catheter (VD 1,2) showing the termination of the narrow QRS complex tachycardia

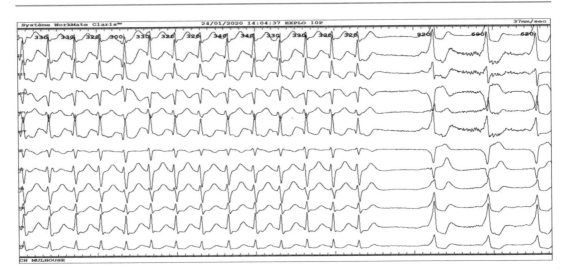

Fig. 18.9 A 12-lead ECG showing spontaneous termination of the tachycardia

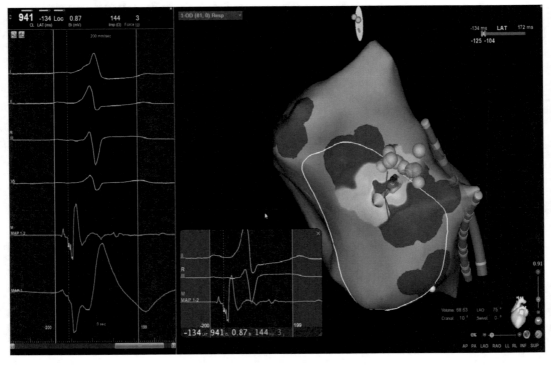

Fig. 18.10 CARTO image in LAO 75° cranial 10° showing the activation map of the right atrium during sinus rhythm, with the earliest local ventricular activation recorded in a narrow area in the parahisian-region, corresponding to the 2 o'clock location at the level of the tricuspid valve, where the earliest local ventricular activation precedes the QRS onset by 25 ms. Left side of the image: surface ECG leads I, II, aVR, V5, and intracavitary recordings from the distal bipolar electrode of the roving/ablation catheter (MAP 1–2), and the unipolar recording from the distal electrode of the roving/ablation catheter (M1), showing a "QS" aspect. The distance from the earliest local ventricular activation and the bundle of His measured 3 mm

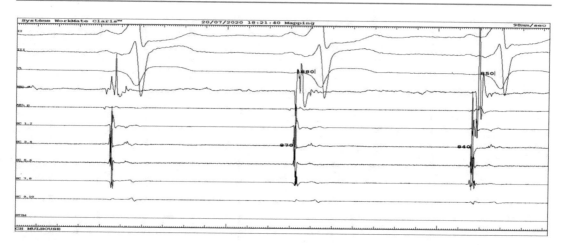

Fig. 18.11 Surface ECG leads II, III, and V1, together with intracavitary leads recorded from the distal and the proximal bipolar electrodes of the ablation catheter (Abl d, Abl p) and from the bipolar electrodes of the coronary sinus catheter (SC 1–2 to S-C 9–10) showing the presence of a short AV interval recorded by the roving ablation catheter at the site of earliest ventricular activation

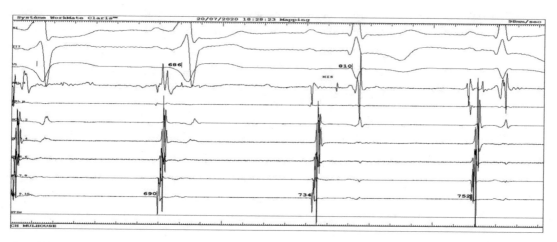

Fig. 18.12 Surface ECG leads II, III, and V1, together with intracavitary leads recorded from the distal and the proximal bipolar electrodes of the ablation catheter (Abl d, Abl p) and from the bipolar electrodes of the coronary sinus catheter (SC 1–2 to S-C 9–10) showing mechanical bumping of the accessory pathway by the ablation catheter at the level of the earliest ventricular activation site, with disappearance of conduction over the accessory pathway and normalization of the HV interval. A pattern of incomplete RBBB can be observed in lead V1

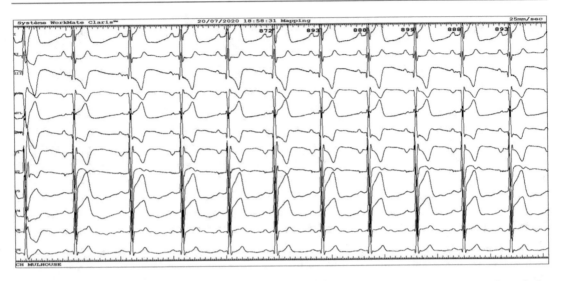

Fig. 18.13 A 12-lead ECG showing sinus rhythm with a heart rate of 67 bpm, QRS axis at +60°, absence of ventricular pre-excitation, incomplete right bundle branch block

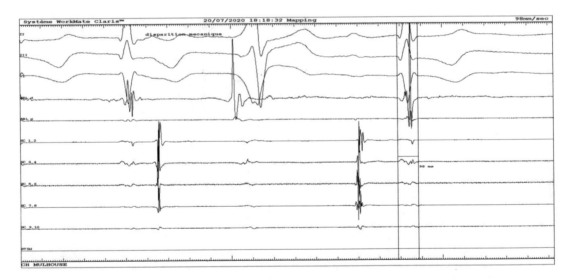

Fig. 18.14 Surface ECG leads II, III, and V1, together with intracavitary leads recorded from the distal and the proximal bipolar electrodes of the ablation catheter (Abl d, Abl p) and from the bipolar electrodes of the coronary sinus catheter (SC 1–2 to S-C 9–10) showing incomplete RBBB after mechanical bump, with a QRS width of 100 ms

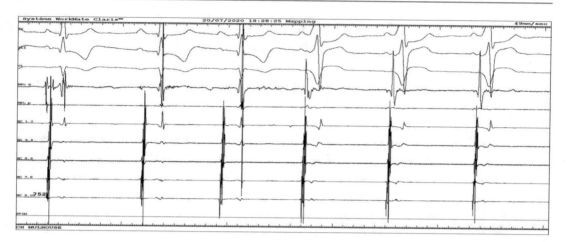

Fig. 18.15 Surface ECG leads II, III, and V1 and intra-cavitary leads recorded from the distal and the proximal bipolar electrodes of the ablation catheter (Abl d, Abl p) and from the bipolar electrodes of the coronary sinus catheter (SC 1–2 to S-C 9–10) showing spontaneous recurrence of conduction over the AP

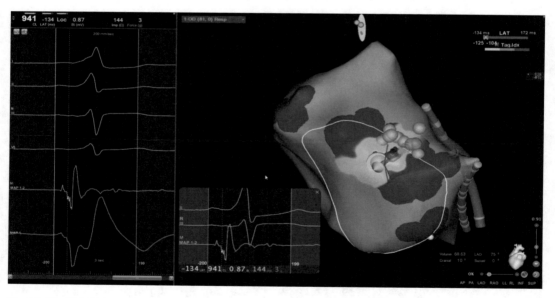

Fig. 18.16 CARTO image in LAO 75° cranial 10° (same as in Fig. 18.7) showing the activation map of the right atrium during sinus rhythm, with the ablation catheter positioned at the level of the earliest local ventricular activation and with a superposed ablation lesion at this level

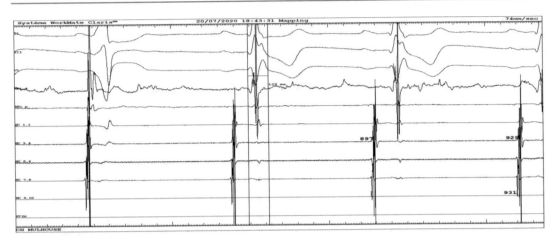

Fig. 18.17 Surface ECG leads II, III, and V1, together with intracavitary leads recorded from the distal and the proximal bipolar electrodes of the ablation catheter (Abl d, Abl p) and from the bipolar electrodes of the coronary

sinus catheter (SC 1–2 to S-C 9–10) showing disappearance of conduction over the accessory pathway were noticed, but with appearance of a complete RBBB pattern. The QRS width is 129 ms

Question 3: What would be your approach at this stage of the procedure, in this situation, for this particular patient?

A. Continue RF application since this is the optimal ablation site, given the elimination of conduction over the accessory pathway, despite creation of a right bundle branch block.

B. Immediately terminate the RF application, since sacrificing conduction over the right bundle for this 18-year-old patients is not the best option.

C. Terminate RF application and switch to cryo ablation.

D. Look for another potential ablation site.

E. Switch to a jugular approach.

Given the young age of the patient, after discussing with the patient the risks and the benefits of the ablation, a decision not to sacrifice conduction over the right bundle was taken. No further RF application was carried out. Conduction over the accessory pathway recurred a few minutes after (Fig. 18.18). The 12-lead ECG at the end of the ablation is shown in Fig. 18.15.

The ECG recorded 24 h after the ablation is shown in Fig. 18.19.

The patient was discharged from the hospital 24 h later on 150 mg of long release flecainide.

ANSWERS TO:

Question 1: E. Parahisian.

Question 2: A. Perform a physical stress test to non-invasively assess the effective refractory period of the AP.

Question 3: open for discussion.

18.3   Commentary

The present case illustrates a catheter ablation procedure of a parahisian accessory pathway and its challenges associated with it.

Non-invasive assessment of the accessory pathway character (benign or malignant) can be performed using an exercise stress test. The sudden disappearance of ventricular pre-excitation at low heart rates during physical effort is a sign of a long refractory period of the accessory pathway and this is associated with a low risk of sudden cardiac death [1]. However, the abrupt disappearance of ventricular pre-excitation during the

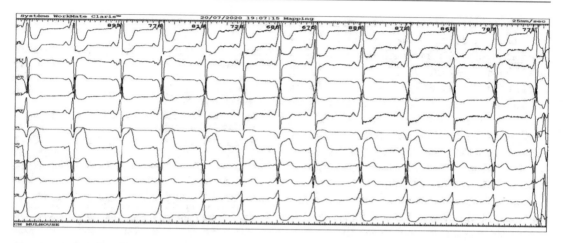

Fig. 18.18 A 12-lead ECG at the end of the ablation procedure showing sinus rhythm with respiratory arrhythmia and ventricular pre-excitation

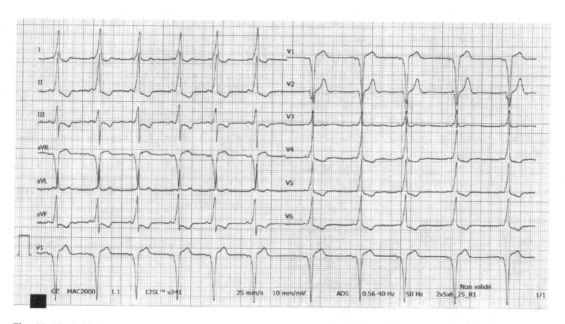

Fig. 18.19 A 12-lead ECG showing sinus rhythm with a heart rate of 75 bpm, QRS axis at +30°, ventricular pre-excitation and sinus arrhythmia

exercise stress test is only seen in a minority of patients with pre-excitation syndrome, between 8% [1] and 20% [2]. Persistence of pre-excitation during exercise stress test, such as in the case in the above-presented patient, does not distinguish malignant from benign accessory pathways. Exercise stress test has a low potential for inducing supraventricular arrhythmias in patients with WPW syndrome [3].

Parahisian AP represents a minority of septal accessory pathways [4]. Catheter ablation of these accessory pathways carries a higher risk of AV block than non-septal AP, due to the vicinity of the conduction system. Complete right bundle branch block is another potential complication of catheter ablation of parahisian AP [5]. Ablation is usually performed using the standard inferior vena cava approach, but ablation from the non-coronary aortic cusp [6] or from the inferior vena cava using a subclavicular vein approach or internal jugular vein approach has been safely and efficiently performed [7]. In their experience, Chokr et al. recommend ablating the parahisian AP from the aortic cusps if the difference between the onset of the earliest local bipolar electrogram recorded in the right atrium and the onset of the delta wave on the 12-lead ECG is less than 23 ms [6] since ablation from the aortic cusps in these cases has a higher success rate.

Catheter ablation can be performed either using radiofrequency or using cryo energy [8]. Radiofrequency can be performed using titration of energy, usually starting at a power of 15 Watts and progressively augmented until the desired effect is obtained. Cryoablation of parahisian AP can have, in experienced hands, an acute success rate of up to 94%, with a very low risk of AV block [8]. In the above-presented case, we chose not to perform RF ablation and sacrifice the right bundle branch, given the young age of the patient (disappearance of pre-excitation was obtained while ablating at low energy, but with RBBB appearance—see Fig. 18.17). A cryoablation procedure might have been a good option, because of the potential reversal effects during the mapping phase at −30° in the case of RBBB.

Learning Point
- Parahisian accessory pathway is characterized by the presence of positive delta waves on the 12-lead ECG in leads II, III, aVF, I, aVL, negative in V1, V2, and a QRS transition in precordial leads in V3 or V4.
- Their ablation is challenging and carry a significant risk of AV block.
- Ablation should be performed at the level of the ventricular insertion of the AP, in order to avoid inadvertent AV node injury.

References

1. Moltedo JM, Iyer RV, Forman H, Fahey J, Rosenthal G, Snyder CS. Is exercise stress testing a cost-saving strategy for risk assessment of pediatric wolff-Parkinson-white syndrome patients? Ochsner J. 2006;6(2):64–7.
2. Jezior MR, Kent SM, Atwood JE. Exercise testing in Wolff-Parkinson-White syndrome: case report with ECG and literature review. Chest. 2005;127(4):1454–7.
3. Strasberg B, Ashley WW, Wyndham CR, Bauernfeind RA, Swiryn SP, Dhingra RC, et al. Treadmill exercise testing in the Wolff-Parkinson-White syndrome. Am J Cardiol. 1980;45(4):742–8.
4. Tai CT, Chen SA, Chiang CE, Lee SH, Chang MS. Electrocardiographic and electrophysiologic characteristics of anteroseptal, midseptal, and para-Hisian accessory pathways. Implication for radiofrequency catheter ablation. Chest. 1996;109(3):730–40.
5. S P. Warren Jackman's Art of War: A Sniper's Approach to Catheter Ablation. 2019.
6. Chokr MO, de Moura LG, Aiello VD, Dos Santos Sousa IB, Lopes HB, do AAL C, et al. Catheter ablation of the parahisian accessory pathways from the aortic cusps-Experience of 20 cases-Improving the mapping strategy for better results. J Cardiovasc Electrophysiol. 2020;31(6):1413–9.
7. Liang M, Wang Z, Liang Y, Yang G, Jin Z, Sun M, et al. Different approaches for catheter ablation of para-hisian accessory pathways: implications for mapping and ablation. Circ Arrhythm Electrophysiol. 2017;10(6):e004882.
8. Swissa M, Birk E, Dagan T, Fogelman M, Einbinder T, Bruckheimer E, et al. Cryotherapy ablation of parahisian accessory pathways in children. Heart Rhythm. 2015;12(5):917–25.

Case 19

Frédéric Halbwachs, Ronan Le Bouar,
Crina Muresan, and Laurent Dietrich

19.1 Case Presentation

A 45-year-old male professional driver with no significant past medical history was addressed to the Cardiology Department by his family physician for a detailed cardiology workup due to the discovery of an old inferior myocardial infarction pattern on his ECG. The patient was asymptomatic and recalls no episode of chest pain. He had no personal history of known heart disease, no family history of sudden cardiac death. He had no cardiovascular risk factors. He was on no chronic medication.

At physical exam, his blood pressure was 120/78 mmHg, heart rate of 78 bpm, SpO_2 98% breathing room air, his weight 74 kg, height 166 cm, BMI of 26.55 kg/m^2, heart sounds were regular, there was no audible heart murmur, there were no signs of heart failure, pulmonary auscultation was normal.

His ECG recorded at admittance to the Cardiology Department is presented in Fig. 19.1.

A transthoracic echocardiography was performed, showing a non-dilated LV, with no global, regional, or segmental kinetic disorder, absence of LV hypertrophy, with a preserved EF% of 63% (Fig. 19.2). It also showed normal diastolic function, a non-dilated left atrium (surface = 19.1 cm^2), absence of significant valve disease, a non-dilated right ventricle, trivial tricuspid regurgitation, absence of pulmonary hypertension, a non-dilated IVC, no pericardial effusion, a non-dilated aorta.

His biological workup showed a Hb level of 13.0 g/dl, leucocytes 6.8×10^9/L, platelets 255×10^9/L, CRP <3 mg/l, BUN 5.0 mmol/l, creatinine 74 μmol/l, glycemia 5.6 mmol/l, Na+ 137 mmol/l, K+ 3.9 mmol/l, total proteins 76 g/l.

> **Question 1: Are there any clues on the 12-lead ECG suggesting a specific diagnosis?**
> A. No. This is a normal ECG.
> B. Yes. Epsilon wave in V1 in favor of arrhythmogenic cardiomyopathy.
> C. Yes. The incomplete right bundle branch block in V1 suggests type 2 Brugada syndrome.
> D. Yes. Short QT interval, in favor of Short QT Syndrome.
> E. Yes. Ventricular pre-excitation.

F. Halbwachs (✉)
Biosense Webster, Mulhouse, France

R. Le Bouar · C. Muresan · L. Dietrich
Cardiology Department, "Emile Muller" Hospital,
Mulhouse, France

© The Author(s), under exclusive license to Springer Nature Switzerland AG 2022
L. Muresan (ed.), *Clinical Cases in Cardiac Electrophysiology: Supraventricular Arrhythmias*,
https://doi.org/10.1007/978-3-031-07357-1_19

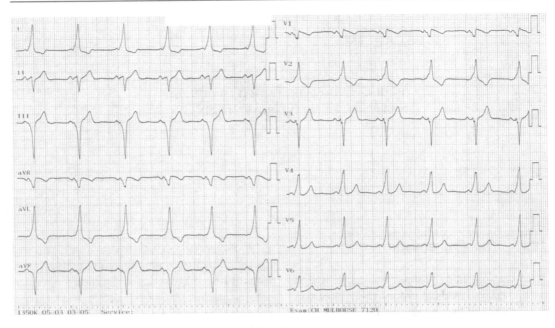

Fig. 19.1 A 12-lead ECG at admittance to the Cardiology Department

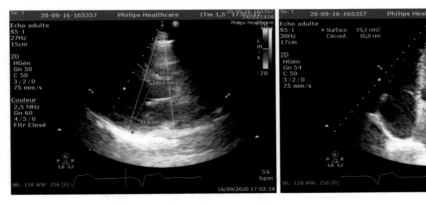

Fig. 19.2 *Left panel:* transthoracic echocardiography image in parasternal long axis showing a non-dilated left ventricle with an end diastolic diameter of 43 mm and with mild LV hypertrophy. *Right panel:* apical 4-chamber view showing a non-dilated left atrium with a surface of 19.1 cm²

Figure 19.1 shows sinus rhythm with a heart rate of 76 bpm, QRS axis at −45°, no LV hypertrophy (R wave of 26 mV in V4), incomplete RBBB, short PR of 120 ms, positive delta wave in V1-V6 and in leads II, negative in lead III, aVF, absence of q waves in V5, V6, in favor of ventricular pre-excitation.

Question 2: Where is the accessory pathway situated?

A. Left lateral.

B. Left postero-septal.

C. Right postero-septal.

D. Right lateral.

E. Right antero-septal.

Given the presence of palpitations and the ECG aspect in favor of ventricular pre-excitation, the diagnosis of WPW syndrome was established. Based on history taking, physical examination, the WPW pattern on the 12-lead ECG and the absence of kinetics disorder with transthoracic echocardiography, the diagnosis of old inferior myocardial infarction was not considered correct. An electrophysiological study was subsequently offered and performed.

19.2   Electrophysiological Study and RF Catheter Ablation Procedure

The electrophysiological study was performed under local anesthesia and conscious sedation. Vascular access was obtained using the modified Seldinger technique, under Doppler ultrasound guidance. A 6F quadripolar steerable catheter (Dynamic Extrem, Microport®) was introduced in a 9F 20 cm vascular sheath and was subsequently advanced via the right common femoral vein up to the bundle of His. Another 6F quadripolar steerable catheter (Dynamic Extrem, Microport®) was introduced in a 6F 20 cm vascular sheath and placed via the right common femoral vein in the coronary sinus, with the distal poles at the level of the lateral mitral annulus. A bipolar non-steerable catheter (Viking, Boston Scientific®) was introduced in a 6F 20 cm vascular sheath and was subsequently advanced via the right common femoral vein up to the right ventricular apex.

Atrial and ventricular pacing were carried out at twice the diastolic threshold using the EP-4™ Cardiac Stimulator (Abbott®) system. Surface ECG and intracavitary ECGs were recorded by the WorkMate Claris™ System (Abbott®).

Radiofrequency ablation was delivered using a Biosense Webster® SmartTouch SF open-irrigated 3.5 mm tip with double curve (D/F). The CARTO ® 3 electro-anatomic mapping system (Biosense Webster, Johnson & Johnson) was used to guide mapping and ablation of the accessory pathway.

The ECG at the beginning of the ablation procedure is presented in Fig. 19.3.

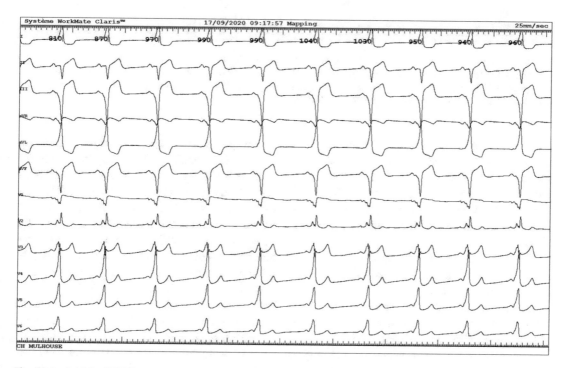

Fig. 19.3   A 12-lead ECG at the beginning of the electrophysiological study

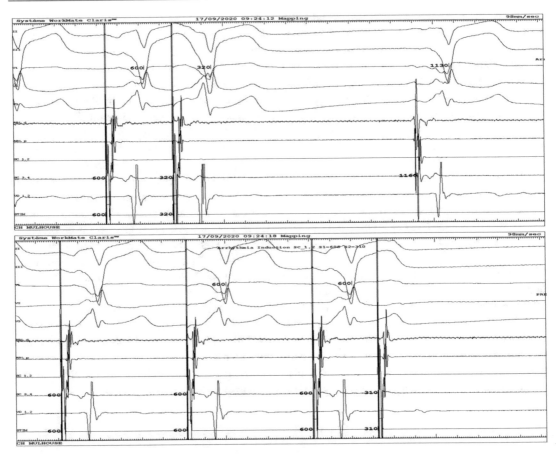

Fig. 19.4 Surface ECG leads II, III, V1, V2, and V3, together with intracavitary leads recorded from the distal and proximal bipolar electrode of the roving/ablation catheter (ABL d, ABL p), distal and proximal coronary sinus (SC 1–2, SC 3–4) and from the right ventricular catheter (VD 1,2) showing the effective antegrade refractory period of the accessory pathway at 310 ms

Baseline AH was 47 ms, the HV interval was -22 ms, confirming the presence of ventricular pre-excitation. The anterior effective refractory period of the accessory pathway was 310 ms during basal conditions while pacing the distal coronary sinus electrodes with a coupling interval of 600 ms (Fig. 19.4).

Programmed atrial stimulation before and after isoprenaline administration did not initiate any sustained arrhythmias.

Given the patient's job, despite the lack of arrhythmia induction, a decision to perform RF ablation was subsequently taken.

Mapping of the right postero-septal region was performed first, during sinus rhythm.

An anatomical map of the right atrium was first created, carefully identifying key structures such as the superior and inferior vena cava, the right atrial appendage, and the bundle of His. The right atrium was non-dilated, with a volume of 60 ml. Subsequently, an activation map of the ventricular myocardium around the tricuspid annulus was then performed, targeting the earliest local ventricular activation site during sinus rhythm. This was found to be at 4 o'clock at the level of the tricuspid valve (Fig. 19.5), where the local ventricular electrogram preceded the onset of the QRS complex by 27 ms. The local AV interval was short, and the local unipolar ventricular electrogram had a "QS" aspect.

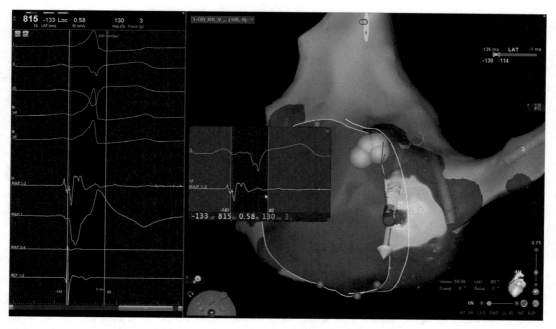

Fig. 19.5 CARTO image in LAO 80° showing the activation map of the right atrium during sinus rhythm, with the earliest local ventricular activation recorded in a narrow area corresponding to the 4 o'clock position at the level of the tricuspid valve, where the earliest local ventricular activation preceded the QRS onset by 27 ms. Left side of the image: surface ECG leads I, II, III, V4, and V5 and intracavitary recordings from the distal bipolar electrode of the roving/ablation catheter (MAP 1–2), and the unipolar recording from the distal electrode of the roving/ablation catheter (M1), showing a "QS" aspect

Target ablation parameters were a power of 30 W, with a target ablation index of 450 s.

Application of RF energy at the site of the earliest local ventricular activation, where the sharp local potential was recorded and eliminated the conduction over the accessory pathway (Figs. 19.6 and 19.7).

During RF delivery at the successful ablation site, junctional beats were also observed (Fig. 19.8), which determined interruption of RF application. The distance from the successful ablation site and the His bundle was 12 mm. Three short additional "consolidation" RF lesions were applied, with no prolongation of the AH or HV interval (Fig. 19.9).

Ventricular pacing after the RF application demonstrated absence of retrograde conduction over the accessory pathway. There was no complication related to the procedure. The 12-lead ECG recorded after the catheter ablation procedure is presented in Fig. 19.10.

The ECG recorded 24 h after the ablation procedure showed sinus rhythm with absence of ventricular pre-excitation (Fig. 19.11).

The patient was discharged from the hospital 24 h later, on no antiarrhythmic medication.

ANSWERS TO:
Question   1:   E.   Yes.   Ventricular pre-excitation
Question 2: C. Right postero-septal

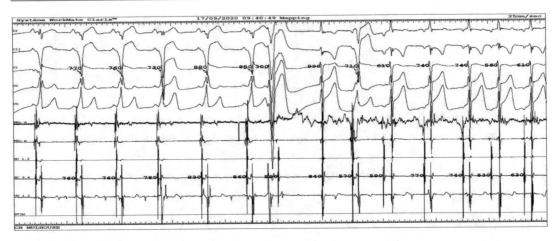

Fig. 19.6 Surface ECG leads II, III, V1, V2, and V3, together with intracavitary leads recorded from the distal and proximal bipolar electrode of the roving/ablation catheter (ABL d, ABL p), distal and proximal coronary sinus (SC 1–2, SC 3–4) and from the right ventricular catheter (VD 1,2) showing disappearance of conduction over the accessory pathway during RF ablation at 4 o'clock position at the tricuspid annulus

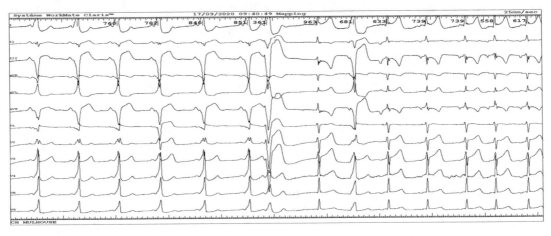

Fig. 19.7 A 12-lead ECG showing disappearance of conduction over the accessory pathway during RF ablation at 4 o'clock position at the tricuspid annulus

19.3   Commentary

The present case presents a catheter ablation procedure of a right postero-septal accessory pathway in a 45-year-old male professional driver with WPW ECG pattern. Several details merit attention and further discussion.

The first aspect that merits discussion is the indication of performing an electrophysiological study in an asymptomatic WPW patient. According to A Systematic Review for the 2015 ACC/AHA/HRS Guideline for the Management of Adult Patients With Supraventricular Tachycardia [1], that analyzed data from several observational studies comprising 883 patients who did not undergo catheter ablation, 9% of patients developed malignant ventricular arrhythmias and 2% developed ventricular fibrillation during the follow-up period. These finding support the performance of an electrophysiological study for risk stratification of patients with asymptomatic WPW syndrome, especially in

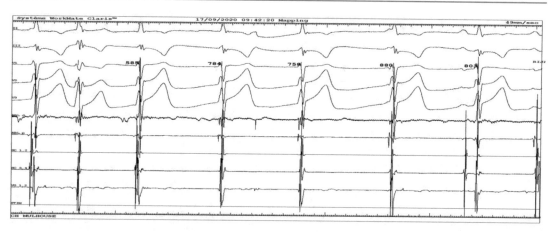

Fig. 19.8 Surface ECG leads II, III, V1, V2, and V3, together with intracavitary leads recorded from the distal and proximal bipolar electrode of the roving/ablation catheter (ABL d, ABL p), distal and proximal coronary sinus (SC 1–2, SC 3–4) and from the right ventricular catheter (VD 1,2) showing the presence of active junctional rhythm during RF ablation at the successful site

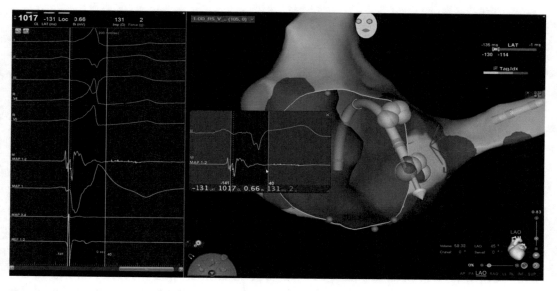

Fig. 19.9 CARTO image in LAO 45 ° showing the activation map of the right atrium during sinus rhythm, with the ablation catheter positioned at the level of the earliest local ventricular activation, recorded in a narrow area corresponding to the 4 o'clock position at the level of the tricuspid valve, where the earliest local ventricular activation preceded the QRS onset by 27 ms. RF ablation lesions were applied at this site (pink and red dots). Left side of the image: surface ECG leads I, II, III, V4, and V5 and intracavitary recordings from the distal bipolar electrode of the roving/ablation catheter (MAP 1–2), and the unipolar recording from the distal electrode of the roving/ablation catheter (M1), showing a "QS" aspect

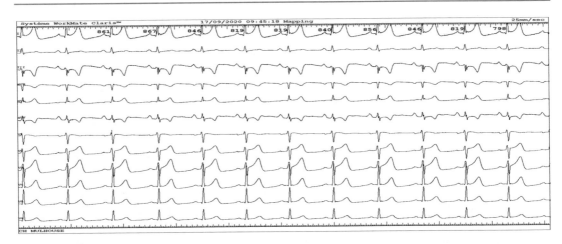

Fig. 19.10 A 12-lead ECG at the end of the ablation procedure showing sinus rhythm with heart rate of 78 bpm, QRS axis at +30°, no LV hypertrophy, incomplete RBBB, negative T waves in lead III and aVF (T wave memory)

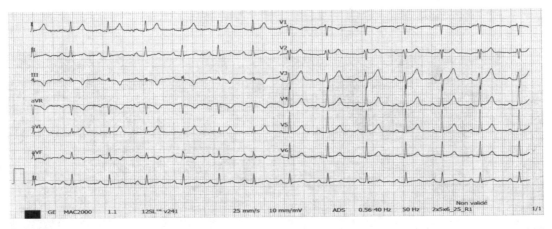

Fig. 19.11 A 12-lead ECG after the ablation procedure showing sinus rhythm with heart rate of 78 bpm, QRS axis at +30°, no LV hypertrophy, incomplete RBBB, negative T waves in lead III and aVF (T wave memory)

those in whom the non-invasive assessment of the accessory pathway (with an exercise stress test) is inconclusive. Another important element to keep in mind when assessing patient with asymptomatic WPW is the fact that 30% of these patients may develop symptoms during the following 10 years after the diagnosis of ventricular pre-excitation [2]. These were arguments that were taken into considerations when ablation of the accessory pathway was offered to the present patient.

A short antegrade effective refractory period of the accessory pathway characterizes its capability to rapidly conduct electrical impulses

from atria to the ventricles. A shorter than 250 ms pre-excited RR interval (SPERRI) during atrial fibrillation was associated in several studies with a higher risk of developing malignant ventricular arrhythmias and is considered a marker of increased arrhythmic risk in WPW syndrome patients [1, 3]. A shorter than 250 ms antegrade ERP was also shown to be a marker of increased risk. As shown by Moore et al., administration of isoprenaline during the electrophysiological study of patients with WPW syndrome is associated with a reduction between 70 and 90 ms in the antegrade ERP of the accessory pathway [4]. This change classified an additional 34% of their studied children with WPW as having a high arrhythmic risk. According to several authors, a fastest manifest conduction over the AP of <220 ms after isoprenaline infusion is associated with a higher risk of malignant ventricular arrhythmias [3, 5–7]. However, this finding had to be put in balance with the fact that no arrhythmia was inducible during the electrophysiological study and that the patient was asymptomatic.

The current studies assessing asymptomatic patients with WPW [1, 8, 9] recommend performing catheter ablation in patients with high risk properties of AP, such as those with a SPERRI of <250 ms. Given the localization of the accessory pathway in the right postero-septal region in our patient, the patient's occupation (professional driver), the utilization of an electroanatomical mapping system, the risk/benefit ratio of an ablation procedure were considered in favor of performing the ablation procedure. This was performed safely and no complication occurred. The decision might have been different though, for other AP localization such as mid-septal or parahisian.

> **Learning Point**
> - Invasive assessment with the electrophysiological study in asymptomatic patients with WPW syndrome is generally recommended.
> - Catheter ablation of the accessory pathway may be performed in those patients with a high future risk of developing malignant ventricular arrhythmias.

References

1. Al-Khatib SM, Arshad A, Balk EM, Das SR, Hsu JC, Joglar JA, et al. Risk Stratification for Arrhythmic Events in Patients With Asymptomatic Pre-Excitation: A Systematic Review for the 2015 ACC/AHA/HRS Guideline for the Management of Adult Patients With Supraventricular Tachycardia: A Report of the American College of Cardiology/American Heart Association Task Force on Clinical Practice Guidelines and the Heart Rhythm Society. J Am Coll Cardiol. 2016;67(13):1624–38.
2. Munger TM, Packer DL, Hammill SC, Feldman BJ, Bailey KR, Ballard DJ, et al. A population study of the natural history of Wolff-Parkinson-White syndrome in Olmsted County, Minnesota, 1953-1989. Circulation. 1993;87(3):866–73.
3. Klein GJ, Bashore TM, Sellers TD, Pritchett EL, Smith WM, Gallagher JJ. Ventricular fibrillation in the Wolff-Parkinson-White syndrome. N Engl J Med. 1979;301(20):1080–5.
4. Moore JP, Kannankeril PJ, Fish FA. Isoproterenol administration during general anesthesia for the evaluation of children with ventricular preexcitation. Circ Arrhythm Electrophysiol. 2011;4(1):73–8.
5. Timmermans C, Smeets JL, Rodriguez LM, Vrouchos G, van den Dool A, Wellens HJ. Aborted sudden death in the Wolff-Parkinson-White syndrome. Am J Cardiol. 1995;76(7):492–4.
6. Bromberg BI, Lindsay BD, Cain ME, Cox JL. Impact of clinical history and electrophysiologic characterization of accessory pathways on management strategies to reduce sudden death among children with Wolff-Parkinson-White syndrome. J Am Coll Cardiol. 1996;27(3):690–5.
7. Paul T, Guccione P, Garson A Jr. Relation of syncope in young patients with Wolff-Parkinson-White syndrome to rapid ventricular response during atrial fibrillation. Am J Cardiol. 1990;65(5):318–21.
8. Mohan S, Balaji S. Management of asymptomatic ventricular preexcitation. Indian Pacing Electrophysiol J. 2019;19(6):232–9.
9. Ksiazczyk TM, Pietrzak R, Werner B. Management of young athletes with asymptomatic preexcitation-a review of the literature. Diagnostics. 2020;10(10):824.

Case 20

Frédéric Halbwachs, Ronan Le Bouar,
Charline Daval, Tarek El Nazer, and Jacques Levy

20

20.1 Case Presentation

A 26-year-old male patient with no known cardiovascular disease presents to the Emergency Department for an episode of syncope that occurred 1 h to his presentation to the hospital, preceded by palpitations with a rapid heart rate. Careful history taking revealed another episode of syncope 2 years prior, while driving, complicated by a car accident, with subsequent chest trauma, fracture of 4 ribs, and fracture of the right tibia. At that time, the loss of consciousness was considered to have occurred as a consequence of the accident and was not investigated any further.

His cardiovascular risk factors were represented by grade 1 obesity. He had no family history of sudden cardiac death. He denied smoking, alcohol consumption, or consumption of illicit drugs. He was on no chronic medication.

At physical exam, his blood pressure was 120/70 mmHg, heart rate of 110 bpm, SpO_2 98% breathing room air, $H = 190$ cm, $W = 110$ kg, BMI = 30.47 kg/m^2, heart sounds were rapid and regular, there was no audible heart murmur, there were no signs of heart failure, pulmonary auscultation was also normal.

His ECG recorded at admittance to the Cardiology Department is presented in Fig. 20.1.

Question 1: Are there any clues on the 12-lead ECG in Fig. 20.2 **suggesting a specific diagnosis?**
A. No. This is a normal ECG.
B. Yes. Incomplete RBBB suggesting type 2 Brugada syndrome.
C. Yes. Delta waves suggesting ventricular pre-excitation.
D. Yes. Q waves in I, aVL, suggesting remote LV posterior wall myocardial infarction.
E. Yes. Incomplete RBBB suggesting arrhythmogenic cardiomyopathy.

Transthoracic echocardiography showed a non-dilated LV with a preserved LV EF% of

F. Halbwachs (✉)
Biosense Webster, Mulhouse, France

R. Le Bouar · C. Daval · T. El Nazer · J. Levy
Cardiology Department, "Emile Muller" Hospital, Mulhouse, France

© The Author(s), under exclusive license to Springer Nature Switzerland AG 2022
L. Muresan (ed.), *Clinical Cases in Cardiac Electrophysiology: Supraventricular Arrhythmias*,
https://doi.org/10.1007/978-3-031-07357-1_20

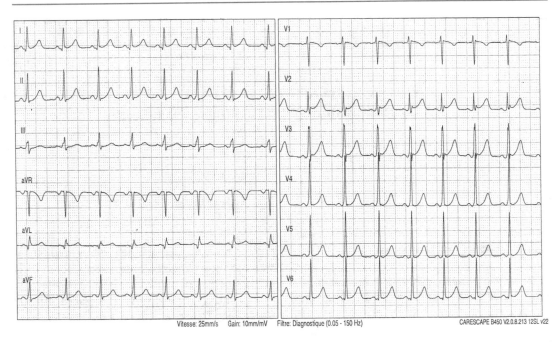

Fig. 20.1 A 12-lead ECG at admittance to the Cardiology Department, showing sinus rhythm with a heart rate of 110 bpm, QRS axis at °, absence of LV hypertrophy, absence of ischemia

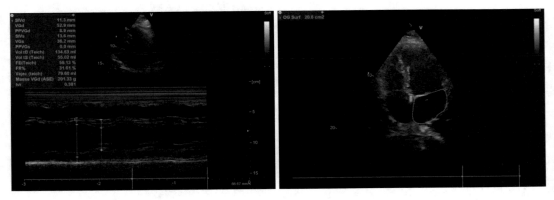

Fig. 20.2 *Left panel:* transthoracic echocardiography image in parasternal long axis view showing a non-dilated LV with an ESD of 48 mm. *Right panel:* apical 4 chamber view showing a LV EF% of 52%

59%, absence of LV hypertrophy, no significant valve disease, non-dilated right ventricle, absence of pericardial fluid (Fig. 20.2).

His biological workup showed a Hb level of 15.5 g/dl, leucocytes 9.34 × 10⁹/L, platelets 250 × 10⁹/L, CRP <3 mg/L, BUN 4.1 mmol/L, creatinine 58 μmol/L, glycemia 5.0 mmol/L, Na⁺ 142 mmol/L, K⁺ 3.8 mmol/L, total proteins 79 g/L, D-dimers 350 ng/ml, TSH 2.22 IU/L, NT pro-BNP 724 pg/ml.

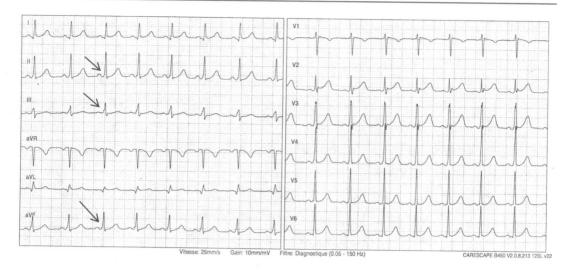

Vitesse: 25mm/s   Gain: 10mm/mV   Filtre: Diagnostique (0.05 - 150 Hz)   CARESCAPE B450 V2.0.8.213 12SL v22

Figure 20.1 (explained). A 12-lead ECG showing sinus rhythm with a heart rate of 97 bpm, QRS axis at +60°, absence of LV hypertrophy, incomplete RBBB, short PR of 120 ms, positive delta wave in V1-V6 and in leads II, III, aVF (red arrows), negative delta waves in V5, V6 (not to be mistaken for q waves suggestive of myocardial necrosis).

Given the presence of syncope preceded by palpitations, the presence of ventricular pre-excitation on the 12-lead ECG, an electrophysiological study was offered and accepted by the patient.

20.2   Electrophysiological Study and RF Catheter Ablation Procedure

The electrophysiological study was performed under local anesthesia and conscious sedation. Vascular access was obtained using the modified Seldinger technique, under Doppler ultrasound guidance. A 6F quadripolar steerable catheter (Dynamic Extrem, Microport®) was introduced in a 9F 20 cm vascular sheath and was subsequently advanced via the right common femoral vein up to the bundle of His. A quadripolar steerable catheter (Dynamic Extrem, Microport®) was introduced in a 6F 20 cm vascular sheath and

placed via the right common femoral vein in the coronary sinus, with the distal poles at the level of the lateral mitral annulus. A bipolar non-steerable catheter (Viking, Boston Scientific®) was introduced in a 6F 20 cm vascular sheath and was subsequently advanced via the right common femoral vein up to the right ventricular apex. Atrial and ventricular pacing were carried out at twice the diastolic threshold using the EP-4™ Cardiac Stimulator (Abbott®) system. Surface ECG and intracavitary ECGs were recorded by the WorkMate Claris™ System (Abbott®).

Radiofrequency ablation was delivered using a Biosense Webster® SmartTouch SF open-irrigated 3.5 mm tip with dual curve (D/F). The CARTO ® 3 electro-anatomic mapping system (Biosense Webster, Johnson & Johnson) was used to guide mapping and ablation of the accessory pathway (Fig. 20.3).

The ECG at the beginning of the electrophysiological study is presented in Fig. 20.4.

Baseline AH was 99 ms, the HV interval was 27 ms, confirming the diagnosis of ventricular pre-excitation.

Retrograde conduction was present, concentric, non-decremental, with the earliest local atrial electrogram recorded at the level of the CS electrodes 7–8.

The effective anterograde refractory period of the accessory pathway at a coupling interval of

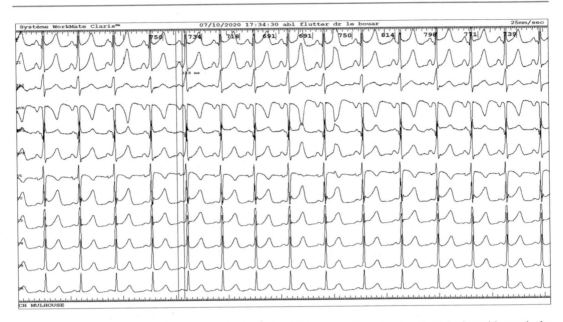

Fig. 20.3 A 12-lead ECG recorded at the beginning at the ablation procedure, showing sinus rhythm with ventricular pre-excitation, with a heart rate of 80 bpm, with a short PR interval of 115 ms

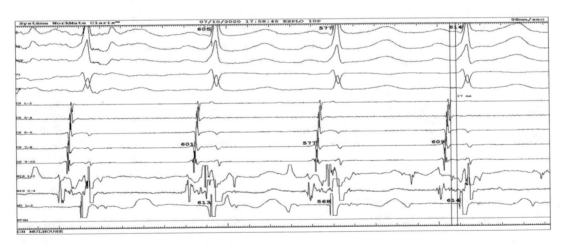

Fig. 20.4 Surface ECG leads I, II, III, V1, V2, and V3 together with intracavitary leads recorded from the bipolar electrodes of the coronary sinus catheter (SC 1–2 to S-C 9–10), the distal and the proximal electrodes of the His catheter (His 1–2, His 3–4), and the bipolar electrodes of the RV apex catheter (VD 1–2) showing a short HV interval of 27 ms, confirming ventricular pre-excitation

600 ms was 220 ms . The effective anterograde refractory period of the accessory pathway at a coupling interval of 400 ms was 210 ms (Fig. 20.5).

Retrograde conduction was present, showing 3 different depolarization sequences (Figs. 20.6, 20.7, and 20.8).

Programmed atrial stimulation initiated the wide QRS complex tachycardia from Fig. 20.9, with a cycle length of 300 ms.

The 12-lead ECG during the antidromic tachycardia is presented in Fig. 20.10.

The diagnostic maneuvers demonstrated this to be an antidromic tachycardia.

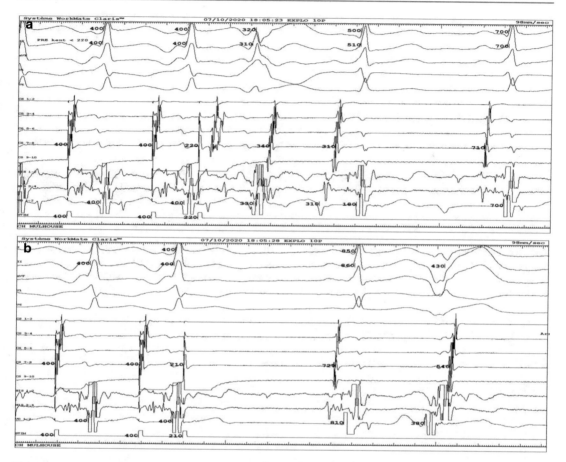

Fig. 20.5 (a) Surface ECG leads I, II, III, V1, V2, and V3 together with intracavitary leads recorded from the bipolar electrodes of the coronary sinus catheter (SC 1–2 to S-C 9–10), the distal and the proximal electrodes of the His catheter (His 1–2, His 3–4), and the bipolar electrodes of the RV apex catheter (VD 1–2) showing the presence of conduction over the accessory pathway at a coupling interval of 220 ms. (b) Surface ECG leads I, II, III, V1, V2, and V3 together with intracavitary leads recorded from the bipolar electrodes of the coronary sinus catheter (SC 1–2 to S-C 9–10), the distal and the proximal electrodes of the His catheter (His 1–2, His 3–4), and the bipolar electrodes of the RV apex catheter (VD 1–2) showing the effective antegrade refractory period of the accessory pathway of <220 ms. The effective antegrade refractory period of the atrium is 210 ms

Figure 20.11 shows degenerating of ART into atrial fibrillation. The shortest recorded RR interval during atrial fibrillation was 255 ms (Fig. 20.12). Conversion of AF to SR is shown in Fig. 20.13.

Given the antegrade refractory period of 210 ms in favor of a malignant accessory pathway and the presence of repeated symptomatic episodes of ART and atrial fibrillation, a decision to ablate the accessory pathway was taken. The aspect during maximal pre-excitation (positive delta waves in leads II, III, aVF, V1-V6, negative delta waves in leads I, aVL) suggested a left lateral origin.

Mapping of the lateral region of the mitral valve was performed first, using the CARTO system.

Access to the mitral valve was obtained using an antegrade approach. A single transseptal puncture was performed under fluoroscopic guidance using an 8.5F 67cm Swartz SL0™ transseptal sheath (Abbott®) and a BRK ™ XS 71 cm needle (Abbott®).

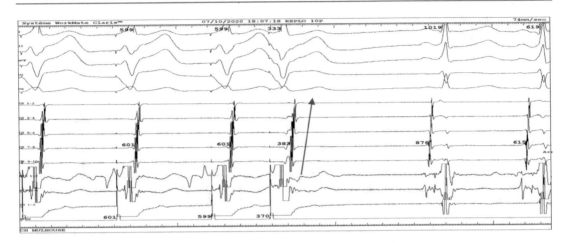

Fig. 20.6 Surface ECG leads I, II, III, V1, V2, and V3 together with intracavitary leads recorded from the bipolar electrodes of the coronary sinus catheter (SC 1–2 to S-C 9–10), the distal and the proximal electrodes of the His catheter (His 1–2, His 3–4), and the bipolar electrodes of the RV apex catheter (VD 1–2) showing a concentric retrograde activation sequence, compatible with conduction over the AV node

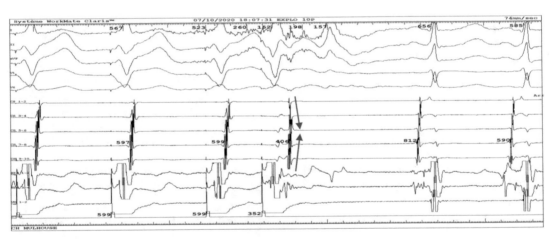

Fig. 20.7 Surface ECG leads I, II, III, V1, V2, and V3 together with intracavitary leads recorded from the bipolar electrodes of the coronary sinus catheter (SC 1–2 to S-C 9–10), the distal and the proximal electrodes of the His catheter (His 1–2, His 3–4), and the bipolar electrodes of the RV apex catheter (VD 1–2) showing a concentric retrograde activation sequence, compatible with fusion, with conduction over both the AV node and an accessory pathway

After the transseptal puncture, anticoagulation was obtained with unfractionated Heparin 70 IU/kg given as bolus, followed by continuous infusion of 12 IU/kg/h, with a target ACT of 300 s.

Once the access to the left atrium was granted, the SmartTouch SF roving/ablation catheter was introduced in the SL0 transseptal sheath, and mapping of the mitral valve was performed. An anatomical map of the left atrium was first created. An activation map targeting the earliest local ventricular activation was subsequently created during atrial pacing, in order

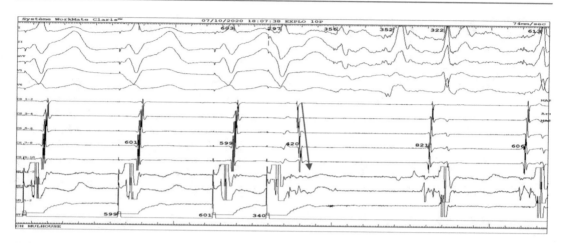

Fig. 20.8 Surface ECG leads I, II, III, V1, V2, and V3 together with intracavitary leads recorded from the bipolar electrodes of the coronary sinus catheter (SC 1–2 to S-C 9–10), the distal and the proximal electrodes of the His catheter (His 1–2, His 3–4), and the bipolar electrodes of the RV apex catheter (VD 1–2) showing an eccentric retrograde activation sequence, compatible with conduction over the accessory pathway

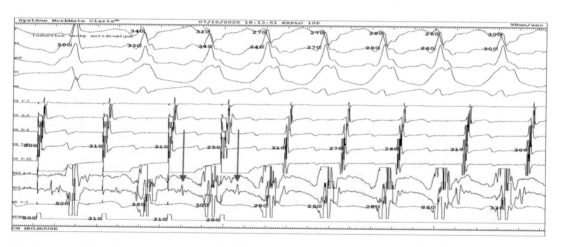

Fig. 20.9 Surface ECG leads I, II, aVF, V1, together with intracavitary leads recorded from the bipolar electrodes of the coronary sinus catheter (SC 1–2 to S-C 9–10) the distal and the proximal electrodes of the His catheter (His 1–2, His 3–4) and the bipolar electrodes of the RV apex catheter (VD 1–2) showing the initiation of a wide QRS complex tachycardia. Note that the His potential is clearly visible during pacing from the coronary sinus electrodes 7–8, but no longer visible after the initiation of the tachycardia

to obtain maximal pre-excitation, with careful analysis of the local ventricular electrograms recorded around the mitral annulus. The earliest local ventricular activation was recorded in the lateral region of the annulus, corresponding to the 2'clock position, where the local ventricular electrogram preceded the onset of the surface QRS complex by 15 ms (Fig. 20.14).

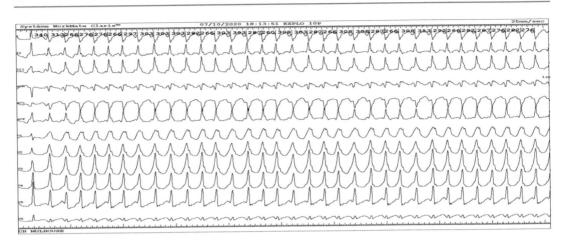

Fig. 20.10 A 12-lead ECG leads showing a wide QRS complex tachycardia with a cycle length of 310 ms. The morphology is not typical of RBBB, excluding a functional RBBB

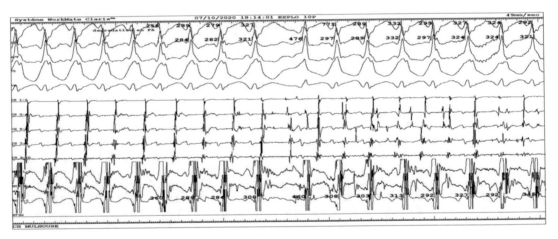

Fig. 20.11 Surface ECG leads I, II, III, V1, V2, and V3 together with intracavitary leads recorded from the bipolar electrodes of the coronary sinus catheter (SC 1–2 to S-C 9–10), the distal and the proximal electrodes of the His catheter (His 1–2, His 3–4), and the bipolar electrodes of the RV apex catheter (VD 1–2) showing the antidromic tachycardia degenerating into atrial fibrillation

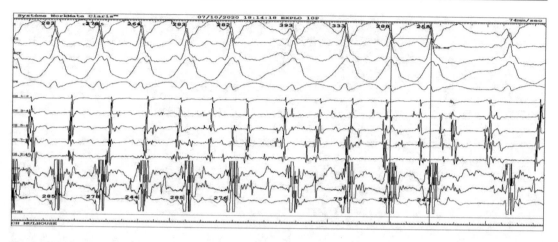

Fig. 20.12 Surface ECG leads I, II, III, V1, V2, and V3 together with intracavitary leads recorded from the bipolar electrodes of the coronary sinus catheter (SC 1–2 to S-C 9–10), the distal and the proximal electrodes of the His catheter (His 1–2, His 3–4), and the bipolar electrodes of the RV apex catheter (VD 1–2) showing the shortest RR interval during atrial fibrillation, measuring 255 ms

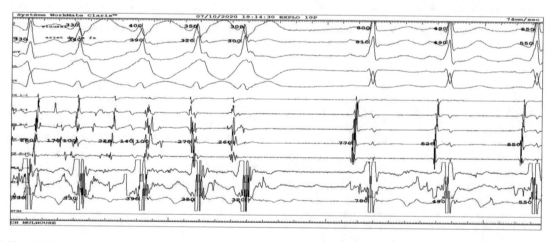

Fig. 20.13 Surface ECG leads I, II, III, V1, V2, and V3 together with intracavitary leads recorded from the bipolar electrodes of the coronary sinus catheter (SC 1–2 to S-C 9–10), the distal and the proximal electrodes of the His catheter (His 1–2, His 3–4), and the bipolar electrodes of the RV apex catheter (VD 1–2) showing spontaneous termination of the atrial fibrillation

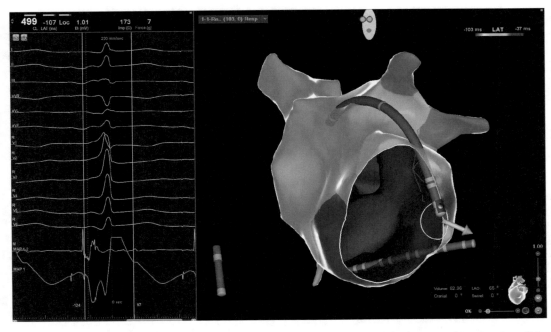

Fig. 20.14 CARTO image in LAO 65° showing the activation map of the left atrium during coronary sinus pacing. The area of the earliest antegrade ventricular activation is recorded in the antero-lateral region of the mitral valve (red area), where the shortest AV was recorded

Question 2: Is this a good ablation site?
A. Yes. The bipolar EGM precedes the surface ECG by 15 ms.
B. Yes. The unipolar EGM shows a "QS" aspect.
C. Yes. The local AV is short.
D. No. The surface ECG suggests a left postero-septal origin.
E. No. The local bipolar EGM is not the earliest local EGM that can be recorded in this patient.

Application of RF energy at this level interrupted the conduction over the accessory pathway 5.5 s after the initiation of RF delivery (Fig. 20.15), with no recurrence of conduction over the accessory pathway.

The 12-lead ECG during RF ablation of the accessory pathway is presented in Fig. 20.16. This was carried out during atrial stimulation from the CS electrodes, in order to increase the degree of pre-excitation. Target ablation parameters were a power of 30 W and an ablation index of 450. Application of RF energy at the site of the earliest local ventricular activation interrupted the conduction over the accessory pathway 5.5 seconds after the application onset (Fig. 20.16).

The ECG at the end of the ablation procedure is shown in Fig. 20.17.

The ECG recorded 24 h after the ablation procedure is shown in Fig. 20.18.

The patient was discharged from the hospital 24 h later.

ANSWERS TO:
Question 1: C. Yes. Delta waves suggesting ventricular pre-excitation.
Question 2:
A. **Yes. The bipolar EGM precedes the surface ECG by 15 ms.**
B. **Yes. The unipolar EGM shows a "QS" aspect.**
C. **Yes. The local AV is short.**

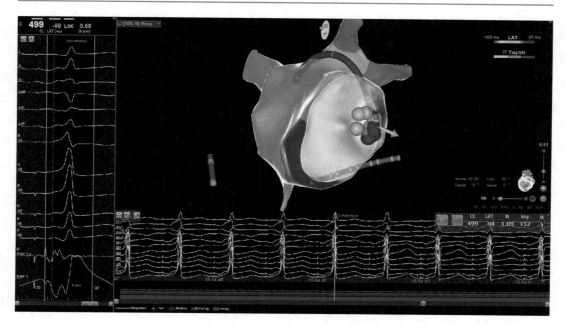

Fig. 20.15 CARTO image in LAO showing the activation map of the left atrium during coronary sinus pacing. The area of the earliest antegrade ventricular activation is recorded in the antero-lateral region of the mitral valve (red area), where the shortest AV was recorded. Left side of the image: 12-lead ECG and intracavitary ECG showing the bipolar (MAP 1–2) and unipolar (MAP 1) local electrograms recorded by the distal pole of the roving/ ablation catheter (blue) at the successful ablation site. The bottom part of the image: surface ECG leads during the first RF application at the site of the earliest antegrade ventricular activation with rapid interruption of the antegrade conduction at the level of the accessory pathway (first QRS complex after the vertical red line). The change in the QRS complex morphology is subtle, but visible in lead I and V1

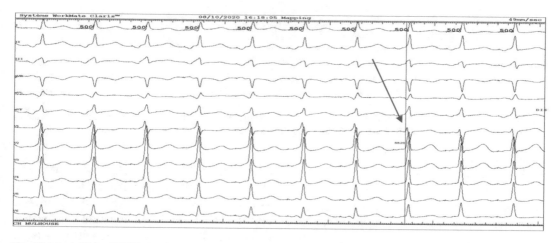

Fig. 20.16 A 12-lead ECG showing disappearance of conduction over the accessory pathway during RF application (red arrow)

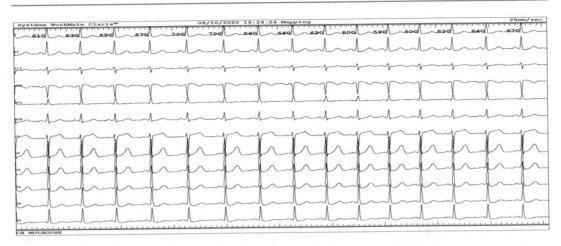

Fig. 20.17 A 12-lead ECG recorded at the end of the ablation procedure, showing sinus rhythm and absence of ventricular pre-excitation

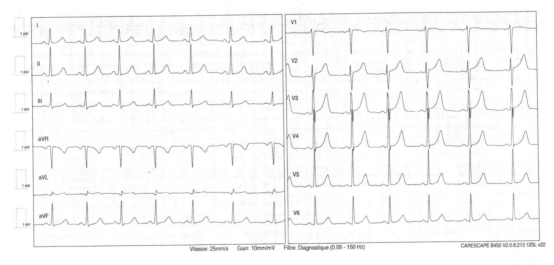

Fig. 20.18 A 12-lead ECG recorded 24 h after the ablation procedure, showing sinus rhythm with a heart rate of 75 bpm, QRS axis at +60°, and absence of ventricular pre-excitation

20.3 Commentary

The present case illustrates a catheter ablation procedure of a left-lateral accessory pathway in a patient with WPW syndrome. Several aspects related to this case merit discussion.

Antidromic tachycardia is a rare type of tachycardia in patients with WPW syndrome, with an incidence of less than 5% in children [1]. In the experience of Ceresnak et al., more than 50% of children with ART from their study had high risk features. Multiple AP were a rare finding in their study; the most common loca-

tions of the AP in their patients with ART were septal and left lateral. ART in children may be associated with an increased risk of adverse events [1]. When taken together (adults and children), ART can be induced in 8% of patients during the electrophysiological study [2]. Brembilla et al. found a higher incidence of atrial fibrillation in patients with inducible ART. However, the incidence of major adverse effects (fast pre-excited AF and death) were not significantly different compared to patients without ART. In adults, it is considered that the prognostic significance of ART is not well known. Atié et al. [3] found an incidence of 10% of ART in their population of patients. Multiple APs were present in 33% of patients with ART. Dizziness and syncope were present in 50% of patients with ART. Atrial fibrillation was documented in 16% and VF in 11%.

Atrial fibrillation occurs in up to 50% of patients with WPW syndrome [4]. As discussed for cases 11, 13, and 14, ablation of the accessory pathway is the treatment of choice for preventing AF recurrence in these patients.

In the above-presented case, both atrial fibrillation and ART were present during the EP study. Interestingly, AF was triggered by ART, as can be seen in Fig. 20.11. AF was symptomatic and self-terminating. Ablation of the accessory pathway was accomplished using the transseptal approach. PVI was not performed since it was not deemed necessary [5, 6].

> **Learning Point**
> - Antidromic tachycardia is a rare form of tachycardia in patients with WPW syndrome.
> - Several types of tachycardias (ORT, ART, atrial fibrillation/flutter, SVT with bystander AP) can coexist in the same patient with WPW syndrome.

References

1. Ceresnak SR, Tanel RE, Pass RH, Liberman L, Collins KK, Van Hare GF, et al. Clinical and electrophysiologic characteristics of antidromic tachycardia in children with Wolff-Parkinson-White syndrome. Pacing Clin Electrophysiol. 2012;35(4):480–8.
2. Brembilla-Perrot B, Pauriah M, Sellal JM, Zinzius PY, Schwartz J, de Chillou C, et al. Incidence and prognostic significance of spontaneous and inducible antidromic tachycardia. Europace. 2013;15(6):871–6.
3. Atie J, Brugada P, Brugada J, Smeets JL, Cruz FS, Peres A, et al. Clinical and electrophysiologic characteristics of patients with antidromic circus movement tachycardia in the Wolff-Parkinson-White syndrome. Am J Cardiol. 1990;66(15):1082–91.
4. Brugada J, Katritsis DG, Arbelo E, Arribas F, Bax JJ, Blomstrom-Lundqvist C, et al. 2019 ESC Guidelines for the management of patients with supraventricular tachycardiaThe Task Force for the management of patients with supraventricular tachycardia of the European Society of Cardiology (ESC). Eur Heart J. 2020;41(5):655–720.
5. Kawabata M, Goya M, Takagi T, Yamashita S, Iwai S, Suzuki M, et al. The impact of B-type natriuretic peptide levels on the suppression of accompanying atrial fibrillation in Wolff-Parkinson-White syndrome patients after accessory pathway ablation. J Cardiol. 2016;68(6):485–91.
6. Wu JT, Zhao DQ, Li FF, Zhang LM, Hu J, Fan XW, et al. Effect of pulmonary vein isolation on atrial fibrillation recurrence after accessory pathway ablation in patients with Wolff-Parkinson-White syndrome. Clin Cardiol. 2020;43(12):1511–6.

Printed in the United States
by Baker & Taylor Publisher Services